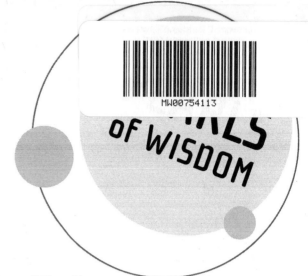

Emergency Medicine
Q&A

Third Edition

Edited by

Joseph Lex, MD, FACEP, FAAEM
Associate Professor
Department of Emergency Medicine
Temple University School of Medicine
Philadelphia, Pennsylvania

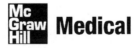 **Medical**

New York Chicago San Francisco Lisbon London Madrid Mexico City Milan
New Delhi San Juan Seoul Singapore Sydney Toronto

Emergency Medicine Q&A: Pearls of Wisdom, Third Edition

First edition copyright by Boston Medical Publications, Boston, Massachusetts.

2 3 4 5 6 7 8 9 0 IBT/IBT 12 11 10 9

ISBN   978-0-07-154469-6
MHID   0-07-154469-0

Notice

This book was set in Adobe Garamond by Aptara®, Inc.
The editors were Kirsten Funk and Robert Pancotti.
The production supervisor was Sherri Souffrance.
Project management was provided by Samir Roy, Aptara®, Inc.
The text designer was Eve Siegel; the cover designer was Handel Low.
Quebecor World Dubuque was printer and binder.

This book is printed on acid-free paper.

Library of Congress Cataloging-in-Publication Data

Lex, Joseph.
   Emergency medicine Q & A / Joseph Lex. – 3rd ed.
      p. ;   cm. – (Pearls of wisdom)
   Includes bibliographical references and index.
   ISBN-13: 978-0-07-154469-6 (pbk. : alk. paper)
   ISBN-10: 0-07-154469-0 (pbk. : alk. paper)   1.   Emergency medicine–Examinations, questions, etc.   I. Title. II. Title: Emergency medicine Q and A. III. Series.
   [DNLM: 1. Emergency Medicine–Examination Questions.   WB 18.2 E5275 2009]
   RC86.9.L49 2009
   616.02′5–dc22
                                                    2008045677

CONTENTS

CONTRIBUTORS

Stephanie Barbetta, MD
Assistant Professor
Department of Emergency Medicine
Temple University School of Medicine
Philadelphia, Pennsylvania
Cutaneous Emergencies
Head, Eye, Ear, Nose, and Throat Emergencies

Jeffrey Barrett, MD, FAAEM
Assistant Professor
Department of Emergency Medicine
Temple University School of Medicine
Philadelphia, Pennsylvania
Traumatic Emergencies

Thomas B. Barry, MD
Department of Emergency Medicine
Temple University School of Medicine
Philadelphia, Pennsylvania
Obstetric and Gynecologic Emergencies

Colin M. Bucks, MD
Department of Emergency Medicine
Albert Einstein Medical Center
Philadelphia, Pennsylvania
Thoracic and Respiratory Emergencies

Thomas G. Costantino, MD
Assistant Professor
Department of Emergency Medicine
Temple University School of Medicine
Philadelphia, Pennsylvania
Medical Imaging

Manish Garg, MD, FAAEM
Assistant Professor and Associate Residency
   Program Director
Department of Emergency Medicine
Temple University School of Medicine
Philadelphia, Pennsylvania
Environmental Emergencies
Psychobehavioral Emergencies

Liza D. Lê, MD
Clinical Instructor
Department of Emergency Medicine
Temple University School of Medicine
Philadelphia, Pennsylvania
Administrative Emergency Medicine, Emergency
   Medical Services, and Ethics

Joseph Lex, MD, FACEP, FAAEM
Associate Professor
Department of Emergency Medicine
Temple University School of Medicine
Philadelphia, Pennsylvania
Abdominal and Gastrointestinal
   Emergencies
Cardiovascular Emergencies
Endocrine and Metabolic Emergencies
Nontraumatic Musculoskeletal
   Emergencies
Neurologic Emergencies

Raemma Paredes Luck, MD, MBA
Director of Research
Department of Emergency Medicine
St. Christopher's Hospital for Children
Associate Professor
Department of Pediatrics and Emergency
   Medicine
Temple University School of Medicine
Philadelphia, Pennsylvania
Pediatric Emergencies

Richard Martin, MD, FAAEM
Assistant Professor
Department of Emergency Medicine
Temple University School of Medicine
Philadelphia, Pennsylvania
Administrative Emergency Medicine, Emergency
   Medical Services, and Ethics

Scott H. Plantz, MD, FAAEM
Associate Clinical Professor of Emergency Services
Rosalind Franklin University of Medicine and Science
Chicago Medical School
Chicago, Illinois
Head, Eye, Ear, Nose, and Throat Emergencies
Administrative Emergency Medicine, Emergency
   Medical Services, and Ethics

Jane M. Prosser, MD
Fellow, Medical Toxicology
New York City Poison Center
New York University Medical Center
New York, New York
Toxicologic Emergencies

Mark Saks, MD, MPH
Assistant Professor
Department of Emergency Medicine
Drexel University College of Medicine
Philadelphia, Pennsylvania
Systemic Infectious Emergencies
Renal and Urogenital Emergencies

Sachin J. Shah, MD, MBA, FAAEM
Assistant Professor
New York Medical College
Attending Physician
Emergency Medical Associates
Westchester Medical Center
Valhalla, New York
Hematologic and Oncologic Emergencies
Immunologic Emergencies

David A. Wald, DO
Associate Professor
Department of Emergency Medicine
Temple University School of Medicine
Philadelphia, Pennsylvania
Resuscitation

EDITORS, SECOND EDITION

Joseph Lex, MD, FACEP, FAAEM
Associate Professor of Emergency Medicine
Temple University School of Medicine
Philadelphia, Pennsylvania

Lance W. Kreplick, MD, MMM, FAAEM
Medical Director of Hyperbaric Medicine
Fawcett Wound Management and Hyperbaric
  Medicine
Company Care Occupational Health Services
President and Chief Executive Officer
QED Medical Solutions, LLC
Port Charlotte, Florida

Scott H. Plantz, MD, FAAEM
Associate Clinical Professor of Emergency
  Services
Rosalind Franklin University of Medicine and
  Science
Chicago Medical School
Chicago, Illinois

Daniel Girzadas, Jr., MD
Department of Emergency Medicine
EHS Christ Hospital and Medical Center
Oak Lawn, Illinois

CONTRIBUTING AUTHORS, SECOND EDITION

Stephanie Barbetta, MD
Tom Barry, MD, FAAEM
Leslie "Toby" Carroll, MD, FAAEM, ABMT
Michael DeAngelis, MD, FAAEM
Manish Garg, MD, FAAEM
Nina Gentile, MD, FAAEM
Sachin Shah, MD, FAAEM

CONTRIBUTING AUTHORS, FIRST EDITION

Dirk H. Alander, MD
Sarah Alander, MD
Edward G. Arevalo, MD

Steven M. Barret, MD
Eric Benink, MD
Tina M.H. Blair, MD
Jack P. Campbell, MD
Robert Cates, MD
Steven G. Chilinski, MD
Woody Chung, MD
Jesse A. Cole, MD
Vernon Cook, Jr., MD
Wesley A. Curry, MD
Irving Danesh, MD
Terry Davis, MD, JD
Charles A. Denton, MD
Bernard J. Feldman, MD
Juan F. Fitz, MD
Denise Fligner, MD
Peter O. Fried, MD
Katherine M. Gillogley, MD
Daniel Girzadas, Jr., MD
William Gossman, MD
Robert C. Harwood, MD
Gabrial Haas, MD
Suchinta Hakim, MD
Bruce S. Heischober, MD
Harold Hirsh, MD, JD
N. Eric Johnson, MD, MPH
Robert Johnson, MD
Kevin M. Kavanaugh, MD
Jane Kreplick, BSN, JD
Jon R. Kroemer, MD
Gordon Larsen, MD
Paul G. Lehmitz, MD
A. S. Lorenzo, MD
Nicholas Y. Lorenzo, MD
Ronald B. Low, MD
Henry C. Maguire, Jr., MD
David L. McCarty, MD
Michael W. Mott, MD
Robert L. Muelleman, MD
Robert K. Nakamura, MD
Carol Newman, MD
Cliff O'Callahan, MD
Joyce O'Shaugnessy, MD
Robert G. Penn, MD
Brian Pierce, MD
Kent Reckewey, MD
Augusta Saulys, MD

Randolph P. Scott, PharmD, PhD, MD

Barbara Shufeldt, MD

Steven Smarcus, MD

Susan K. Sucha, MD

James Sullivan, MD

Peter C. Valco, MD

Richard A. Walker, MD

H. Neil Wigder, MD

Lyle W. Williams, MD

Thomas N. Wise, MD

INTRODUCTION

Emergency Medicine Q&A: Pearls of Wisdom has been designed to provide physicians with a comprehensive, relevant, and convenient instrument for self-evaluation and review. The question type is in accordance with the format of the American Board of Emergency Medicine certification examination. Although this book should be helpful to residents preparing for the certification examination, it should also be useful for physicians in practice who are interested in maintaining a high level of competence in emergency medicine. Study of this review book should help to (1) identify areas of relative weakness; (2) confirm areas of expertise; (3) assess knowledge of the sciences fundamental to emergency medicine; (4) assess clinical judgment and problem-solving; and (5) introduce recent developments in emergency medicine.

Each question in the book is accompanied by an answer and a paragraph of explanation. A bibliography listing the sources used in the book follows the last chapter.

Perhaps the most effective way to use this book is to allow yourself one minute to answer each question in a given chapter. As you proceed, indicate your answer beside each question. When you have finished answering the questions in a chapter, you should then spend time verifying your answers and carefully reading the explanations. Although you should pay special attention to the explanations for the questions you answered incorrectly, you should read every explanation. The authors of this book have designed the explanations to reinforce and supplement the information tested by the questions. If, after reading the explanations for a given chapter, you feel that you require more information regarding the material covered, you should consult and study the references listed in the bibliography.

Joseph Lex, MD, FACEP, FAAEM

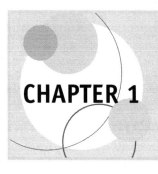

CHAPTER 1 Resuscitation

David A. Wald, DO

1. A previously healthy 54-year-old man presents to the emergency department complaining of chest pain. His EKG shows an acute inferior wall myocardial infarction. His blood pressure is 90/60 mm Hg. On physical examination, he has jugular vein distention and clear lungs. You should treat him immediately with which of the following:

   a. Intravenous fluids.
   b. Norepinephrine.
   c. Dopamine.
   d. Nesiritide.
   e. Nitroprusside.

   The answer is a. This patient's presentation is consistent with a right ventricular infarction complicating an inferior myocardial infarction (MI). Approximately one-third of patients with acute inferior wall MIs are complicated by a right ventricular infarct. The appropriate initial treatment is to "fill the tank"—intravenous fluids.

2. When considering the diagnosis of acute aortic dissection, which of the following statement is true:

   a. Associated syncope occurs in up to 15% of patients.
   b. Neurologic symptoms occur in less than 5% of cases.
   c. Proximal dissections involving left coronary artery are most common and occur in approximately 10% of cases.
   d. Aortic dissection is rare in patients younger than 40 years.
   e. An extremity pulse deficit occurs in up to 30% of cases.

   The answer is d. The incidence of syncope in patients with aortic dissection occurs in up to 9% of cases. Neurologic symptoms including focal deficits and or altered mental status has been noted to occur in up to 17% of cases of aortic dissection. Proximal dissections involving the ostium of a coronary artery are rare, occurring in up to 3% of cases. When present, it most frequently involves the right coronary artery. An extremity pulse deficit (upper) has been known to occur in up to 15% of cases.

3.   **A 54-year-old man presents with two episodes of hematemesis since yesterday. The most likely cause of this patient's upper gastrointestinal bleeding is:**

   a. Gastritis.
   b. Esophagitis.
   c. Esophageal varices.
   d. Peptic ulcer disease.
   e. Mallory-Weiss tear.

   The answer is d. Listed in decreasing frequency, the causes of upper GI bleeding are peptic ulcer disease, gastric erosions, esophageal varices, Mallory-Weiss tear, esophagitis, and duodenitis.

4.   **Regarding outcomes after resuscitation from prehospital cardiac arrest:**

   a. 60% of patients successfully resuscitated will survive to hospital discharge.
   b. Survival rates are the same in prehospital systems using only basic emergency medical technicians versus those systems using paramedics.
   c. Early in-hospital deaths are attributed to complications of sepsis.
   d. Late in-hospital deaths are attributed to complications of anoxic encephalopathy.
   e. Less than 10% of patients surviving to hospital discharge have persistent neurologic deficits.

   The answer is d. Less than 50% of patients successfully resuscitated will survive to hospital discharge. Resuscitation and survival rates are the highest in prehospital systems that employ paramedics. Early in-hospital deaths are attributed to cardiogenic shock and dysrhythmias. Of patients surviving to hospital discharge, one-third have persistent neurologic deficits.

5.   **Succinylcholine:**

   a. Is associated with catecholamine release leading to sinus tachycardia.
   b. Is associated with life-threatening hyperkalemia in patients with an acute burn injury.
   c. Exerts its effects by binding competitively with acetylcholine receptors on the motor end plate.
   d. Should be avoided in patients suspected of having reduced cholinesterase activity, such as in pregnancy or in liver disease.
   e. Retains more than 90% of its original activity when stored at room temperature for up to 3 months.

   The answer is e. Although at times it is difficult to distinguish the effects of succinylcholine from the effects of laryngoscopy and intubation, it causes cardiac muscarinic receptor stimulation leading to bradycardia. Acute trauma such as burn injuries is not a contraindication to the use of succinylcholine. The effects of succinylcholine are exerted by its noncompetitive binding with acetylcholine receptors on the motor end plate. It is not necessary to avoid succinylcholine in any patient suspected of having reduced pseudocholinesterase activity.

6.   **Shortly after delivery, a newborn was noted to have good muscle tone and movement of all extremities, a heart rate of 90/min, sneezing, coughing, a loud cry, and pink color over the entire body. Her Apgar score is:**

   a. 6.
   b. 7.
   c. 8.
   d. 9.
   e. 10.

Table 1–1 Apgar Scoring Method for Condition of a Newborn Infant

Sign	0 Points	1 Point	2 Points
Activity (muscle tone)	Absent	Arms and legs flexed	Active movement
Pulse	Absent	<100 bpm	>100 bpm
Grimace (reflex irritability)	None	Grimace	Sneeze, cough, pulls away
Appearance (color)	Blue-gray, pale	Normal, except for extremities	Normal over entire body
Respirations	Absent	Slow, irregular	Good, crying

The answer is d. Apgar scores (named after Virginia Apgar, who first described them) are taken at 1 minute and 5 minutes, and repeated every 15 minutes if the score is less than 7. Table 1–1 shows the scoring method.

7. **The medication of choice to treat a patient in torsades de pointes is:**
    a. Epinephrine.
    b. Flecainide.
    c. Calcium gluconate
    d. Magnesium sulfate.
    e. Procainamide.

The answer is d. Torsades de pointes is a form of polymorphic ventricular tachycardia. Most episodes are associated with an acquired form of QT prolongation. Many of these cases can be treated medically with intravenous magnesium sulfate. Class IA and IC antiarrhythmic agents are contraindicated, they may worsen the dysrhythmia by further prolonging ventricular repolarization.

8. **A 45-year-old man is brought to the ED after suffering a 40% body surface area partial- and full-thickness burn. His estimated body weight is 80 kg. Using the Parkland fluid resuscitation formula, how much lactated Ringer's (LR) solution would you administer to this patient in the first 8 hours postburn?**
    a. 4400 mL.
    b. 5400 mL.
    c. 6400 mL.
    d. 7400 mL.
    e. 8400 mL.

The answer is c. The Parkland fluid resuscitation formula for burn patients is used as follows: LR solution (4 mL/kg/% total body surface area burned) is administered intravenously in the first 24 hours, half of the volume is to be given in the first 8 hours and the other half over the next 16 hours. In this case, 40% × 4 mL/kg × 80 kg = 12,800 mL, half 6,400 mL over the first 8 hours.

9. **You are caring for a patient with severe COPD who will require intubation and mechanical ventilation. To limit or prevent the development of dynamic hyperinflation, your next step should be:**
    a. Increase the minute ventilation.
    b. Increase the expiratory flow rates of the ventilator.
    c. Increase the I–E ratio of the ventilator.
    d. Reduce the F_{IO_2}.
    e. Intubate with a small diameter endotracheal tube.

    The answer is c. Dynamic hyperinflation can occur in patients with COPD because of inadequate expiratory time leading to air trapping. This dynamic hyperinflation can result in an increased work of breathing for the patient. Ways to counteract this can include minimizing the tidal volume to reduce exhaled volume, increase the expiratory flow rates, increase the I–E ratio of the ventilator, the use of bronchodilators and corticosteroids may also be of help. Externally applied PEEP may also be of assistance in counteracting the intrinsic PEEP (auto PEEP).

10. **A 4-year-old boy is in severe respiratory distress after a motor vehicle crash. He was ejected from the vehicle and has major facial and head trauma. When managing his airway, you should:**
    a. Use an appropriately sized laryngeal mask airway to limit the likelihood of aspiration.
    b. Perform a needle cricothyrotomy rather than a formal surgical cricothyrotomy if you cannot intubate or ventilate.
    c. Extend the neck to improve visualization of the airway structures.
    d. Attempt blind nasotracheal intubation with an appropriate size endotracheal tube.
    e. Avoid succinylcholine because of the acute trauma.

    The answer is b. Laryngeal mask airways may be used as a rescue device in this age, but they do not protect against aspiration of stomach contents. Needle cricothyrotomy is preferred over formal surgical cricothyrotomy in young children because of the size of the small cricothyroid membrane. The tracheal opening is located more anterior and superior than in adults. In this case, hyperextension of the neck is contraindicated because of the potential for cervical spine injury after trauma. Blind nasotracheal intubation is not performed in young children, especially in patients after head and facial trauma. Succinylcholine is not contraindicated in acute trauma.

11. **A 32-year-old woman complains of near syncope and lightheadedness. Her heart rate is 186/min and her blood pressure is 132/76 mm Hg. She has a history of Wolff-Parkinson-White syndrome. Her EKG shows a wide complex irregular tachycardia with ventricular preexcitation. The medication of choice is:**
    a. Adenosine.
    b. Propranolol.
    c. Diltiazem.
    d. Digoxin.
    e. Procainamide.

    The answer is e. This patient is presenting with atrial fibrillation with WPW. All AV nodal blocking agents are contraindicated in this case, including beta-blockers, calcium channel blockers, digoxin, and adenosine. Use of these agents may accelerate conduction through the accessory pathway and increase the ventricular response, leading to ventricular fibrillation. The medication of choice is procainamide.

12. **A 6-month-old infant is brought to the ED because of poor feeding. The infant is listless, but responds to pain. There are no palpable pulses and the cardiac monitor shows a narrow complex tachycardia with a rate of 250. The child weighs 8 kg. Your next step should be:**

    a. Administer verapamil 0.1 mg/kg slow IV push.

    b. Administer digoxin 0.02 mg/kg IV.

    c. Cardiovert immediately with 16 J.

    d. Cardiovert immediately with 8 J.

    e. Defibrillate immediately with 16 J.

    The answer is d. This unstable patient requires immediate cardioversion using 0.5–1 J/kg. In a stable child, you can try adenosine 0.05–0.1 mg/kg IV. Intravenous digoxin may be used to treat SVT in the nonemergent situation, as it may take hours to be effective. Verapamil is contraindicated in children younger than 2 years because it can cause irreversible cardiovascular collapse. Defibrillation with 2 J/kg and standard pharmacologic therapy are used for treatment of VT.

13. **A 62-year-old woman presents with an altered mental status. She is responsive to painful stimuli and has a Glasgow Coma Scale score of 11. Blood pressure is 100/60 mm Hg and heart rate is 100/min. Physical examination reveals poor skin turgor and dry mucus membranes. EKG shows QT interval shortening. Laboratory findings are serum calcium 14.2 mg/dL, serum phosphorus 2.9 mg/dL, serum potassium 3.9 mEq/L, and creatinine 1.9 mg/dL. Your initial treatment should include:**

    a. Magnesium sulfate 2 gm slow IV push.

    b. Pamidronate 60 mg IV.

    c. Calcitonin 4 IU/kg.

    d. Furosemide 60 mg IV after saline resuscitation.

    e. Immediate hemodialysis.

    The answer is d. The initial treatment of choice in this patient with severe hypercalcemia and dehydration is aggressive administration of saline and furosemide diuresis. Subsequent therapy is dictated by the cause and severity. The biphosphonates (pamidronate) and calcitonin are also effective in treating hypercalcemia, but they are usually not used in the ED, and would not be instituted until after the patient is rehydrated with IV fluids. Patients with renal failure and hypercalcemia may require dialysis.

14. **Which of the following statement regarding the use of cardiac markers in the evaluation of a patient with an acute coronary syndrome is true:**

    a. Myoglobin levels are not affected by renal failure.

    b. A single troponin measurement on presentation can effectively rule out myocardial infarction.

    c. Cardiac troponins are the best markers for identifying myocardial cell injury.

    d. Total CPK levels are as specific as cardiac troponins in identifying myocardial cell injury.

    e. CPK-MB fraction is not associated with false-positive test results.

    The answer is c. Myoglobin levels are often elevated in patients with renal failure because of decreased clearance. A single troponin measured on ED presentation of a patient has limited utility in excluding an acute MI. Cardiac troponins have no ability to exclude unstable angina without myocardial infarction because cell injury is required to elevate the troponin and because of the time delay associated with the rise in levels. Total CPK levels are not as specific as cardiac troponins for identifying myocardial cell injury. CPK-MB fraction is associated with false-positive test results, and may occur in certain clinical conditions such as pericarditis and myocarditis.

15.   **The initial management of a patient in hemorrhagic shock should consist of:**

   a. Rapid infusion of isotonic crystalloid fluids.
   b. Ensuring adequate oxygenation and ventilation.
   c. Pharmacologic support to maintain stable hemodynamics.
   d. Stabilization of all long bone fractures.
   e. Immediate transfusion of uncrossmatched blood.

   The answer is b. As in most patients, the initial management revolves around evaluating and ensuring that the patient has adequate oxygenation and ventilation. The rapid infusion of isotonic crystalloids is part of the standard management after the airway is managed. Pharmacologic agents to support hemodynamics play essentially no role in the face of hemorrhagic shock. Stabilization of all long bones fractures is a secondary priority. The transfusion of uncrossmatched blood is often used in the scenario of refractory hypotension after crystalloid resuscitation.

16.   **The Combitube airway device:**

   a. Is an acceptable alternative to endotracheal intubation as a primary airway management device.
   b. Is the preferred method of airway management in the prehospital setting.
   c. Is one of several rescue devices to be considered in the difficult airway.
   d. Will pass blindly into the tracheal most of the time.
   e. Placement cannot be confirmed by end-tidal CO_2 detectors, as it is unreliable in this device.

   The answer is c. The esophageal tracheal Combitube does have a role in emergency airway management. Its role is primarily a substitute for endotracheal intubation by non-ETT-trained personnel; however, it may have a role as a primary intubating device in the prehospital setting. The Combitube has been used as a rescue device or as a primary intubating device in difficult airways. In the emergency department, its use should be restricted to a rescue device after failed oral intubation. The Combitube has virtually no role in the emergency department as a primary airway management device except in cardiopulmonary arrest when expertise for endotracheal intubation is not available.

17.   **You are preparing to intubate an obese patient (body weight 127 kg) with a history of sleep apnea. What would be the approximate desaturation time ($SaO_2 < 90\%$) for this patient after paralysis if he was fully preoxygenated with an FiO_2 of 1.0:**

   a. 1 minute.
   b. 3 minutes.
   c. 5 minutes.
   d. 7 minutes.
   e. 9 minutes.

   The answer is b. All patients undergoing rapid sequence intubation should undergo preoxygenation if possible. The administration of 100% oxygen for 3 minutes of normal, tidal volume breathing in a healthy adult results in the establishment of an adequate oxygen reservoir to permit approximately 8 minutes of apnea before oxygen desaturation to less than 90% occurs. However, the time to desaturation to less than 90% in children, obese adults, late-term pregnant women, and patients with significant comorbidity is considerably less.

18. **The benefits associated with the use of nitroglycerin in patients with acute coronary syndromes result primarily from:**

    a. Pulmonary artery vasoconstriction.

    b. Decreasing myocardial preload.

    c. Increasing afterload.

    d. Coronary vasoconstriction.

    e. Inotropic support.

    The answer is b. Nitroglycerin provides benefit to patients with an acute coronary syndromes by decreasing myocardial preload and to a lesser extent afterload. Nitroglycerin increase venous capacitance leading to venous pooling, a decrease in preload and myocardial oxygen demand. Coronary vasodilation may improve blood flow to ischemic myocardium.

19. **You are managing a patient who is hypotensive, refractory to intravenous fluids. You decide to use a pure alpha-adrenergic agent, so choose:**

    a. Dopamine.

    b. Dobutamine.

    c. Amrinone.

    d. Isoproterenol.

    e. Phenylephrine.

    The answer is e. Adrenergic agents are divided into pure alpha-agents (phenylephrine), mixed alpha- and beta-agents (epinephrine, norepinephrine), and pure beta- or primarily beta-agonists (isoproterenol, dobutamine, dopamine). The alpha-receptors are found primarily in blood vessels, where alpha stimulation causes vasoconstriction. Beta-agonists work primarily on the heart and promote increased heart rate, increased contractility, and increased myocardial oxygen consumption. Beta$_2$ receptors are in smooth muscle of the bronchi, blood vessels, and uterus.

20. **While caring for a patient with suspected pericardial tamponade, you would expect to find:**

    a. Equalization of right and left ventricular pressures.

    b. Isolated systolic hypertension.

    c. A hyperdynamic precordium.

    d. Poor R wave progression on the 12-lead electrocardiogram.

    e. Mitral regurgitation.

    The answer is a. Findings of cardiac tamponade may be influenced by volume and rate of accumulation. The classic physical examination finding is Beck's triad of jugular venous distention, hypotension, and muffled heart sounds. Echocardiography can confirm the diagnosis when paradoxical systolic wall motion abnormalities are seen in a patient with a pericardial effusion. A Swan-Ganz catheter can also be diagnostic when demonstrating equalization of right and left ventricular pressures.

21. **The most common diagnosis identified by computed tomography (CT) of the thorax in patients undergoing an evaluation for pulmonary embolism is:**

    a. Pneumonia.

    b. Unsuspected pericardial effusion.

    c. Mass suggesting new carcinoma.

    d. Aortic dissection.

    e. Pneumothorax.

    The answer is a. Frequency of potentially important non-PE diagnoses disclosed on computed tomography: pneumonia (6%), unsuspected pericardial effusion (1%), mass suggesting new carcinoma (1%), aortic dissection (0.5%), and pneumothorax (0.5%).

22. **A 49-year-old dialysis patient presents with generalized weakness. His EKG shows peaked T waves and a widened QRS complex. The most appropriate initial therapy should include:**

    a. Intravenous glucose and insulin.

    b. Intravenous sodium bicarbonate.

    c. Intravenous calcium gluconate.

    d. Nebulized albuterol.

    e. Oral or rectal sodium polystyrene sulfonate (Kayexalate).

    The answer is c. While nebulized albuterol will reliably lower the serum potassium rapidly, calcium salts act immediately by stabilizing cell membranes and is the recommended first line agent in the setting of a wide QRS complex. The duration of action of the calcium is approximately 20–40 minutes. Bicarbonate should not be used unless the patient is acidemic. The other therapies will reduce the serum potassium level but have longer onsets of action.

23. **You are managing a patient who is in acute pulmonary edema, with cool clammy skin. His blood pressure is 84/56 mm Hg. The medication of choice in this patient would be:**

    a. Epinephrine.

    b. Dobutamine.

    c. Vasopressin.

    d. Phenylephrine.

    e. Norepinephrine.

    The answer is b. This patient is presenting with cardiogenic shock. In this case, to improve myocardial contractility, dobutamine and dopamine are the agents of choice begun in order at the same doses used for septic shock.

24. **A 72-year-old man with a history of COPD presents to the emergency department with a complaint of progressive shortness of breath. His preintubation arterial blood gas analysis on a non-rebreather face mask shows a pH of 7.22, a P_{CO_2} of 71 mm Hg, and a P_{O_2} of 68 mm Hg. Suggested initial ventilator settings in this patient would be:**

    a. Tidal volume 6 mL/kg and respiratory rate 6/min.

    b. Tidal volume 8 mL/kg and respiratory rate 10/min.

    c. Tidal volume 10 mL/kg and respiratory rate 12/min.

    d. Tidal volume 12 mL/kg and respiratory rate 12/min.

    e. Tidal volume 12 mL/kg and respiratory rate 14/min.

The answer is b. This patient with COPD has arterial blood gas values that support the diagnosis of acute on chronic respiratory acidosis. Initial ventilator settings in patients with COPD should include tidal volume (5–10 mL/kg) and respiratory rate (10–12/min).

25. **The vascular access which is least desirable in a patient of cardiac arrest is the:**
    a. Peripheral antecubital vein.
    b. Subclavian vein.
    c. Internal jugular vein.
    d. Brachial vein
    e. Femoral vein.

    The answer is e. A peripheral vein should be the first choice for IV access in patients with cardiac arrest. Central venous access is an alternative, and if performed, preferred site would be the internal jugular vein to limit interruption of CPR that at times occurs with the insertion of a subclavian line. Because subdiaphragmatic flow is minimal, femoral vein cannulation should be avoided.

26. **The recommended initial therapy for a patient suffering a severe allergic reaction to a bee sting is:**
    a. Albuterol.
    b. Cimetidine.
    c. Dopamine.
    d. Epinephrine.
    e. Norepinephrine.

    The answer is d. Epinephrine is the hallmark of anaphylaxis management. Cold compresses, antihistamines, nonsteroidal anti-inflammatory agents, and corticosteroids are indicated in localized reactions from hymenoptera stings.

27. **Prehospital caregivers can shorten door-to-balloon time for patients with an acute myocardial infarction by:**
    a. Administering aspirin to patients with chest pain.
    b. Establishing intravenous access during transport.
    c. Determining prior allergy to lytic agents.
    d. Transmitting the ECG while en route to the ED.
    e. Using lights and siren while transporting the patient.

    The answer is d. Transmitting the ECG has been shown to be the most effective way of reducing door-to-balloon time in a patient arriving from the prehospital setting.

28.   Diagnostic criteria for sepsis include suspected infection plus:

a. Serum bicarbonate $\geq$ 16 mEq/dL.

b. Core temperature < 36°C (96.8°F).

c. Respiratory rate < 12/min.

d. Plasma glucose < 60 mg/dL.

e. Altered mental status.

The answer is b. Sepsis is defined as systemic inflammatory response syndrome (SIRS) with a presumed infectious cause. SIRS is defined by two or more of the following findings:

- Temperature greater than 38°C or less than 36°C.
- Heart rate of more than 90/min.
- Respiratory rate of more than 20/min or a $Paco_2$ level of less than 32 mm Hg.
- Abnormal white blood cell count (>12,000/μL or <4,000/μL or >10% bands).

29.   The estimated relative risk for venous thromboembolism is greatest in the presence of:

a. Obesity.

b. Cancer.

c. Protein C deficiency.

d. Age > 50.

e. Oral contraceptive use.

The answer is c. The estimated relative risk for various risk factors: obesity (1–3), cancer (5), protein C deficiency (10), age > 50 (5), and oral contraceptive use (5).

30.   You are managing a trauma patient with a flail chest who is in respiratory distress. Indications for mechanical ventilation would include:

a. Respiratory rate > 25/min.

b. Respiratory rate < 12/min.

c. Pao_2 < 70 mm Hg at Fio_2 > 0.5.

d. $Paco_2$ > 55 mm Hg at Fio_2 > 0.5.

e. Alveolar–arterial oxygen gradient > 350.

The answer is d. Indications for treatment of flail chest with mechanical ventilation include respiratory failure, manifested by one or more of the following criteria: clinical signs of respiratory fatigue (respiratory rate > 35/min or < 8/min, Pao_2 < 60 mm Hg at Fio_2 = 0.5, $Paco_2$ > 55 mm Hg at Fio_2 = 0.5, alveolar–arterial oxygen gradient > 450); clinical evidence of severe shock; associated severe head injury with lack of airway control or need to ventilate, or severe associated injury requiring surgery.

31.   A crucial part of the evaluation of a patient with a community-acquired pneumonia is to determine whether the patient should be admitted to a hospital or if he/she can be cared for as an outpatient. The comorbid illness that contributes most to the Pneumonia Outcomes Research Team (PORT) scoring system is:

a. Renal disease.

b. Cerebrovascular disease.

c. Congestive heart failure.

d. Liver disease.

e. Neoplastic disease.

The answer is e. Scoring System for Pneumonia Mortality Prediction, comorbid illness: neoplastic disease, 30; liver disease, 20; congestive heart failure, 10; cerebrovascular disease, 10; renal disease, 10.

32. **You are caring for a 58-year-old man in septic shock. Despite aggressive crystalloid fluid resuscitation, he remains hypotensive. Your vasopressor of choice would be:**

    a. Dopamine.

    b. Dobutamine.

    c. Milrinone.

    d. Nordopamine.

    e. Epinephrine.

    The answer is a. In cases of septic shock refractory to resuscitation with crystalloid fluids, dopamine is a rational first-line vasopressor to be administered. Dopamine can be started at 5 to 15 μg/kg/min and titrated to urine output greater than 1 mL/kg/h and mean arterial BP (two-thirds diastolic plus one-third systolic) greater than 70 mm Hg.

33. **A 67-year-old man complains of weakness and dizziness after three episodes of coffee ground hematemesis in the last 6 hours. His blood pressure is 92/58 mm Hg and his heart rate is 117/min. He is no longer actively bleeding. After initial crystalloid resuscitation, his hemoglobin is 6.7 mg/dL. How many units of packed red blood cells would you anticipate needing to transfuse to raise this patient's hemoglobin to approximately 10 mg/dL:**

    a. 1 or 2 units.

    b. 3 or 4 units.

    c. 5 or 6 units.

    d. 7 or 8 units.

    e. At least 10 units.

    The answer is b. Packed red blood cells (PRBCs) are used to crystalloid fluid resuscitation. In an average adult, 1 unit of PRBCs increases the hemoglobin by approximately 1 g/dL or the hematocrit by approximately 3%.

34. **Of postresuscitative efforts listed below, the one shown to have efficacy in the cardiac arrest patient who has demonstrated return of spontaneous circulation (ROSC) is administration of:**

    a. Glutamate antagonists.

    b. Calcium channel antagonists.

    c. Free radical scavengers.

    d. Insulin to control hyperglycemia.

    e. Sodium channel antagonists.

    The answer is d. In observational studies, survivors of cardiac arrest with hyperglycemia after brain ischemia will have worse outcomes whether diabetic or nondiabetic. To date, the best available evidence supports active treatment of hyperglycemia after global brain ischemia.

35.   Choose the correct statement concerning cyanosis:

a. The presence of cyanosis depends upon the quantity of deoxyhemoglobin in the blood rather than the amount of oxyhemoglobin.

b. The earlobes and palpebral conjunctivae are the most sensitive sites for observing central cyanosis.

c. Patients with polycythemia vera and cyanosis are invariably hypoxemic.

d. Symptomatic sulfhemoglobinemia may be treated with IV methylene blue.

e. In peripheral cyanosis caused by cold exposure in an otherwise healthy patient, analysis of arterial blood gases usually demonstrates decreased arterial oxygen saturation.

The answer is a. Cyanosis is either peripheral or central, and the result of deoxygenated hemoglobin or abnormal hemoglobin. The degree of cyanosis depends on many factors, including blood flow and skin pigments. The most reliable site for detecting central cyanosis is the tongue; other sites such as nail beds and conjunctivae can be unreliable. Cyanosis depends upon the absolute amount of reduced hemoglobin in the blood. An anemic patient may be severely hypoxemic, but not cyanotic. A polycythemic patient may not be hypoxemic, but display cyanosis because of the total amount of deoxygenated hemoglobin. Cyanosis unrelieved by administration of oxygen should lead you to suspect methemoglobinemia. Treatment includes IV methylene blue. Sulfhemoglobinemia is not reversible with methylene blue.

36.   In treating a patient with cardiogenic shock:

a. Dopamine preserves renal blood flow but can cause a reflex bradycardia.

b. Dobutamine increases myocardial contractility and reduces afterload.

c. You should avoid fluid challenges in all hypotensive patients in cardiogenic shock.

d. Furosemide causes venodilatation and decreases afterload more than preload.

e. The optimal filling pressure for a patient in cardiogenic shock ranges from 18 to 20 mm Hg.

The answer is b. Hypoxia and hypotension require aggressive treatment. If the mean arterial pressure drops below 70 mm Hg then underperfused myocardium results. Patients in cardiogenic shock without pulmonary edema may first be given fluid boluses of 150–200 mL. With blood pressure above 100 mm Hg, dobutamine is indicated. If blood pressure is below 90 mm Hg, dopamine is indicated for its pressor effects. Furosemide reduces preload by virtue of its diuretic effect and a direct venodilating effect.

37.   The leading cause of death in patients who are resuscitated from cardiorespiratory arrest is:

a. Myocardial contusion and right-sided heart failure.

b. Recurrent cardiopulmonary arrest.

c. Pneumonia.

d. Anoxic encephalopathy.

e. Hemorrhage from gastric perforation and liver lacerations.

The answer is d. Early complications of correctly performed CPR include myocardial contusion, liver lacerations, pericardial effusions, and gastric rupture. Late complications include pneumonia, recurrent cardiopulmonary arrest, GI bleeding, and pulmonary edema. These are attributable to their morbid conditions rather than to direct complications of CPR.

38. **Choose the correct statement concerning neuromuscular blocking agents:**

   a. Succinylcholine is contraindicated in patients who are allergic to mycins.

   b. Pancuronium bromide is associated with bradycardia.

   c. Vecuronium bromide is reversible with atropine and neostigmine.

   d. Pancuronium or succinylcholine should be avoided in patients with long-bone fractures.

   e. Pancuronium may cause hyperpyrexia.

The answer is c. Succinylcholine (1.5 mg/kg) is a rapid depolarizing neuromuscular blocking agent. Paralysis occurs within 3 minutes after injection. It has a short duration of action unless there are low plasma levels of pseudocholinesterase. The drug may cause muscle fasciculations and bradycardia can occur due to muscarinic blockade. Contraindications to its use include renal failure, myopathies, muscle trauma, or burns more than 24 hours old. Malignant hyperthermia is a rare complication (dantrolene may relieve muscular rigidity). Nondepolarizing agents include pancuronium and vecuronium. The former is associated with a prominent tachycardia from its vagolytic action, and both may cause hypotension. Their duration of action is approximately 30 minutes. These agents are reversible with anticholinesterases (neostigmine, edrophonium). A small dose can be used prior to the use of a depolarizing agent to block muscle fasciculations. Paralyzed patients should receive a sedative agent concomitantly and analgesia as indicated.

39. **Choose the correct association:**

   a. Hypocalcemia and digitalis—cardiac arrest.

   b. Hypermagnesemia—wide QRS, prolonged PR and QT intervals, ST-segment depression with T-wave inversion.

   c. Renal failure and peptic ulcer disease being treated with calcium-based antacid—loss of deep tendon reflexes, hypotension, respiratory failure.

   d. Renal failure and cardiac arrest—empiric intravenous calcium chloride.

   e. Hypermagnesemia (>10 mEq/mL)—hemodialysis.

The answer is d. The most common cause of hypermagnesemia in patients with renal failure is the indiscriminate use of magnesium-containing antacids. Increasing magnesium levels progressively reduce neuromuscular irritability and deep tendon reflexes. Deep tendon reflexes are lost prior to hypotension, cardiac abnormalities, or paralysis. IV calcium can counter the neuromuscular paralysis induced by hypermagnesemia. The primary treatment is saline and furosemide-assisted diuresis (contraindication: renal failure). Magnesium and calcium are poorly dialyzed. Hypomagnesemia may be secondary to chronic diuretic therapy, alcoholism, malnutrition, and diarrhea. Physical findings are similar to those of hypocalcemia and are predominantly neuromuscular (hyperreflexia, tetany, weakness, paresthesias, and carpopedal spasm), CNS (ataxia, confusion, seizures, and coma), and cardiac (arrhythmias, heart failure, and hypotension). When treating hypokalemia-associated arrhythmias, hypomagnesemia should be considered as well. IV administration of calcium is indicated in cardiac arrest secondary to hyperkalemic states.

40. **A 45-year-old man is brought to the ED after being struck by lightning. He has no intravenous access and the medics were unable to intubate him, but they have good bilateral breath sounds with bag-valve mask. Your next step should be:**

a. Immediately intubate orotracheally.

b. Immediately intubate nasotracheally.

c. Insert a central venous catheter.

d. Apply quick-look paddles and defibrillate with 200 J if in asystole.

e. None of the above.

The answer is e. Airway control is sufficient for the time being. The next step is to confirm the presence or absence of pulses. A quick-look paddle or cardiac monitor can check the cardiac rhythm. The myocardium is most likely to be successfully defibrillated in the early stages of cardiac arrest. Asystole is not an indication for defibrillation. Epinephrine may be administered intravenously or via the endotracheal tube per ACLS protocol.

41. **An 8-year-old boy is in respiratory arrest after a motor vehicle crash. He was propelled through the car's windshield and has major facial and head trauma. When obtaining airway control in this patient, you know that:**

a. Needle cricothyrotomy is preferred over surgical cricothyrotomy.

b. Inadequate extension of the neck is the most common cause of intubation failure.

c. When in doubt, a smaller laryngoscope blade and a larger endotracheal tube should be selected for intubation.

d. The tracheal opening is located more posteriorly and inferiorly than in adults.

e. Succinylcholine in contraindicated.

The answer is a. Needle cricothyrotomy is preferred over surgical cricothyrotomy in children younger than 12 years. The tracheal opening is located more anterior and superior than in adults. Because hyperextension of the neck may kink the soft tracheal cartilage, the child's head should be positioned in mild hyperextension. A straight laryngoscopic blade is preferred for use in children. The most common reasons for failure to intubate are improper patient positioning and inadequate preparation of equipment.

42. **After you successfully cannulate the right internal jugular vein in a comatose 25-year-old hypotensive intravenous drug addict with numerous neck scars, your initial central venous pressure (CVP) measurement is 20 cm H$_2$O. Your differential diagnosis should include:**

a. Acute aortic insufficiency.

b. Acute tricuspid insufficiency.

c. Anaphylaxis.

d. Opiate-induced coma.

e. Hypocalcemia.

The answer is b. CVP measurements provide valuable information; however, technical artifacts (catheter or stopcock malposition, erroneous zero point, and the Trendelenburg position) may alter readings. A patient with a normal CVP (5–15 cm H$_2$O) and hypotension should receive saline fluid challenges. The response in CVP guides further therapy. Although hypovolemia would be expected to cause a low CVP, in the presence of coexisting conditions, it may be accompanied by a normal or high CVP. Endocarditis can result in tricuspid insufficiency. Common causes of a high CVP include right ventricular failure secondary to left ventricular failure, pulmonary embolism, right ventricular infarction, cor pulmonale, and tension pneumothorax.

43. **Choose the correct statement concerning cardiac pacing:**

a. Transvenous pacemakers are usually inserted using the right internal jugular vein.

b. Transcutaneous pacing should be temporarily discontinued when physical contact with the patient is necessary.

c. Insertion of a transvenous pacemaker catheter is contraindicated in the pulseless patient.

d. Transcutaneous pacing should be discontinued as soon as the patient regains consciousness.

e. The pads for a transcutaneous pacemaker should be placed at the base and the apex of the patient's heart.

The answer is a. The transcutaneous pacemaker is the easiest pacing device to use in an emergency setting. Patient contact can be maintained during its use. Muscle contractions caused by the pacer may be uncomfortable for the awake patient, but do not contraindicate its use in this setting. For best capture, one pad should be placed on the chest directly over the heart and the other placed on the back in the same approximate location. Transvenous catheters are more easily inserted prior to cardiac arrest. The standard approach is via the right internal jugular. The presence of hemodynamic deterioration after insertion of a pacemaker could indicate cardiac tamponade or tension pneumothorax must be considered.

44. **Choose the correct statement concerning acute coronary syndromes:**

a. Fewer than 10% of patients with unstable angina or acute myocardial infarction have "heartburn" as their chief complaint.

b. The poorly localized, indistinct pain from myocardial ischemia is a result of visceral pain fibers of the sympathetic nervous system.

c. Typical angina is episodic, usually lasts less than 5 minutes, is provoked by exertion, and relieved by nitroglycerin; 90% of patients report a retrosternal component and more than 50% report no radiation of the discomfort.

d. Patients with rest angina or angina of changing character are at no higher risk of infarction and sudden death compared to patients with exertional symptoms.

e. Prinzmetal's angina is characterized by frequently coexistent conduction abnormalities in addition to provocation by exertion and resistance to nitroglycerin.

The answer is b. Prinzmetal's variant angina occurs without provocation, often while the patient is at rest. It is typically relieved by nitroglycerin. Prinzmetal's angina results from coronary artery vasospasm; one-third of cases occur in people with otherwise normal coronary arteries. ST-segment elevation, tachyarrhythmias, and other transient conduction abnormalities may occur during attacks. Unstable angina is defined as (1) new onset angina, (2) crescendo angina, or (3) rest angina. It is important to recognize that these patients have a higher risk of infarction and sudden death. Anginal pain lasting longer than 15 minutes, unrelieved by nitroglycerin, or accompanied by other signs such as diaphoresis, nausea, or dyspnea suggests AMI. Approximately 30% of patients with unstable angina or acute myocardial infarction have "heartburn" as their chief complaint. Remember in the diagnosis of AMI the old adage "Absence of proof is not proof of absence." AMI may be atypical, particularly in diabetic patents and the elderly. The diagnosis of AMI is not ruled out by a normal EKG and initial normal cardiac marker profile.

45. **A 2-month-old infant is brought to the ED by her mother. The mother relates that the baby was found in its crib an hour ago with blue skin. Her husband was out in the cornfield at the time, and she picked up the baby to administer mouth-to-mouth breathing. The infant immediately awoke and began to cry. The child had been breastfed until 3 days ago when the mother voluntarily discontinued. The child is now on formula mixed with well water. Physical examination reveals a mildly cyanotic infant in no distress. Arterial blood gas on room air shows PO_2, 90; saturation, 92%; pH, 7.39, PCO_2, 32; HCO_3, 23. There is no change in the infant's color after administration of oxygen. Hgb, 16.2; Hct, 47; WBC, 5.8. The next step would be to:**

    a. Obtain an echocardiogram to rule out cyanotic heart disease.

    b. Repeat the arterial blood gas.

    c. Order a lung scan to rule out pulmonary embolus.

    d. Order a stat chest x-ray.

    e. None of the above.

    The answer is e. Cyanosis that is unresponsive to oxygen but with normal arterial blood gas measurements suggests abnormal hemoglobin. Many ABG analyzers do not report abnormal hemoglobin. Methemoglobinemia may be inherited or acquired. Benzocaine, nitrates, and certain poisonous mushrooms can cause this disorder. In methemoglobinemia, the pulse oximeter will overestimate the oxygen saturation, and the ABG will show a normal PO_2, a normal calculated oxygen saturation, and a decrease in the measured oxygen saturation. Symptoms are secondary to hypoxia. Well water that has been contaminated with nitrates from farm fertilizer has been shown to cause methemoglobinemia.

46. **A patient in cardiogenic shock who would benefit most from the placement of an intra-aortic counterpulsation balloon pump is one with:**

    a. Left mainstem coronary disease and a poor response to intravenous dopamine.

    b. A prior history of cardiogenic shock, with new Q waves and pulmonary edema.

    c. Anteroseptal myocardial infarction and the new onset of a cooing, systolic murmur at the left sternal border.

    d. Hypotension, distended neck veins, and muffled heart tones after blunt chest trauma.

    e. None of the above.

    The answer is c. The balloon pump is most useful with the stabilization of patients with surgically correctable lesions that are causing the failure, such as a ruptured papillary muscle and acute mitral regurgitation. The balloon pump should be considered in patients unresponsive to all forms of pharmacologic management. Patients with a history of severe, preexisting cardiac disease and a new MI have a poor prognosis. The balloon pump is not indicated as a treatment for pericardial tamponade.

47. **Choose the true statement about pulmonary artery catheters and CVP lines:**

    a. The pulmonary artery occlusion pressure directly measures left ventricular filling pressure, and thus preload.

    b. In the absence of structural heart disease, a pulmonary artery occlusion pressure higher than the diastolic pulmonary artery pressure is probably an artifact.

    c. The CVP is as accurate as a pulmonary artery catheter for monitoring volume replacement in a young healthy patient.

    d. Pericardial tamponade may be differentiated from tension pneumothorax using pulmonary artery catheter pressures and waveform characteristics.

    e. Placement of a pulmonary artery catheter in the elderly hypotensive patient with known cardiac disease must be performed prior to instituting pressor or volume therapy in the emergency department (ED) setting.

The answer is b. The pulmonary artery occlusion (wedge) pressure (PAWP) measures left atrial pressure, which is an indirect measurement of left ventricular filling pressure. Preload is defined as the left ventricular end-diastolic volume, not pressure. In general, the pulmonary artery (PA) diastolic pressure is 1 to 5 mm Hg higher than the wedge pressure and approximates the PAWP. A wedge pressure higher than the PA diastolic pressure might signify mitral regurgitation. Otherwise suspect an artifact, as a PAWP greater than PA diastolic pressure would mean that blood flow through the heart is reversed! Pericardial tamponade and tension pneumothorax would both result in a flattening of the waveforms and equalization of chamber pressures.

48. **Under normal circumstances, the largest drop in blood pressure in the systemic circulatory system occurs in the:**
    a. Vena cava.
    b. Small and large veins and venules.
    c. Aorta.
    d. Small arteries and arterioles.
    e. Capillaries and venules.

    The answer is d. The small arteries and arterioles have the highest resistance and therefore cause the largest drop in pressure along this segment of the vascular system.

49. **The most important principle in the management of severe hemorrhagic shock is to:**
    a. Obtain blood for possible type-specific transfusion.
    b. Place CVP lines early for fluid resuscitation and monitoring.
    c. Rapidly infuse colloid fluids.
    d. Apply MAST garment.
    e. Secure the airway and adequate ventilation.

    The answer is e. ABCs apply to all acute life-threatening processes. Identification and control of the bleeding source may be performed simultaneously with IV access and fluid resuscitation. Type-specific or O-negative blood should be given for the treatment of hemorrhagic shock if hemodynamic instability persists after 2 L of crystalloid infusion.

50. **Choose the true statement about septic shock:**
    a. Gram-positive organisms do not cause septic shock, because they lack the cell-wall endotoxin.
    b. Leukopenia is not a feature of septic shock.
    c. The second most common source of Gram-negative bacteremia is the urinary tract.
    d. *Escherichia coli* is the second most common organism identified in Gram-negative bacteremia.
    e. The toxic effects of Gram-negative endotoxin appear to be the result of the abnormal activation of normal physiologic pathways.

    The answer is e. Gram-negative and Gram-positive organisms can cause septic shock. The agent responsible for Gram-negative sepsis is the cell-wall lipopolysaccharide endotoxin—the lipid A component. The urinary tract is the most common source for bacteremia (34%). Unknown sites of origin are the second most common source (30%). *E. coli* is the most common organism identified in Gram-negative septicemia. Endotoxin apparently activates the complement, coagulation, and inflammatory pathways.

51.   What will be the 24-hour fluid and caloric requirement for a 51-lb child?

    a. 1600 mL fluid, 1600 calories.

    b. 1800 mL fluid, 1800 calories.

    c. 1600 mL fluid, 1800 calories.

    d. 1525 mL fluid, 1525 calories.

    e. 1525 mL fluid, 1325 calories.

The answer is a. The formula for calculating basal fluid and caloric requirements in children and adults is:

First 0 to 10 kg: 100 cal/kg/24 h

Next 10 to 20 kg: 50 cal/kg/24 h

From 20 to 70 kg: 20 cal/kg/24 h

Note that caloric requirements and fluid requirements are equal in the unstressed child (such as fever). In children maintained only on IV fluid (NPO), approximately 20% of the caloric requirement should be replaced with glucose, which equals 5 g/100 mL of fluid in the patient except the newborn. The normal daily requirement for sodium is 3 mEq/kg. The daily requirement for potassium is 2 mEq/kg.

52.   In a patient with hemorrhagic shock, cerebral blood flow will be maintained by:

    a. Autoregulation.

    b. Reactive hyperemia.

    c. Active hyperemia.

    d. Increased metabolism

    e. The diving reflex.

The answer is a. The brain, more than almost any other organ, has the inherent ability to autoregulate its blood flow. Although active and reactive hyperemia and increased metabolism can increase cerebral blood flow, autoregulation is by far the most dominant mechanism.

53.   The most important factor that influences the outcome of penetrating cardiac injuries is:

    a. Comminuted tear of a single chamber.

    b. Number of chambers injured.

    c. Coronary artery injury.

    d. Coronary sinus injury.

    e. SA or AV node injury.

The answer is c. Multiple studies have shown that injuries to the coronary arteries are the most important factor in determining outcome after penetrating cardiac injury. Injury to a single chamber (even if comminuted) or to multiple chambers is less likely to be fatal than injuries that involve a major coronary artery.

54.   Match the radiographic finding with the appropriate diagnosis:

    a. "Thumbprint" appearance of the epiglottis in a 34-year-old—sublingual abscess.

    b. Anterior displacement of C2 on C3 in toddler—locked facets.

    c. "Steeple"-shaped trachea in toddler—epiglottitis.

    d. Prevertebral space swelling of neck in an asymptomatic infant—artifact.

    e. Air in intestinal wall of newborn—intussusception.

The answer is d. Epiglottitis is not only a disease of children. Older patients and adults may present with a history of sore throat, fever, dysphagia, and hoarseness, without pharyngitis or neck tenderness. Epiglottitis is caused by a variety of organisms including *Haemophilus influenzae* and *Streptococcus* species. The infection can progress to an epiglottic abscess. In laryngotracheobronchitis, AP views of the trachea often show subglottic narrowing (the steeple sign). Lateral neck films may demonstrate a widened hypopharynx. Retropharyngeal swelling is often an artifact: expiration causes the prevertebral soft tissue to widen. In the symptomatic child, usually from age 6 months to 3 years, such swelling is diagnostic for a retropharyngeal abscess. Pneumatosis intestinalis is diagnostic of necrotizing enterocolitis in the premature or stressed neonate.

55. **Choose the correct statement about the oxygen–hemoglobin dissociation relationship:**

    a. Increasing P_{CO_2} results in shift of dissociation curve to left.
    b. Decreasing 2,3-DPG results in shift of dissociation curve to left.
    c. Decreasing hydrogen ion concentration results in shift of dissociation curve to right.
    d. Increasing F_{IO_2} results in shift of dissociation curve to right.
    e. Increasing temperature results in shift of dissociation curve to left.

    The answer is b. The inspired oxygen concentration has no direct effect on the oxygen–hemoglobin dissociation curve. Increasing P_{CO_2}, increasing temperature, increasing hydrogen ion concentration (decreasing pH), and increasing 2,3-DPG shifts the curve to the right and results in an increase in oxygen tissue delivery.

56. **Choose the correct statement regarding the pathogenesis of cerebral ischemic injury:**

    a. Most structural damage occurs during reperfusion.
    b. Decreased intracellular calcium is an important contributor to neuronal cell death.
    c. Xanthine oxidase, which produces oxygen free radicals, is protective against cerebral damage.
    d. Excess protein synthesis contributes to ischemic injury.
    e. Restoring blood flow to an ischemic area lessens the chance of cerebral damage.

    The answer is a. High cytosolic calcium is a major event leading to cell death. Calcium activates membrane phospholipases and contributes to degradation of both membrane and DNA. The presence of xanthine oxidase, an enzyme that produces oxygen free radicals, contributes to irreversible cell death. Suppression of protein synthesis contributes to ischemic injury. Restoring blood flow to an ischemic area contributes to neuronal injury and cell death.

57. **Nitroglycerin relaxes vascular smooth muscle. At low doses, its effects are best seen in:**

    a. Coronary arteries.
    b. Veins.
    c. Large arteries.
    d. Small arteries.
    e. Capillaries.

    The answer is b. At lower dosages, nitrates are primarily venodilatators. They effectively decrease pulmonary artery occlusion pressures (PAOP) and are therefore very effective in the initial therapy of acute pulmonary edema. At higher dosages IV nitroglycerin also causes arteriolar dilatation that results in decreased blood pressure and afterload. The afterload reduction effect appears to be more pronounced in hypertensive patients. Nitrates act as an exogenous source of nitric oxide, which causes vascular smooth muscle relaxation and may have a modest effect on platelet aggregation and thrombosis.

58.   The therapeutic goal in treating a patient with shock is to:

a. Establish a normal CVP pressure.

b. Replace the estimated blood loss with 3 times the volume of crystalloid.

c. Obtain a normal urine output of 0.5–1.0 mL/kg/h.

d. Obtain a blood pressure >120/80 mm Hg.

e. None of the above.

The answer is e. The treatment goal for shock is to restore adequate tissue perfusion. This can only be judged by the effects of therapy on all the major body organs: brain (CNS function); vascular system (blood pressure, pulse pressure, skin color); and kidneys (urine output). No single organ system should be used as the determinant of adequate tissue perfusion. Other factors may mask abnormal function, such as glycosuria increasing urine output or intoxication masking CNS function. Failure to respond to therapy or clinical deterioration should lead one to suspect complicating factors (unrecognized coexistent disease, hypoadrenalism, gastric distension, pneumothorax, cardiac tamponade, etc.).

59.   Prolonged hypoxia can result in:

a. Pulmonary vasodilation.

b. Reduced proportion of pulmonary blood flow to the lung apex.

c. Coronary vasoconstriction.

d. Decreased right ventricular end diastolic pressure.

e. Increased mean circulatory filling pressure.

The answer is e. Hypoxia causes a sustained generalized pulmonary vasoconstriction that increases pulmonary arterial pressure. This increased pulmonary arterial pressure tends to increase perfusion in the lung apex by minimizing the effects of gravity on pulmonary perfusion. Increased pulmonary vasoconstriction initially decreases cardiac output, leading to reflex increases in salt and water retention, leading to increased extracellular volume and subsequent increase in mean circulatory filling pressure, which contributes to an increase in right ventricular end diastolic pressure and an increased preload that helps the right ventricle compensate for the increased afterload. Prolonged hypoxia also causes vasodilation.

60.   Properly performed closed-chest cardiac massage provides approximately what percentage of prearrest cardiac output?

a. 15%.

b. 25%.

c. 45%.

d. 60%.

e. 85%.

The answer is b. Cardiac output declines by 75% during CPR. Diastolic blood pressure, which is the main determinant of coronary blood flow, falls from 40 to 20 mm Hg. Epinephrine increases vasomotor tone and helps preserve diastolic pressure. Coronary and cerebral blood flow during properly performed CPR are reduced to 5% and 10%, respectively, of prearrest blood flow.

61.　A 33-year-old man presents comatose with no available history. You secure the airway, check blood glucose (90 mg/dL), administer naloxone, and assess for trauma. You receive the following laboratory results: sodium, 148 mEq/L; chloride, 125 mEq/L; HCO$_3$, 17 mEq/L; potassium, 5.8 mEq/L; BUN, 18 mg/dL; creatinine, 1.1 mg/dL; serum osmolarity, 305. His condition is most likely due to:

a. Addisonian crisis.

b. Methanol ingestion.

c. Salicylate ingestion.

d. Cyanide ingestion.

e. Alcohol ingestion.

The answer is a. Calculation of the anion gap [$Na^+ - (Cl^- + HCO_3)$] helps differentiate metabolic acidosis. A normal anion gap is less than 12. Causes of normal anion gap acidosis include renal tubular acidosis, Addison's disease, diarrhea, and ureterosigmoidostomy. Causes of a high anion gap acidosis include methanol, uremia, DKA, paraldehyde, isoniazid, lactic acidosis, ethanol, salicylates, and cyanide.

62.　A 65-year-old man is receiving a fibrinolytic agent for an acute anterior wall myocardial infarction. He develops a wide complex regular ventricular rhythm with a rate of 90/min. His blood pressure is 120/80 mm Hg and he is asymptomatic. You should now:

a. Continue close monitoring, but give no medication.

b. Give intravenous lidocaine 100 mg followed by a drip.

c. Cardiovert at 100 J.

d. Give intravenous procainamide 20 mg/min until resolution.

e. Arrange for rescue angioplasty.

The answer is a. This patient has an accelerated idioventricular rhythm, commonly seen during lytic therapy. If he remains stable, this rhythm requires no treatment. In fact, lidocaine may precipitate asystole. If the patient becomes hypotensive, temporary pacing may be tried.

63.　When resuscitating a patient in pulseless electrical activity (PEA), your options include:

a. Fluid challenge.

b. Intravenous calcium chloride.

c. Intravenous lidocaine.

d. Intravenous calcium gluconate.

e. Intravenous nitroglycerin.

The answer is a. The differential diagnosis of PEA includes, but is not limited to, hypoxia, hypovolemia, cardiac tamponade, acidosis, tension pneumothorax, and pulmonary embolus. Pacing is not effective. There is no evidence that calcium is of any therapeutic value. Epinephrine is the recommended pharmacologic therapy.

64.   **A 62-year-old man with an unknown past medical history is brought to the ED after successful prehospital resuscitation. He is intubated and normotensive but remains poorly perfused. The most appropriate pressor agent to use in this situation is:**

a. Epinephrine at 0.05–1.0 μg/kg/min.

b. Dobutamine at 5–20 μg/kg/min.

c. Dopamine at 5–10 μg/kg/min.

d. Dopamine at 2–5 μg/kg/min.

e. Norepinephrine at 4 μg/kg/min.

The answer is b. Dobutamine may be an effective agent in the normotensive postarrest patient who remains poorly perfused. Dobutamine tends to decrease systemic vascular resistance (SVR), which is not helpful in the hypotensive patient.

65.   **The highest level of ventilatory assistance is provided by placing a patient on:**

a. Synchronized intermittent mandatory ventilation (SIMV).

b. Assist-control mode (AC).

c. Continuous positive airway pressure (CPAP).

d. Positive end-expiratory pressure (PEEP).

e. Intermittent positive pressure breathing (IPPB).

The answer is b. The assist-control (AC) mode provides the highest level of ventilatory assistance. The physician sets the tidal volume (Vt), respiratory rate (RR), inspiratory flow rate (IFR), fraction of inspired oxygen (F_{IO_2}), and PEEP. The trigger that initiates inspiration can be either a patient's inspiratory effort or a time interval based on the set respiratory rate. If the patient is breathing below the set respiratory rate, mandatory breaths are interspersed among the patient's breaths. If the patient's respiratory rate is at or above the set rate, all breaths are patient initiated. When either event occurs, the machine cycles on and provides the tidal volume.

66.   **The first maneuver to correct respiratory alkalosis in a patient on mechanical ventilation should be:**

a. Paralysis.

b. Increase tidal volume.

c. Sedation.

d. Increase respiratory rate.

e. Decrease respiratory rate.

The answer is e. Initial maneuvers should be performed to decrease ventilation and, therefore, relieve hypocapnia, which results from blowing off CO_2 during hyperventilation. This should include maneuvers to decrease the respiratory rate and decrease the tidal volume.

67. A 72-year-old man with a history of chronic obstructive pulmonary disease (COPD) presents to the emergency department with a complaint of progressive shortness of breath. He has an arterial blood gas analysis on room air with a pH of 7.26, a PCO_2 of 52 mm Hg, and a PO_2 of 48 mm Hg. An arterial blood gas analysis performed 6 months ago, when the patient was in stable condition, showed a pH of 7.40, PCO_2 of 43 mm Hg, and a PO_2 of 72 mm Hg. Oxygen is started at 4 L via facemask. A repeat arterial blood gas drawn 30 minutes later shows a pH of 7.22, a PCO_2 of 65 mm Hg, and a PO_2 of 70 mm Hg. The most likely cause of this patient's worsening hypercapnia is:

    a. Worsening shunt.

    b. Increased ventilation–perfusion mismatch.

    c. Anxiety.

    d. Worsening diffusion abnormality.

    e. Oxygen toxicity.

    The answer is b. Hypercapnia in COPD has multiple factors. These factors include decreased responsiveness to hypoxia and hypercapnia (which can complicate treatment options), increased ventilation–perfusion mismatch leading to increased dead-space ventilation, and decreased diaphragm function secondary to fatigue and hyperinflation. In patients receiving oxygen therapy with a subsequent worsening of hypercapnia, increased ventilation–perfusion mismatch is the most likely cause of worsening hypercapnia.

68. A 39-year-old woman presents with acute hypoxemic respiratory failure. A chest x-ray shows a diffuse interstitial infiltrate. Physical examination shows a fever and a rash described by a central vesicle surrounded by erythema. The most likely cause of her infection is:

    a. Mycoplasma pneumonia.

    b. Pulmonary sarcoidosis.

    c. Legionella pneumonia.

    d. Aspiration pneumonia.

    e. Varicella pneumonia.

    The answer is e. Varicella pneumonia always should be suspected when a patient has fever, pneumonia, and a characteristic skin rash. The varicella rash is unique (described as a dew drop on a rose petal) and parallels pneumonia. Varicella also causes chickenpox and shingles.

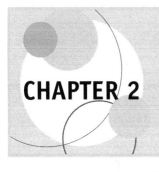

CHAPTER 2

Abdominal and Gastrointestinal Emergencies

Joseph Lex, MD, FACEP, FAAEM

1. **A 10-year-old boy swallowed a Canadian dollar ("Loonie") almost 12 hours ago. He complains of difficulty swallowing solids, but not liquids. Chest radiograph shows a round, flat, metallic object at the level of the aortic arch. He has no respiratory difficulty. At this point, you should:**

   a. Extract the coin using a Foley catheter.

   b. Perform imaging study using a water-soluble contrast agent, followed by extraction of the foreign body with a Foley catheter.

   c. Extract the coin using a Foley catheter, then follow with a barium swallow to rule out esophageal injury.

   d. Arrange immediate endoscopic consultation.

   e. Discharge home and instruct the parents to observe for passage of the coin.

   The answer is d. This esophageal foreign body has not progressed distally for several hours. A contrast study is unnecessary, as the chest radiograph has identified the foreign body and its location. Passing the distal tip of a balloon-tipped catheter past the foreign body, inflating the balloon, and then trying to pry the foreign body proximally carries the risk of aspiration and perforation. Endoscopy is the best method for removal of esophageal foreign bodies.

2. **Most patients with appendicitis have:**

   a. Pyuria.

   b. Nausea and vomiting, but not diarrhea.

   c. A temperature greater than 39.4°C (102.9°F).

   d. Leukocytosis above 20,000 WBC/mm^3.

   e. Appendicolith on plain abdominal radiographs.

   The answer is b. Patients with appendicitis frequently run a low-grade fever, between 37.7°C and 38.3°C (100°F and 101°F), but fever may be absent in more than half the patients with peritoneal signs. Plain abdominal radiographs lack the sensitivity and specificity to be helpful in making the diagnosis, although some experts consider the finding of an appendicolith to be pathognomonic. While many patients with appendicitis complain of constipation, a few do have one or two diarrheal stools, although far from a majority. Pyuria is an infrequent finding.

3.   **A 60-year-old woman complains of diarrhea and weight loss for the past several weeks. She also complains of "hot flashes" similar to what she underwent 10 years ago during menopause. You notice several "spider veins" on her nose and cheeks. On physical examination, you hear a heart murmur, which gets louder when she takes a deep breath. The most helpful test you can order to confirm your suspected diagnosis is:**

   a. Serum serotonin level.

   b. Liver ultrasound.

   c. Serum sodium bicarbonate level.

   d. Plasma chromogranin A (CgA) level.

   e. Stool for *Clostridium difficile*.

   The answer is d. The syndrome strongly suggests a carcinoid tumor, which accounts for up to one-third of small intestine tumors. Carcinoid involvement of the heart resulting in right-sided valvular lesions is a late manifestation of metastatic disease. The most sensitive screening test for small intestine carcinoids is a CgA level, which is elevated in almost 90% of patients with advanced small bowel carcinoid. Urinary 5-HIAA or platelet serotonin levels are also elevated in patients with metastatic carcinoid, but are less sensitive than CgA.

4.   **Choose the correct statement concerning the treatment of suspected infectious diarrhea in adults:**

   a. Only patients who have a positive Wright stain for fecal white blood cells seem to benefit from antibiotic therapy.

   b. Only patients who have a positive stool culture for pathogens seem to benefit from antibiotic therapy.

   c. Trimethoprim/sulfamethoxazole (Bactrim DS) is more efficacious than ciprofloxacin in treating suspected infectious diarrhea, but should be avoided since it prolongs the carrier state.

   d. Combination treatment with trimethoprim/sulfamethoxazole (Bactrim DS) and loperamide (Imodium) has been proven to be both safe and effective in treating traveler's diarrhea.

   e. Diphenoxylate/atropine (Lomotil) and loperamide (Imodium) have been shown equally effective in treating diarrhea, but loperamide should be avoided in patients with a history of cardiac disease.

   The answer is d. For adults with diarrhea in whom the origin is felt to be infectious, antibiotics (500 mg of ciprofloxacin by mouth as a single dose for onset of travelers' diarrhea or twice daily for 3 days) shorten the duration of illness by approximately 24 hours, regardless of the causative agent. Trimethoprim/sulfamethoxazole (one tablet of Bactrim DS by mouth as a single dose or twice daily for 3 days) also shortens the duration of infectious diarrhea in adults but is inferior to ciprofloxacin. Regardless of the causative agent, all patients (even those with negative Wright stain and negative stool culture) improve on ciprofloxacin. Combination treatment with Bactrim and loperamide is both safe and effective in treating traveler's diarrhea. Lomotil, a combination of diphenoxylate and atropine, was first approved by the FDA in 1960. Diphenoxylate is an oral, synthetic opiate agonist structurally related to meperidine. Atropine is added in small quantities to discourage deliberate abuse or overdosage of diphenoxylate. Despite its long-term availability, there is little data about comparative safety of Lomotil, although some experts suggest that it should be avoided in patients with a history of cardiac disease.

5.   **The age group experiencing the highest incidence of rotavirus-induced diarrhea is:**

   a. Neonates.

   b. Infants.

   c. School-age children.

   d. Adults.

   e. Elderly.

The answer is b. In the United States, rotavirus predominantly affects infants between ages 3 and 15 months. The peak incidence is in the winter months, and rotavirus accounts for as much as 50% acute diarrhea in winter. Enteric adenoviruses are the second most common viral pathogen in infants. Bacteria, including *Escherichia coli*, *Salmonella*, and *Shigella*, cause most cases of diarrhea in summer.

6. **A 70-year-old woman complains of several hours of lower abdominal cramping and massive rectal bleeding. Nasogastric aspirate shows bile but no blood. Her most likely diagnosis is:**

    a. Diverticulitis.
    b. Peptic ulcer disease.
    c. Internal hemorrhoids.
    d. Diverticulosis.
    e. Ischemic bowel.

The answer is d. The most common cause of apparent massive lower gastrointestinal bleeding (LGIB) remains upper gastrointestinal bleeding, which must be excluded in all patients. The most common cause of documented LGIB in the elderly is diverticulosis, although angiodysplasia, especially of the right colon, is also a common etiology. Hemorrhoids are the most common cause of rectal bleeding but rarely cause massive blood loss. Ischemic colitis usually does not result in massive bleeding. Colon carcinoma is usually manifested by occult blood.

7. **Choose the correct statement concerning hepatitis B:**

    a. The highest rates of hepatitis B virus (HBV) infection are among intravenous drug users and homosexual men.
    b. Hepatitis B surface antigen (HBsAg) has been detected in saliva, semen, stool, and urine, but not in tears or vaginal secretions.
    c. The typical interval between exposure and onset of clinical illness is between 1 and 3 weeks.
    d. Approximately 25% of adults infected with HBV become chronic carriers of HBsAg.
    e. Health care workers who routinely come in contact with blood have a prevalence of HBsAg of more than 5%.

The answer is a. Hepatitis B virus (HBV) is principally transmitted by parenteral exposure but can also be transmitted by intimate contact, with highest rates of infection among IV drug users and men who have sex with men. HBsAg has been detected in saliva, semen, stool, tears, urine, and vaginal secretions. The typical interval between exposure and onset of clinical illness is between 60 and 90 days, but serologic markers of infection generally appear within 1–3 weeks. Approximately 10% of adults and 90% of neonates who are infected with HBV become chronic HBsAg carriers. Health care workers who routinely come in contact with blood have a prevalence of HBsAg of 1–2%.

8. **Mechanical obstruction of the large bowel is most commonly caused by:**

    a. Adhesions.
    b. Carcinoma.
    c. Diverticulitis.
    d. Hernia.
    e. Volvulus.

The answer is b. Colon carcinoma is the most common cause of mechanical obstruction of the colon; it is followed in frequency by sigmoid diverticulitis and volvulus, with these three accounting for more than 90% of cases of colonic obstruction. While adhesions and hernia account for more than 75% of small bowel obstructions, they are uncommon causes of large bowel obstruction.

9.   **At 35 weeks gestation, a G2P1 woman complains of right lower quadrant pain, nausea, and loss of appetite. Her heart rate is 95/min. She is tender in the right lower abdomen, but has no peritoneal signs. Laboratory studies show a WBC 18,500/mm^3 and a C-reactive protein of 1.2 mg/dL. Her urine shows pyuria without bacteriuria. The finding most helpful in diagnosing appendicitis is the:**

   a. Anorexia.

   b. Elevated WBC count.

   c. Right lower quadrant abdominal tenderness.

   d. Relative tachycardia.

   e. Elevated C-reactive protein.

   The answer is a. Physiologic changes of pregnancy include 45% plasma volume expansion (leading to dilutional anemia); increased leukocyte counts (to 180,000/mm^3 or higher) and increased C-reactive protein increase. Heart rate increases 15–20 beats above baseline by the end of term, and systolic and diastolic pressures decrease by 15–20 mm Hg. Although anorexia is a very common symptom of appendicitis, its absence does not exclude appendicitis from the differential diagnosis of RLQ pain. While the classic teaching is that enlargement of the uterus may change the location of the appendix, a recent study found that even when appendicitis occurred in the third trimester, the vast majority of patients still had right lower quadrant pain.

10. **A 75-year-old woman passed out in church. She is presently pale and clammy. Her physical examination is otherwise unremarkable except for burgundy-colored stool in her rectal vault. Her heart rate is 80/min, and her blood pressure is 100/50 mm Hg. Her hemoglobin is 4.7 mg/dL. Your most appropriate approach should be to:**

   a. Resuscitate with crystalloid and blood, order contrast-enhanced CT scan of the abdomen, and consult general surgeon.

   b. Resuscitate with crystalloid and blood; insert a nasogastric tube. If positive, consult endoscopist, if negative, arrange for angiography or technetium-tagged red blood cell scan.

   c. Resuscitate with crystalloid only, consult diagnostic and therapeutic endoscopist for esophagogastroduodenoscopy (EGD).

   d. Resuscitate with crystalloid and blood, consult general surgeon for laparotomy.

   e. Resuscitate with crystalloid only, obtain surgical consultation.

   The answer is b. Blood per rectum can signal either upper or lower GI bleeding. Placement of a nasogastric tube with lavage can rule out bleeding proximal to the pylorus. If blood is found, then EGD is the diagnostic and therapeutic maneuver of choice. If no blood is found (but bile is aspirated), then a lower GI source of bleeding is more likely. Angiography sometimes can detect the site of bleeding, but requires a relatively brisk bleeding rate (0.5–2.0 mL/min) to be diagnostic. Technetium-labeled red cell scintigraphy is even more sensitive than angiography and can localize the site of bleeding at a rate of 0.1 mL/min. The hemoglobin is critically low, and blood transfusion should be started along with crystalloid infusion. CT scan has only a minimal role in the management of GI bleeding. Laparotomy is not indicated until the bleeding is localized by other tests to the upper or lower GI system.

11. **A 54-year-old man with long history of alcohol abuse and prior history of pancreatitis complains of severe upper abdominal pain and numerous episodes of nonbloody, nonbilious vomiting after a weekend binge of drinking. His serum amylase level is within normal range, but you still suspect acute pancreatitis, knowing that amylase may be falsely depressed in a patient with concomitant:**

   a. Hypercholesterolemia.

   b. Hypertriglyceridemia.

   c. *Helicobacter pylori* infection.

   d. Hypocalcemia.

   e. Occult gastrointestinal bleeding.

   The answer is b. While serum amylase is a reasonable screening tool for acute pancreatitis, it is not perfect. If you can exclude intestinal perforation or infarction from the differential (both of which cause a rise in amylase), then a level >300 U/dL is present in 85% of patients within the first 24 hours of symptoms. Reasons for incorrect normal values include extensive pancreatic necrosis, infarction, and pseudocyst formation. Both serum amylase and serum lipase can be falsely low in patients with hypertriglyceridemia. False lows are also reported in patients with chronic pancreatitis.

12. **A 50-year-old man complains of abdominal pain and a 1-week history of black bowel movements, weakness, nausea, and dark colored urine. He reports heavy alcohol consumption. His gait is ataxic. His temperature is 37.9°C, heart rate 70/min, respiratory rate 18/min, and blood pressure 140/60 mm Hg. He is disoriented and has a tender enlarged liver, guaiac-positive stool, and mild ascites. Laboratory test results: WBC, normal; PT and INR, mildly prolonged; AST, 3 times normal; total bilirubin, 2.0; alkaline phosphatase, moderately elevated. Immediate management should include:**

   a. Rectal lactulose.

   b. Abdominal CT with contrast.

   c. Percutaneous liver biopsy.

   d. Diagnostic paracentesis.

   e. Bedside ultrasound.

   The answer is d. Alcoholic hepatitis is often associated with additional complicating disease: meningitis, pneumonia, subdural hematomas, peritonitis, and GI bleeding. Hepatic encephalopathy may account for neuropsychiatric symptoms. Treatment is supportive, and unless the disease is clearly mild, hospital admission is justified. Blood cultures should be ordered to evaluate for sepsis. A paracentesis is needed to evaluate for spontaneous bacterial peritonitis. If indicated, a liver biopsy may be performed on an elective basis, but certainly not before reversal of the abnormal coagulation status.

13. **A 50-year-old man complains of abdominal pain. He recently underwent open cholecystectomy and exploration of the common bile duct for gallstone pancreatitis. He is afebrile and has epigastric tenderness. You palpate a vague mass in the right upper quadrant. Bile drains from the T-tube. You should now order:**

    a. HIDA scan.

    b. Full obstruction series.

    c. Abdominal CT scan with oral and intravenous contrast.

    d. Chest radiograph to rule out free air.

    e. Upper GI series with barium.

The answer is c. CT scan in a patient with suspected pancreatitis helps to rule out other causes of abdominal pain and evaluates potential peripancreatic complications such as hemorrhage, pseudocyst, abscess, or vascular abnormalities. It is also quite accurate at determining the amount of pancreatic necrosis. The Atlanta International Symposium recommends CT in patients with (1) an uncertain diagnosis; (2) severe clinical pancreatitis, abdominal distention, tenderness, temperature higher than 102°F, and leukocytosis; (3) a Ranson score of more than 3 or APACHE score of more than 8; (4) no improvement within 72 hours; and (5) acute deterioration. The main indication for obtaining a CT scan in the emergency department is to exclude other diagnoses; however, if the patient is significantly ill and can tolerate the procedure, early CT may help determine whether complications are already present.

14. **The most sensitive and specific test to confirm the diagnosis of acute cholecystitis is:**

    a. Oral cholecystogram.

    b. HIDA radioisotope scan.

    c. Ultrasound.

    d. Plain film of the abdomen.

    e. The triad of fever, elevated bilirubin, and elevated alkaline phosphatase.

The answer is b. Ultrasonography has an unadjusted 94% sensitivity and 78% specificity for the diagnosis of acute cholecystitis. The 50% sensitivity of CT scanning is insufficient for it to be used in place of ultrasonography. Technetium-iminoacetic acid analogue-based radioisotope scintigraphy (HIDA) has 97% sensitivity and 90% specificity. Within 1 hour of injection, a normal patient will have a clearly outlined gallbladder and cystic duct. Failure to demonstrate the gallbladder within this time frame is consistent with cystic duct obstruction.

15. **A 39-year-old woman complains difficulty swallowing, predominantly with liquids, and regurgitation of foul-tasting food. She had an esophagram a few days ago, and you obtain the results, which show a flaccid, dilated esophagus with a sharply tapered narrowing at the gastroesophageal junction. She has:**

    a. Esophageal colic.

    b. Esophageal malignancy.

    c. Reflux esophagitis.

    d. Scleroderma.

    e. Achalasia.

The answer is e. Achalasia is a disorder of esophageal motility and incomplete relaxation of the lower esophageal sphincter (beaking of LES). In contrast to mechanical narrowing, the dysphagia is often temperature-dependent and improves with warm food. Radiologically, it may be confused with malignancy. Reflux esophagitis and peptic stricture do not result in a significantly dilated esophagus. Scleroderma causes a rigid, aperistaltic esophagus; the LES is not beaked.

16. **A 37-year-old woman with extensive past medical history now has acute cholecystitis. You suspect cholesterol gallstones because of her past history of:**

    a. Hypertriglyceridemia.

    b. Hypercholesterolemia.

    c. G6PD deficiency with recent inadvertent use of sulfa-containing antibiotic.

    d. Sickle cell trait.

    e. Surgical resection of the ileum.

    The answer is e. Obesity, clofibrate therapy, age, and oral contraceptive use contribute to the formation of cholesterol gallstones, by increasing biliary cholesterol excretion. Ileal resection leads to malabsorption of bile salts, depletion of bile acid pool, and an inability to micellize cholesterol, resulting in an increased risk of gallstone formation. There is no correlation between serum cholesterol level and biliary cholesterol stone formation. Cholesterol gallstones can also form during gallbladder hypomotility, such as occurs with parenteral nutrition, fasting, or pregnancy. While hemoglobinopathies, such as sickle cell disease or hemolytic anemias, can lead to gallstone formation, these are pigment gallstones, not cholesterol stones.

17. **A 45-year-old man with a history of alcoholism complains of 12 hours of severe, painful hemorrhoids. Past medical history is significant for upper gastrointestinal bleeding due to alcoholic gastritis. He has not consumed alcohol for 2 years. He has a nontender, protuberant abdomen with shifting dullness. Rectal examination reveals a severe prolapsed internal hemorrhoid with a thrombosis and a large thrombosed external hemorrhoid. The best treatment plan is to:**

    a. Discharge home on stool softeners, sitz baths, and opioid pain relief.

    b. Incise the hemorrhoid, evacuate the clot, discharge home on stool softener, sitz bath, and pain medicine.

    c. Consult and admit to surgical service.

    d. Do a coagulation profile; if normal, evacuate the clot of the external hemorrhoid; and discharge home on stool softener, sitz bath, and pain medicine.

    e. Do a coagulation profile; if normal, then only evacuate the clot of the internal hemorrhoid; and discharge home on stool softener, sitz bath, and pain medicine.

    The answer is c. Portal hypertension may cause severe hemorrhoids. Bleeding from this site can be difficult to control. This particular patient requires a surgeon's expertise and his management is beyond the scope of customary treatment in an emergency department.

18. **A 63-year-old woman complains of severe abdominal pain and diarrhea. She has a history of congestive heart failure (CHF) and atrial fibrillation. She is allergic to shrimp. Medications include furosemide and digitalis. Physical examination reveals a soft abdomen with mild tenderness and guarding; bowel sounds are hypoactive; and the remainder of her examination is unremarkable. Vital signs are: temperature, 36.2°C (97.2°F); heart rate, 100/min; respiratory rate, 30/min. Laboratory studies show: WBC, 19,500/mm^3; potassium, 3.0 mEq/dL; arterial pH, 7.27; arterial P_{CO_2}, 27. Abdominal radiographs show an adynamic ileus, but no free air. She has no acute EKG findings. Your next step is to order:**

    a. Emergent angiography.

    b. Four-hour intravenous potassium replacement.

    c. Admission to an observation unit.

    d. Ultrasound of gallbladder to rule out atypical cholecystitis.

    e. Digitalis FAB fragments.

    The answer is a. The diagnosis of exclusion is mesenteric ischemia; clues include abdominal pain out of proportion to physical findings, a history of cardiac disease, digitalis use, and acidosis. Atypical cholecystitis in the elderly population does not present this way. Physical findings are vague because the visceral pain fibers of the ischemic bowel do not result in stimulating muscle spasm, as in peritonitis. Mesenteric ischemia requires angiography. An allergy to shrimp is not an absolute contraindication to emergency angiography. The administration of FAB fragment is not indicated in this particular patient.

19. **Choose the correct statement about laboratory studies available to test hepatic function:**

    a. AST is more specific than ALT as a marker of hepatocyte injury.

    b. Prothrombin time and albumin reflect hepatocyte synthetic function.

    c. Elevated alkaline phosphatase (AP) reflects catabolic function of the liver.

    d. Lactate dehydrogenase (LDH) elevation is highly specific for hepatocyte damage.

    e. Elevated serum ammonia levels reliably correlate with acute worsening of hepatic function.

    The answer is b. Laboratory tests for hepatobiliary disease can be divided into three general categories: (1) markers of acute hepatocyte injury and death, including aspartate aminotransferase (AST or SGPT), alanine aminotransferase (ALT or SGOT), and alkaline phosphatase; (2) measures of hepatocyte synthetic function, including prothrombin time and albumin; and (3) indicators of hepatocyte catabolic activity, including direct and indirect bilirubin, and ammonia. AST is nonspecific as it also found in heart, smooth muscle, kidney, and brain tissues; ALT is a more specific marker of hepatocyte injury. Moderate elevations of LDH are seen in all hepatocellular disorders and cirrhosis, but may also become significantly elevated as a result of hemolysis. Ammonia levels do not correlate accurately to clinical status.

20. **In diagnosing a patient with peptic ulcer disease or gastritis, the most helpful symptom is:**

    a. Pain at night.

    b. Food intolerance.

    c. Pain made worse by food.

    d. Belching.

    e. Nausea.

    The answer is a. Although no symptoms allow complete discrimination, peptic ulceration is more likely than nonulcer dyspepsia or cholelithiasis in the presence of night pain; pain relieved by food, milk, or antacids; and a shorter duration of pain. Postprandial pain, food intolerance, nausea, retrosternal pain, and belching are not related to peptic ulcer disease.

21. **Melena:**

    a. Is present in 95% of patients with upper gastrointestinal bleedings (UGIB).
    b. Is from blood that has been in the GI tract for at least 24 hours.
    c. Is present in approximately one-third of lower gastrointestinal bleedings (LGIB).
    d. May occur from as little as 10 mL of blood in the GI tract.
    e. Will remain black and tarry for no more than 24 hours after bleeding stops.

    The answer is c. Melena (from the Greek melaina, meaning "black") or black tarry stools occurs from approximately 150–200 mL of blood in the GI tract. Melena is present in approximately 70% of patients with upper GI bleed and 33% of patients with lower GI bleed. Black nontarry stool may result from as little as 60 mL of blood. Blood from the jejunum or duodenum must remain in the GI tract for at least 8 hours before it turns black. Stool may remain black and tarry for several days after bleeding has stopped.

22. **A 58-year-old man complains of difficulty swallowing. He has a peculiar habit of making two or three attempts to swallow his saliva as he speaks. He appears nervous. The most likely site of esophageal dysfunction in this patient is at the:**

    a. Gastroesophageal junction.
    b. Level of the left mainstem bronchus.
    c. Level of the frontal cortex.
    d. Level of the third cranial nerve brainstem nucleus.
    e. Level of the cricopharyngeus.

    The answer is e. Dysphagia is the awareness that something is wrong with swallowing. Globus hystericus is the sensation of a lump in the throat from emotional causes (**c**). This patient's symptoms are characteristic of transfer dysphagia, or the inability to initiate swallowing, and may be caused by mechanical or neuromuscular disorders. Causes of transfer dysphagia include pharyngitis, tonsillar abscesses, monilial or herpetic infection, foreign bodies, epiglottitis, and carcinoma of the base of the tongue or pharynx. Neuromuscular causes may be associated with nasopharyngeal regurgitation and aspiration; stroke, polymyositis, and bulbar palsies (**d**) are among the causes. Esophageal body dysphagia (**a** and **b**) is associated with retrosternal pain and regurgitation. In this patient, without other evidence of disease, choice e is the best answer. Zenker's diverticulum should also be suspected.

23. **The majority of esophageal perforations are:**

    a. Spontaneous.
    b. Iatrogenic.
    c. Traumatic.
    d. Caused by caustic ingestion.
    e. Idiopathic.

    The answer is b. Spontaneous esophageal perforation accounts for only 15% of cases, with iatrogenic injuries accounting for most of the remainder. These usually occur as a complication of upper endoscopy, dilation, sclerotherapy, or other GI procedures.

24.   Ciguatera fish poisoning classically causes:

a. Perioral, hand, and foot paresthesias.

b. Painless hematuria.

c. Wheezing and cyanosis.

d. Chest pain and palpitations.

e. A generalized maculopapular rash.

The answer is a. Vomiting and diarrhea occur 2–30 hours after ingestion of contaminated grouper, snapper, or kingfish from tropical and subtropical waters. Subsequently, the patient develops neurologic manifestations such as myalgias, weakness, paresthesias of the perioral region and distal extremities, and severe burning sensations of the hands and feet. Treatment is supportive care. The disease usually lasts for several days, but symptoms may persist for months.

25.   The most common cause of acute diarrheal disease is:

a. Food intolerance.

b. Toxic contaminants.

c. Bacterial disease.

d. Parasitic contaminants.

e. Viral illness.

The answer is e. Most cases of acute diarrheal illness are caused by viral infections (Norwalk virus, rotavirus, enteroviruses, and adenoviruses). Other etiologies of diarrhea include antibiotic-induced colitis, inflammatory bowel disease, lactose intolerance, obstruction (paradoxical diarrhea from impaction), bacterial toxins, food toxins (mushrooms, ciguatera), individual sensitivity to food, and systemic illnesses (malabsorption and malignancy).

26.   In differentiating a patient with cholangitis from one with simple cholecystitis, the most helpful finding is:

a. Fever.

b. Hyperlipasemia.

c. Jaundice.

d. Murphy's sign.

e. Elevated serum aminotransferases.

The answer is c. Although patients with cholangitis, in general, will have a higher fever and appear more ill than those with cholecystitis, there can be considerable variability and overlap. The presence of jaundice is the clinical sign most helpful in differentiating these two disorders. An elevated bilirubin is characteristic of cholangitis and uncommon in cholecystitis. Elevated serum aminotransferases may be found in both conditions.

27.   The most frequent cause of acute pancreatitis in patients older than 50 years presenting to community hospitals is:

a. Gallstones.

b. Alcohol.

c. Carcinoma of the pancreas.

d. Viral infection.

e. Trauma.

The answer is a. Biliary pancreatitis is the most common cause of acute pancreatitis in patients older than 50 years in the community hospital setting. Alcohol is a more common cause in patients younger than 50 years in urban areas. Trauma, viral infection, and pancreatic carcinoma are less common causes of acute pancreatitis.

28. **The most common indication for surgery secondary to acute diverticulitis is:**

   a. Abscess.
   b. Hemorrhage.
   c. Perforation.
   d. Fistula formation.
   e. Obstruction.

The answer is a. While all of these complications are reported with diverticular disease, the most common indication for surgery is abscess formation, accounting for up to 50% of complications. Obstruction accounts for another 10–30%, while free perforation can occur in 10–15% of complicated cases of diverticulitis. Fistula formation is uncommon, and bleeding almost always occurs in the absence of inflammation.

29. **Radiation proctocolitis is a common side effect of radiation therapy. Choose the correct statement about this troublesome condition:**

   a. Acute radiation proctocolitis requires aggressive therapy with high-dose steroids.
   b. More than half of patients with pelvic radiation develop chronic radiation proctocolitis.
   c. Chronic radiation proctocolitis can begin anytime up to 2 years after the end of radiation therapy.
   d. Symptoms of chronic radiation proctocolitis are easily distinguished from infectious or ischemic colitis.
   e. Massive rectal bleeding requiring transfusion and surgery is common with both presentations.

The answer is c. Radiation proctocolitis occurs in 50–75% of patients receiving radiation to the pelvis. Acute radiation proctocolitis begins during or shortly after a course of radiation therapy, usually is easily diagnosed, and is self-limited. Chronic radiation proctocolitis typically begins anytime up to 2 years after the end of radiation therapy, although 10% of cases have onset delayed beyond 2 years. Approximately 5–10% of patients with pelvic radiation develop chronic radiation proctocolitis. Bleeding can occur but is usually not hemodynamically significant. Symptoms of chronic radiation proctocolitis generally are clinically indistinguishable from other causes of bowel inflammation including IBD, infectious colitis, and ischemic colitis.

30. **Formation of a pilonidal sinus is best characterized as:**

   a. An acquired problem that has a high rate of recurrence despite surgical treatment.
   b. An acquired problem that rarely recurs after surgical excision.
   c. A congenital problem that commonly recurs after surgical excision.
   d. A congenital problem that rarely recurs after surgical excision.
   e. A congenital problem that is best treated with antibiotics.

The answer is a. Once considered a congenital problem, the formation of a pilonidal sinus is now considered to be an acquired problem. Incision and drainage with packing is adequate initial therapy; clumps of hair and detritus should be removed. Antibiotics are not necessary unless cellulitis is present or the patient is immunocompromised. The condition has a relatively high recurrence rate.

31.   **A 48-year-old woman complains of epigastric and right upper quadrant pain and jaundice. She has a fever of 39.5°C (103.1°F) with chills. She probably has:**

    a. Viral hepatitis.

    b. Alcoholic hepatitis.

    c. Pancreatitis.

    d. Ascending cholangitis.

    e. Acute cholecystitis.

The answer is d. Charcot triad consists of fever with chills, right upper quadrant pain, and jaundice. A purulent infection extends into the liver. Ascending cholangitis is a surgical emergency and carries a high mortality.

32.   **Acute mesenteric ischemia is most commonly caused by:**

    a. Arterial thrombosis.

    b. Arterial embolus.

    c. Venous occlusion.

    d. Hypercoagulable state.

    e. Nonocclusive vascular disease.

The answer is b. Although all of the above can cause acute mesenteric ischemia, the most common cause is an arterial embolus.

33.   **In predicting severity of illness for a patient with acute pancreatitis, useful findings in the emergency department include:**

    a. Lactate dehydrogenase level.

    b. Serum calcium level.

    c. Serum lipase level.

    d. Hematocrit.

    e. Serum amylase level.

The answer is a. Ranson's criteria are used to predict in-hospital mortality. Useful presentation criteria include the patient's age, WBC, AST (SGOT), amylase, and LDH levels at the time of admission. After 48 hours, the criteria include a falling hematocrit, rising BUN and low calcium. Serum lipase is a more specific indicator of acute pancreatitis than serum amylase, but it is not included in Ranson's criteria.

34.   **Choose the correct statement about foreign bodies of the esophagus:**

    a. Button battery ingestion in a child always mandates endoscopic removal.

    b. Proteolytic enzymes are the initial treatment of choice in a patient with esophageal food impaction from a piece of chicken meat with bone.

    c. Refusal to eat in an otherwise healthy child suggests an esophageal foreign body.

    d. Smooth muscle relaxers, such as tolteridine (Detrol), have proven useful.

    e. Radiographs generally show a stuck coin to be sideways on the AP view.

The answer is c. Esophageal perforation is a known complication of using papain to dissolve an esophageal meat bolus. Furthermore, if aspirated, papain may result in hemorrhagic pulmonary edema. Glucagon can be used to try and relieve a food impaction by acting to relax the esophagus. Children may only present with the inability to swallow (drooling) in cases of ingestion of a foreign body. Ingested button batteries must be removed from the esophagus only if they do not spontaneously pass into the stomach. The mnemonic to remember coin orientation on radiographs: Is it SAFE? Sideways–Airway; Face–Esophagus.

35. **Cecal volvulus:**

    a. Is common in infants.
    b. Is the most common cause of bowel obstruction in pregnancy.
    c. Occurs more frequently in the obese.
    d. Rarely leads to gangrene.
    e. Is common in the elderly, debilitated patient.

    The answer is b. Volvulus of the cecum occurs in all ages but is most common in persons 25–35 years of age. Unlike in sigmoid volvulus, severe, chronic constipation is not an underlying factor, and there is no association with psychiatric or neurologic diseases. Cecal volvulus is the most common cause of bowel obstruction in pregnancy, accounting for approximately 12% of all cases. Bowel gangrene is common and occurs in 20% of patients with cecal volvulus.

36. **The most common parasitic cause of diarrhea in the United States is:**

    a. *Entamoeba histolytica.*
    b. *Cryptosporidium.*
    c. *Giardia duodenalis.*
    d. *Naegleria.*
    e. *Trichomonas gastrointestinalis.*

    The answer is c. Symptoms of giardiasis are abdominal pain and distension, postprandial defecatory urgency, and fatty, foul smelling stools as in pancreatic insufficiency. The causative agent recently underwent a name change, from *Giardia lamblia* to *Giardia duodenalis*. Diagnosis is by antigen testing of stool or by examination of at least three stool specimens for ova and parasites. Duodenal aspirate may be necessary. Metronidazole is still the first drug of choice for treatment, although resistant strains are being reported more frequently. Newer, more expensive medications such as nitazoxanide (Alinia) or tinidazole (Tindamax) may be needed in resistant cases. *Cryptosporidium* is a common cause of diarrhea in preschoolers and immunosuppressed patients and is diagnosed by acid-fast stain of the stool.

37.   **A 23-year-old woman who has had an appendectomy is complaining of pain of the right lower quadrant, fever, anorexia, and dysuria. She vomited once, but denies diarrhea or constipation. Her last menstrual period was 12 days ago, and she takes oral contraceptives. Her temperature is 38.2°C (100.1°F). The examination shows tenderness of the right lower quadrant with local peritoneal signs, slight cervical motion tenderness, and right adnexal tenderness without mass. Laboratory test results show WBC, 12,500/mm³ with 18% immature forms. Urinalysis shows 5–10 WBCs and 10 RBCs per high-power field. Her pregnancy test is negative. The most likely diagnosis is:**

a. Regional enteritis.

b. Pylephlebitis.

c. Pyelonephritis.

d. Acute salpingitis (PID).

e. Regenerative appendicitis.

The answer is a. Regional enteritis, like appendicitis, can cause inflammation of the ureter and result in pyuria and hematuria. The inflammatory process may lie next to the uterus and bladder, causing symptoms of dysuria and pelvic tenderness. Pyelonephritis may mimic appendicitis, although its presence is less likely without flank pain. Acute salpingitis may present with the same symptoms but is more likely to occur within 7 days of the last menses, and nausea, vomiting, and anorexia are less likely to occur. One or more episodes of acute salpingo-oophoritis usually precedes tubo-ovarian abscess. Pylephlebitis is septic thrombosis of the portal vein and the least likely diagnosis in this patient.

38.   **A newly hired nurse is accidentally stuck with a hollow needle, which she had just used to start an intravenous line on a patient known to have chronic hepatitis B. She has not yet started her primary hepatitis prophylaxis series. You decide to:**

a. Send antibody levels (HBsAg) on the employee and determine treatment based on the results.

b. Give her hepatitis B immune globulin (HBIG) 0.06 mL/kg and start the hepatitis B vaccine series, with the first shot in the buttock.

c. Give her hepatitis B immune globulin (HBIG) 0.06 mL/kg and start the hepatitis B vaccine series, with the first shot in the deltoid.

d. Give her hepatitis B immune globulin (HBIG) 0.6 mL/kg and start the hepatitis B vaccine series, with the first shot in the buttock.

e. Give her hepatitis B immune globulin (HBIG) 0.6 mL/kg and start the hepatitis B vaccine series, with the first shot in the deltoid.

The answer is c. HBV immune globulin (HBIG) is recommended for immediate passive immunization in individuals not previously immunized but exposed to potentially infective material. HBIG alone diminishes the risk of HBV infection by 75%. Unvaccinated, exposed people should receive HBIG 0.06 mL/kg intramuscularly (IM) in addition to the HB vaccine. Centers for Disease Control and Prevention (CDC) data suggest that optimal immunologic response results from deltoid injection.

39.   **Choose the correct statement concerning Crohn's disease:**

a. There is no known hereditary predisposition to developing Crohn's disease.

b. Juvenile and adult onset follow different courses and are treated differently.

c. It may involve the small bowel only, the colon only, or both (as in ileocolitis).

d. It involves continuous lesions of the superficial bowel layers.

e. Psychogenic factors play a major causative role.

The answer is c. Crohn's disease involves all the layers of bowel and is discontinuous ("skip" lesions). In 50% of patients with Crohn's disease, both the small and large bowels are affected. Disease localized to the colon occurs in 20% of patients. There is little data to support psychogenic factors as a cause of Crohn's disease. The disease is apparently one of a disordered immune response, but the exact pathophysiology is not understood. With the exception of retardation of growth, the course is similar in adults and children.

40. **A 35-year-old woman complains of severe pain during and for several hours postdefecation. Visual inspection of the anus shows a single midline anterior hemorrhoid. She refuses further examination. The next most appropriate step is to:**

    a. Explain that without examination, treatment cannot be prescribed.
    b. Treat with analgesic ointments and hydrocortisone cream.
    c. Inquire about symptoms of neoplasm, Crohn's disease, syphilis, and tuberculosis.
    d. Recommend surgical excision.
    e. Advise sitz baths and bulk laxatives.

    The answer is e. Severe pain on defecation, refusal to allow a rectal examination, and a midline pile (usually posterior, though it may be anterior in women) are diagnostic of anal fissure. Nonmidline fissures suggest another process, such as Crohn's disease. Analgesic ointments and steroid creams may delay healing. Softening the stool with a high-fiber diet and sitz baths provide relief and aid healing. If this fails, surgical excision is necessary.

41. **You have just seen three teenagers from the same 10th grade class of a school who have apparent appendicitis—right lower abdominal pain, anorexia, nausea, and low-grade fever. You realize this is an incredible coincidence and call local hospitals, to find that six of their colleagues are being seen for similar symptoms, and two have already gone to the operating room for appendectomy. You now suspect that rather than appendicitis, they may be infected with:**

    a. *Bacillus cereus.*
    b. *E. coli* 0157:H7.
    c. *Cryptosporidiosis.*
    d. Group D *Streptococcus.*
    e. *Yersinia enterocolitica.*

    The answer is e. The initial clinical picture of Yersinia enterocolitis resembles that of infection by other invasive intestinal organisms: fever; colicky abdominal pain; watery, greenish, and sometimes bloody diarrhea; and constitutional symptoms of anorexia, vomiting, and malaise. A substantial number of patients with yersiniosis, in particular adolescents and young adults, develop an ileocecitis. In these cases, lower abdominal pain with little or no diarrhea predominates and may perfectly mimic acute appendicitis. Large gastrointestinal outbreaks have been traced to contaminated milk, largely because physicians noticed an extraordinary jump in the number of negative appendectomies.

42. **Lactulose removes ammonia ions from the gut by:**

a. Being converted to lactic acid by colonic bacteria; this acidifies the feces, resulting in the trapping of ammonia as ammonium in the stool.

b. Causing ammonia to be transmitted to the intracellular region through the sodium–potassium membrane pump, where it is safely used in the tricarboxylic acid cycle.

c. Forcing renal excretion of chloride, leading to compensatory hyperpnea and respiratory alkalosis, which keeps ammonia nontoxic.

d. Providing a protective coating on the gut's brush border, which blocks ammonia absorption.

e. Mycelizing preammonia prior to its harmonic conversion.

The answer is a. Lactulose is a poorly absorbed sugar metabolized by colonic bacteria yielding lactic acid. The salutary effects of this agent are related both to the acidification of the fecal stream, resulting in the trapping of ammonia as ammonium in the stool, and to its cathartic action. The usual dosage of lactulose is 15–30 mL orally 3 or 4 times daily or in a quantity sufficient to result in several loose bowel movements daily. The principal adverse effect is excessive diarrhea, with resultant fluid and electrolyte imbalance.

43. **The most acutely devastating complication of ulcerative colitis is probably:**

a. Massive bleeding.

b. Mesenteric ischemia.

c. Protein-calorie wasting syndrome.

d. Malabsorption and electrolyte abnormalities.

e. Toxic megacolon.

The answer is e. Toxic megacolon occurs in up to 5% of cases of ulcerative colitis and usually occurs during the initial acute episode. The patient will appear septic, apathetic, and lethargic, with high fever, chills, tachycardia, and progressive abdominal pain, tenderness, and distention. The cause of toxic dilation is unknown, but precipitating factors may include use of antidiarrheal agents, vigorous use of cathartics or enemas, or barium enema examinations. Toxic dilation occurs predominantly in the transverse colon, probably because in the supine position air collects in the transverse colon.

44. **A patient with a thrombosed hemorrhoid:**

a. Requires a "rubber band tourniquet" treatment.

b. Will need incision and drainage in all cases, as there is only rarely spontaneous remission.

c. Should undergo excision and take sitz baths at home following the procedure.

d. Must avoid beets to prevent future episodes.

e. Should not be given opioid analgesics, as the resultant constipation can cause recurrence.

The answer is c. A thrombosed external hemorrhoid can be extremely painful. Surgical excision may require parenteral opioids or benzodiazepines for patient comfort. The best pain relief will be achieved if the thrombosis is excised rather than incised. If the hemorrhoid is very large, one-third or greater of the anal circumference, it is best to excise the middle third of the hemorrhoid leaving as much anoderm as possible to prevent the wound healing with a stricture. If the external hemorrhoid is not tense and the patient can tolerate the pain, conservative management with pain medication, sitz baths, and stool softeners is indicated.

45. **A 34-year-old man complains of repeated emesis and diarrhea, tingling around his mouth and fingers, and a burning sensation when he washes his hands in cold water. He ate a fish dinner of grouper 12 hours ago. He probably is suffering from:**

    a. Scombroid poisoning.

    b. Ciguatera poisoning.

    c. Food allergy.

    d. *Clostridium perfringens* food poisoning.

    e. *Staphylococcus aureus* food poisoning.

    The answer is b. The patient's symptoms are most consistent with ciguatera poisoning. The classic complaint is burning of the extremities on exposure to cold. Scombroid poisoning presents with nausea, diarrhea, pruritus and urticaria. *S. aureus* causes vomiting and diarrhea and is the most common cause of food poisoning. *Clostridium perfringens* causes diarrhea. Neither *S. aureus* nor *Clostridium perfringens* are associated with neurologic or allergic signs or symptoms.

46. **An otherwise healthy 50-year-old man underwent general anesthetic with isoflurane for an inguinal hernia repair 5 days ago. He now presents to the emergency department with fever, jaundice, and malaise. The most likely etiology is:**

    a. Halothane hepatitis.

    b. Preexisting viral hepatitis.

    c. Hypoxic liver injury.

    d. Sepsis.

    e. Prolonged hypotension.

    The answer is b. Halothane hepatitis after isoflurane has an incidence of less than 1 case per 1 million patients. Prolonged hypoxia or hypotension to a degree that would cause liver dysfunction is extremely unlikely in an uneventful instance of anesthetic use in minor surgery. Sepsis would likely be associated with hemodynamic instability. Preexisting viral hepatitis can have an incidence as high as 1 case per 700 surgical patients, with a third of these patients eventually developing jaundice.

47. **An 89-year-old nursing home patient is treated for pneumonia with a series of antibiotics. Twelve days after starting the treatment, he develops severe, watery diarrhea with hematochezia and dehydration. He probably has:**

    a. Amebic colitis.

    b. Staphylococcal pseudomembranous enterocolitis.

    c. *Clostridium difficile* colitis.

    d. Ulcerative colitis.

    e. Ischemic colitis.

    The answer is c. *C. difficile* is the most common cause of pseudomembranous colitis, which is the most likely diagnosis in this patient. Chronic antibiotic use or use of multiple antibiotics is a significant predisposing factor for this condition.

48. **A 22-year-old woman presents with the chief complaint of several days of nausea and vomiting. She has no significant medical history. Upon physical examination, her height is 5 ft 7 in with a weight of 100 lb. Her supine blood pressure is 100/70 mm Hg, and her standing blood pressure is 70/50 mm Hg. Her supine pulse rate is 100 beats per minute (bpm), and her standing pulse rate is 130 bpm. She is afebrile. Her mucous membranes are dry and you notice significant tooth erosions. The remainder of her physical examination, including the abdominal examination, is unremarkable. Laboratory studies show: hemoglobin/hematocrit, 12/35; WBC count, 8000; sodium, 135 mEq/L; potassium, 2.8 mEq/L; chloride, 80 mEq/L; bicarbonate, 32 mEq/L; BUN, 4 mg/dL; and serum creatinine, 0.6 mg/dL. You admit her to your short stay observation unit for rehydration and a diagnosis of gastritis. She is started on intravenous 5% dextrose in isotonic sodium chloride solution with 40 mEq potassium chloride at 125 mL/h. Twelve hours after admission she is confused and disoriented. When you reexamine her she is still afebrile, and the rest of her examination findings are unchanged. She has no focal neurologic findings and no nuchal rigidity. Funduscopic examination findings are normal. She has probably developed:**

a. Acute hyposmolar syndrome.

b. Acute viral meningitis.

c. Acute hypophosphatemic syndrome.

d. Alcohol withdrawal.

e. Acute hypokalemia.

The answer is c. This young woman presents with some classic features of anorexia/bulimia, i.e., a history of nausea and vomiting, markedly low body weight for height, and tooth erosions. Her electrolyte values are consistent with her history of nausea and vomiting. Most comprehensive biochemical panels do not routinely include serum phosphate determination, and it is likely that her phosphate concentration upon admission would have been within reference ranges. However, treatment with dextrose should stimulate insulin secretion, driving phosphate into the cells. In a normally nourished individual, the drop in serum phosphate would be mild and would result in no symptoms. However, in a chronically malnourished patient, the drop can be profound and can lead to delirium, heart failure, and rhabdomyolysis, i.e., the acute hypophosphatemic syndrome. She had a borderline hyponatremia upon admission, but treatment with isotonic sodium chloride solution would be expected to increase, not decrease, her serum sodium level. Thus, her osmolality would increase. The absence of fever, nuchal rigidity, or any neurologic signs or symptoms upon admission make the diagnosis of viral meningitis less likely. Alcohol withdrawal can also manifest as acute confusion, but it is not commonly observed in persons of this age group and this patient has no history of alcohol abuse. Acute hypokalemia generally does not produce confusion.

49. **Rovsing's sign is:**

a. Pain produced by internal rotation of the flexed right hip.

b. Pain produced by external rotation of the flexed right hip.

c. Pain produced by extension of the right hip with the patient in the left lateral decubitus position.

d. Sensation of pain in the right lower quadrant with palpation of the left lower quadrant.

e. Pain produced by the patient coughing.

The answer is d. The obturator sign is the elicitation of pain as the right hip is flexed and internally rotated. Other clinical signs of acute appendicitis include the psoas sign (increase of pain when the psoas muscle is stretched as the patient is asked to extend his/her right hip), and Rovsing's sign (referred right lower quadrant pain with palpation on the left lower quadrant).

50. **Pseudomembranous colitis:**

   a. Has a carrier rate of 35% in healthy individuals.

   b. Can be found in patients who have not been exposed to antibiotics.

   c. Is best diagnosed by stool culture.

   d. Is commonly caused by organisms other than *Clostridium difficile.*

   e. Is treated best with intravenous antibiotics.

   The answer is b. Conditions other than antimicrobial administration could predispose to *C. difficile* pseudomembranous colitis and thus, at times, this can be a tricky diagnosis. Such conditions include bowel ischemia, recent bowel surgery, uremia, dietary change, change in bowel motility, malnutrition, chemotherapy, shock, and Hirschsprung disease. The carrier rate in healthy adults is 3–5%. Stool culture is difficult, not specific, and requires a few days. *C. difficile* is the most common organism. Oral antibiotics are associated with the highest luminal drug concentration and the most favorable results.

51. **Jaundice is visible in the eyes before the skin because:**

   a. Scleral tissue has a high collagen content than skin, allowing more efficient accumulation of bilirubin.

   b. Scleral tissue is supplied with nutrients by perfusion rather than direct circulation, allowing a more highly concentrated accumulation of bilirubin.

   c. Sclera are lighter than skin.

   d. Scleral tissue is high in elastin content, and elastin has a high affinity for bilirubin.

   e. Bilirubin is secreted by the lacrimal glands and directly absorbed into the sclera.

   The answer is d. The higher the elastin content of a tissue, the greater its bilirubin content and the more intense the icteric discoloration. The innermost layer of conjunctiva (the subepithelial lamina propria) and its contiguous, most superficial aspect of the sclera (the episclera) are abundantly endowed with elastin fibers. The sclera proper contains far less elastin tissue.

52. **A 60-year-old man says he has not visited a physician in more than 20 years, but comes to see you because of watery diarrhea for several months which "I just can't take any more." His wife comments that he cannot drive at night any more because "He can't see right, doctor." The patient is slender, pale, and looks sick. His abdominal examination is unremarkable and his rectal swab is negative for blood. He probably has:**

   a. A colon tumor.

   b. Crohn's disease.

   c. Laxative abuse.

   d. Inflammatory bowel disease.

   e. A malabsorption syndrome.

   The answer is e. Anemia combined with nyctalopia, or night blindness, suggests a vitamin A deficiency, leading you to work him up for a malabsorption syndrome. While a colon tumor and inflammatory bowel diseases can lead to anemia, you would expect to find occult blood in the stool. Laxative abuse would not lead to a vitamin A deficiency.

53.   **In treating a patient with diarrhea, you must recall that loperamide:**

a. Is an opioid with moderate to high abuse potential.

b. Can reduce symptoms by 1 day when combined with an appropriate antibiotic.

c. Is less effective than bismuth subsalicylate.

d. Requires a triplicate prescription.

e. Cannot be used in patients with a penicillin allergy.

The answer is b. Loperamide, the antimotility agent of choice for adults, inhibits intestinal peristalsis and has antisecretory properties, but unlike other opiates (such as codeine, diphenoxylate, and paregoric), it does not penetrate the nervous system and has no substantial potential for addiction. When it is used with antibiotics for traveler's diarrhea or bacillary dysentery, it may reduce the duration of diarrhea by as much as 1 day.

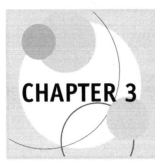

CHAPTER 3

Cardiovascular Emergencies

Joseph Lex, MD, FACEP, FAAEM

1. A 68-year-old woman complains of 45 minutes of crushing retrosternal chest pain. Her past history is significant for borderline diabetes and hypertension, but she has needed no treatment for either. She fell while jogging 3 months ago and required a total hip replacement. She appears anxious and acutely ill. Vital signs: heart rate, 120/min; respiratory rate, 18/min; blood pressure, 140/90 mm Hg; pulse oximetry, 98% on room air. Lung fields are clear; heart rhythm is regular with normal S1 and S2, loud S4, and no murmurs. You see no jugular venous distension. Her EKG shows sinus tachycardia with 2 mm ST elevation in leads II, III, and AVF. An absolute contraindication for use of a fibrinolytic agent is:

    a. Rectal examination showing frankly bloody stool.
    b. Recent use of aspirin for residual hip pain.
    c. Nosebleed last week.
    d. Hip surgery 3 months ago.
    e. Allergy to peanuts.

    The answer is a. Current approaches to fibrinolytic therapy of acute myocardial infarction (AMI) often refer to the first hour after onset of chest pain as the "golden hour," when patients are likely to receive the maximum benefit from fibrinolysis. Absolute contraindications to fibrinolytic therapy include active internal bleeding, ischemia stroke within the prior 6 months, hemorrhagic stroke at any time, central nervous system neoplasm or aneurysm, diastolic blood pressure greater than 120 mm Hg after conservative therapy, pregnancy, major surgery within the prior 2 weeks, and known bleeding disorder.

2.   **Choose the patient who is paired with the most appropriate drug treatment:**

  a. 42-year-old man with acute myocardial infarction, now pain free, with frequent premature atrial contractions, heart rate 80/min; blood pressure 120/70 mm Hg → intravenous propranolol.

  b. 67-year-old woman with a history of congestive heart failure, now with mild breathlessness; takes "heart pill and water pill"; heart rate 100/min; blood pressure 100/70 mm Hg; cardiac monitor shows junctional tachycardia → intravenous digitalis.

  c. 52-year-old man with acute anterior myocardial infarction, allergy to meperidine and morphine, continued pain; heart rate 90/min; blood pressure 130/90 mm Hg → intravenous pentazocine.

  d. 60-year-old woman with acute myocardial infarction, hemodynamically stable → oxygen by nasal cannula at 4 L/min.

  e. 45-year-old man with acute anterior myocardial infarction, heart rate 100/min; blood pressure 170/110 mm Hg. One minute after fibrinolytic infusion begins, heart rate 48/min; blood pressure 80/50 mm Hg → intravenous atropine.

  The answer is d. Nitroglycerin is of benefit in treating a patient with an acute ischemic coronary event, and oral doses may be given repetitively at 3- to 5-minute intervals as needed as long as systolic BP is greater than 100 mm Hg (120 in hypertensive patients). Intravenous nitroglycerin is started at 10 μg/min and titrated to symptoms. Oxygen should be used at 4–6 L/min. Asymptomatic PACs and junctional tachycardias do not require treatment. Pentazocine elevates preload/afterload, decreases contractility, increases oxygen demand, and should not be used in patients with acute MI.

3.   **A 42-year-old previously healthy man complains of 2 hours of severe retrosternal chest pain. Heart rate 92/min, respiratory rate 16/min, blood pressure 120/80 mm Hg. His neck veins are distended to the angle of the mandible, but his lung and heart examinations are unremarkable. His initial EKG shows ST elevation of 2–3 mm in leads II, III, and AVF, and ST-segment depression in the anterior precordial leads. While you are contacting your interventional cardiologist, the patient becomes confused and agitated, and his blood pressure is now palpable at 58 mm Hg. The monitor shows a narrow complex at 135/min. His heart sounds are diminished. You should now:**

  a. Perform pericardiocentesis to relieve the occult pericardial tamponade from rupture of the ventricular free wall.

  b. Arrange for emergent placement of intra-aortic balloon pump to maximize coronary artery perfusion and treat his cardiogenic shock.

  c. Administer a 300 mL normal saline fluid bolus because of suspected inadequate left ventricular filling pressures from a right ventricular infarction.

  d. Immediately administer intravenous metoprolol to decrease the sinus tachycardia in the face of acute myocardial infarction, thus improving left ventricular filling and decreasing myocardial oxygen demand.

  e. Place the patient in Trendelenburg position and remove 500 mL of blood to reduce afterload.

  The answer is c. You should suspect right ventricular infarction in this patient because of the elevated jugular venous pulsations, clear lung fields, and onset of hypotension. Expansion of intravascular volume will normalize right ventricular filling pressures and help reverse the systemic hypotension. Inotropic support may be indicated. Ventricular wall rupture is unusual in AMI and is not seen until 3–5 days following infarction. Cardiogenic shock requiring placement of a balloon is unusual in the setting of acute myocardial infarction, and this treatment is not an appropriate first step in the management of hypotension. Fibrinolytic therapy may be indicated after treatment of the hypotension. The use of a beta-blocker, diuretic, or nitroglycerin would be disastrous.

4. **The most important process in the pathophysiology of acute myocardial infarction is:**

    a. Intracoronary artery thrombosis.

    b. Coronary artery embolism.

    c. Coronary artery spasm.

    d. Progression of coronary artery atherosclerotic narrowing.

    e. Subintimal hemorrhage at the site of a preexisting atherosclerotic narrowing.

    The answer is a. While all the choices listed play a role in the pathophysiology of acute infarction, intracoronary thrombosis is the immediate cause of obstruction in the majority of patients. Furthermore, this observation forms the pathophysiologic basis for the current therapeutic approach to AMI with fibrinolytic therapy.

5. **Choose the correct statement about congestive heart failure (CHF):**

    a. Symptoms of left-sided heart failure include dyspnea, facial flushing, and increased urine output.

    b. Symptoms of right-sided heart failure include dyspnea on exertion and paroxysmal nocturnal dyspnea.

    c. The earliest finding of CHF on chest radiograph is cardiomegaly.

    d. Left atrial myxoma is the most common tumor to cause heart failure.

    e. 5-year survival for patients with good management of their chronic CHF is approximately 75%.

    The answer is d. Left-sided heart failure can present with symptoms related to impaired systemic perfusion (altered mental status or decreased urine output) or elevated pulmonary venous pressure (dyspnea, orthopnea, PND). Right-sided heart failure may cause edema of the gastro-intestinal tract resulting in nausea and vomiting. The earliest radiographic findings of CHF are cephalization and Kerley B lines. Hepatic edema may cause right upper quadrant pain. The 5-year survival in chronic CHF is 50%, with many deaths attributable to arrhythmias.

6. **A 63-year-old man presents with a 24-hour history of progressive dyspnea. Vital signs: respiratory rate 28/min; heart rate irregular at 110/min; blood pressure 110/80 mm Hg. You notice decreased carotid upstroke and you hear bibasilar rales. You hear a prominent S3 and a grade 3/6, late peaking crescendo-decrescendo murmur at the right second intercostal space. Chest radiograph shows a normal heart size and pulmonary congestion. EKG shows left ventricular hypertrophy (LVH) with atrial fibrillation. You recognize that:**

    a. Without treatment, his life expectancy is less than 2 years.

    b. He will require higher than average doses of diuretics to control his symptoms.

    c. Appropriate medical therapy includes sublingual captopril to decrease afterload.

    d. Acute and chronic vasodilator therapy will be beneficial.

    e. Bedside ultrasound will show a hypodynamic right ventricle.

    The answer is a. The findings are typical for valvular aortic stenosis (AS). The three most common presenting signs are syncope, angina and heart failure. Untreated, the prognosis for AS presenting with angina or syncope is less than 5 years; however, heart failure worsens the prognosis and lowers the average survival to less than 2 years. Atrial fibrillation and other tachyarrhythmias are poorly tolerated and may result in acute deterioration. Specific treatment in this patient would be to control his ventricular rate. Because these patients are dependent on an adequate filling pressure, administering diuretics may be hazardous. Vasodilators are often not tolerated, as they can increase the gradient across the valve and worsen left ventricular function.

7.   **Choose the most correct pairing of therapy with hypertensive condition:**

   a. Eclampsia → phenytoin + acetazolamide.
   b. Thoracic aortic dissection, type 1 → diltiazem.
   c. Acute cardiogenic pulmonary edema → nitroglycerin.
   d. Pheochromocytoma → propranolol.
   e. Hypertensive encephalopathy → furosemide + hydralazine.

   The answer is c. Hypertensive emergencies require blood pressure reduction within 60 minutes to halt target organ damage. Definitive treatment of eclampsia is delivery. Temporizing measures include magnesium sulfate, hydralazine or labetalol. In a patient with aortic dissection and hypertension, labetalol, a combined alpha- and beta-blocker, is given with nitroprusside to reduce the blood pressure and aortic pressure wave. Nitroglycerin for hypertension associated with pulmonary edema lowers blood pressure and preload while dilating coronary arteries. Nitroprusside has been described as having a coronary steal phenomenon, which makes it less attractive in this setting. Nitroprusside however is the drug of choice for hypertensive encephalopathy. Pheochromocytoma requires both alpha and beta blockade to lower blood pressure, and propranolol would result in unopposed alpha stimulation, paradoxically increasing the blood pressure.

8.   **In a patient with peripheral vascular disease, the principal source of distal emboli is the:**

   a. Aorta.
   b. Femoral artery.
   c. Heart.
   d. Iliac artery.
   e. Popliteal artery.

   The answer is c. An embolus is the most common cause of an acute arterial occlusion in the limb and originates from the heart in 80–90% of cases of embolism. The two primary causes of mural thrombus within the heart are atrial fibrillation and recent myocardial infarction.

9.   **Which statement concerning arterial disease is true?**

   a. To develop an acutely ischemic limb, either thrombosis in situ or embolic obstruction must occur.
   b. You must start anticoagulant therapy in all patients who present with acute limb ischemia.
   c. 90% of emboli causing acute lower extremity ischemia arise in the abdominal aorta.
   d. The most common site of an embolus of an upper extremity is the distal radial artery.
   e. The diagnosis of arterio-arterial emboli may be confused with a vasculitis.

   The answer is e. Low cardiac output may result in acute extremity ischemia without initial thrombosis or embolus. The duration of symptoms is an important prognostic determinant. Limb salvage is poor if ischemic sensory-motor deficits have been present for more than 3 hours. Antithrombotic therapy is not indicated for the nonsalvageable or gangrenous limb. Up to 90% of peripheral emboli arise in the heart. The most common upper extremity vessel involved is the brachial artery. Aneurysms of the aorta or major vessels may dislodge arterio-arterial microemboli, resulting in muscle tenderness from infarcts, skin lesions, and gangrenous toes. Endocarditis and systemic vasculitis have a different distribution of lesions and physical signs.

10. **Choose the true statement concerning venous thromboembolic disease:**

    a. The most frequent source of pulmonary embolism is the deep calf veins.

    b. The most common symptom of pulmonary embolism is hemoptysis.

    c. The most common sign of pulmonary embolism is tachycardia.

    d. Most cases of pulmonary embolism are idiopathic.

    e. A normal ventilation–perfusion lung scan virtually excludes the diagnosis.

    The answer is e. Thrombosis of deep calf veins is not considered to be a source of pulmonary embolism (PE). However, it is associated with thrombosis of the popliteal and deep femoral veins, which together account for 70–90% of PE. Shortness of breath is the most common symptom, with chest pain almost as common; tachypnea is the most frequent sign. Syncope is an uncommon but important sign. Patients with PE nearly always have an identifiable risk factor. The risk factors of Virchow's triad are: stasis (heart disease, immobilization), hypercoagulability (contraceptives, pregnancy, malignancy, polycythemia, postoperation), and vessel wall trauma. A normal ventilation–perfusion scan virtually excludes the diagnosis. Multibeam helical computerized tomographic pulmonary angiography (HCTPA) is replacing standard pulmonary angiography as the study of choice, although the literature is still unclear about how accurate this study may be for small distal clots, or the significance of missing those clots.

11. **As with all valvular diseases, exertional dyspnea is the most common presenting symptom in patients with mitral stenosis, occurring approximately 80% of the time. A symptom relatively specific to patients with mitral stenosis is:**

    a. Hemoptysis.

    b. A pulsating tongue.

    c. Transient visual changes.

    d. Syncope.

    e. Headache.

    The answer is a. Patients with hemodynamically significant mitral stenosis often complain of dyspnea on exertion, orthopnea, and hemoptysis, all of which result from left ventricular failure and pulmonary hypertension. Occasionally there is massive hemoptysis from rupture of pulmonary bronchial venous connections.

12. **Choose the true statement about prosthetic heart valves:**

    a. In a patient with a porcine aortic or mitral valve, the acute onset of heart failure is likely to be related to valve failure.

    b. The porcine mitral valve is associated with a diastolic rumble.

    c. Hemolysis of red blood cells implies valve dysfunction.

    d. Embolic complications occur more commonly with bioprostheses than with mechanical prostheses.

    e. Bacterial endocarditis within 2 months of surgery is most likely to be caused by staphylococci sp. or *Streptococcus viridans*.

    The answer is b. There are four main types of prosthetic valves: caged-ball (Starr-Edwards); disk (Bjork-Shiley); bileaflet (St. Jude's); and porcine heterograph. The porcine grafts usually do not require anticoagulation if the patient has sinus rhythm, but thrombosis can occur and lead to acute heart failure. Normally functioning valves may be associated with a variety of murmurs, depending on the valve and anatomic location. Only the mitral bioprosthesis is normally associated with a diastolic rumble. Acute endocarditis is usually from *S. aureus* or *S. epidermidis*. Subacute endocarditis is secondary to *S. viridans*, *Serratia*, or *Pseudomonas*. Embolic complications occur with mechanical prosthetic valves at a rate of 1% a year. Bioprostheses have a lower incidence of emboli formation.

13. **In 2007, revised guidelines for prophylaxis against infective endocarditis were developed and endorsed by the American Dental Association, the Infectious Diseases Society of America, and the American Academy of Pediatrics. According to these latest guidelines:**

a. All patients with porcine valve replacements should now routinely receive prophylaxis against methicillin-resistant *Staphylococcus aureus* (MRSA) prior to dental procedures.

b. Genitourinary or gastrointestinal operations or procedures require less intense prophylaxis than do oral or respiratory procedures.

c. In patients with prosthetic heart valves, the number needed to treat (NNT) to prevent one case of infective endocarditis is less than 1000.

d. Patients with hypertrophic cardiomyopathy are at higher risk than previously thought.

e. High-risk adults with penicillin allergy may receive cephalexin 2 g, clindamycin 600 mg, or either azithromycin or clarithromycin 500 mg.

The answer is e. Prophylactic antibiotics are recommended for high-risk patients undergoing "procedures that involve manipulation of gingival tissue or the periapical region of teeth or perforation of the oral mucosa." Such high-risk patients include those with (1) prior infective endocarditis, (2) prosthetic cardiac valves, (3) unrepaired cyanotic congenital heart defects, including palliative shunts and conduits, (4) congenital heart defects completely repaired with prosthetic material or a device, whether placed by surgery or by catheter intervention, during the first 6 months after the procedure, (5) repaired congenital defects with residual defects at the site or adjacent to the site of a prosthetic patch or prosthetic device, and (6) cardiac transplants with development of cardiac valvulopathy. Patient groups that may have received routine antibiotic prophylaxis in the past but are no longer candidates for it include those with mitral and aortic valve disease, rheumatic heart disease, or structural disorders like ventricular or atrial septal defects or hypertrophic cardiomyopathy, according to the AHA statement. Amoxicillin at a dose of 2 g (or 50 mg/kg in children) is recommended for most patients requiring antibiotics. This medication should be given to patients 30–60 minutes before the procedure. High-risk adults with penicillin allergy may receive cephalexin 2 g; clindamycin 600 mg; or either azithromycin or clarithromycin 500 mg. Routine antibiotic prophylaxis is not necessary before routine gastrointestinal or genitourinary procedures, including esophagogastroduodenoscopy or colonoscopy, but antibiotics may be considered prior to procedures designed to treat infections in the gastrointestinal or genitourinary tracts.

14. **Which statement is true concerning abdominal aortic aneurysms?**

a. A nonpulsatile abdominal mass in a patient with acute abdominal pain excludes the diagnosis of an expanding or ruptured aneurysm.

b. Since aneurysms less than 3 cm are usually treated expectantly, these patients who present with back pain may be treated symptomatically.

c. Most patients who present with an expanding or rupturing aneurysm are hypotensive.

d. If aortography is not available, the diagnosis of an expanding abdominal aortic aneurysm should always be confirmed by contrast-enhanced CT scan.

e. Fewer than 20% of patients with abdominal aortic aneurysms present with symptoms attributable to the aneurysm.

The answer is e. Eighty percent of patients with an abdominal aortic aneurysm (AAA) are asymptomatic when first diagnosed. A ruptured or leaking aneurysm may be confined to the retroperitoneum and compress somatic nerves. The pain will be well localized but referred to the thigh, perineum, back, groin, or abdomen. Although a 3 cm aneurysm is less likely to rupture, any patient with a known AAA and acute abdominal pain or a palpable abdominal mass (whether pulsatile or not) should be presumed to have an expanding or rupturing aneurysm. Seventy percent of patients with symptomatic AAA are normotensive at the time of presentation. A plain abdominal film may show the characteristic eggshell calcification. Limit diagnostic delays and obtain prompt surgical consultation.

15. **A 49-year-old man complains of acute tearing chest pain radiating to his back and abdomen. His blood pressure is 200/110 mm Hg. Chest x-ray shows a widened aortic knob. His past history is significant for high blood pressure. He now complains of leg pain, and his femoral pulses are no longer palpable; his legs are pale and he says that he cannot move his toes. At this point, you should:**

    a. Begin fibrinolytic therapy.

    b. Keep systolic blood pressure above 150 mm Hg to ensure adequate distal circulation.

    c. Avoid pain medicine as it will make blood pressure monitoring difficult.

    d. Administer a 10,000 unit bolus of heparin and begin an infusion at 1000 U/h.

    e. Arrange for immediate surgery or interventional radiology.

    The answer is e. An aortic dissection may cause acute lower extremity ischemia from obstruction. Anticoagulation would ensure catastrophic results. The treatment is immediate surgery. Acute extremity ischemia secondary to an embolus or thrombosis requires heparinization. The initial treatment goal for an aortic dissection is blood pressure reduction. Nitroprusside and propranolol are the agents of choice.

16. **In evaluating a patient who has suffered syncope, the most sensitive and specific tests are:**

    a. Complete blood count and basic metabolic panel.

    b. Electrocardiogram and echocardiogram.

    c. Head CT and carotid Doppler ultrasound.

    d. History and physical examination.

    e. Cardiac monitor and postural (orthostatic) vital signs.

    The answer is d. The cause of syncope can be determined by thorough history and physical examination in 50–85% of patients. No other laboratory examination has greater diagnostic efficacy. A detailed account of the event must be obtained from the patient. This must include the circumstances surrounding the episode, precipitant factors, activity, and position. Head CT is not part of the workup in a patient with simple syncope.

17. **A 47-year-old man with no significant past history complains of 4 hours of nausea and a dull chest pain radiating to his back. He thought it was indigestion, but he is not improving with antacids or over-the-counter medicines. He is a slender, athletic-appearing man in no distress. Heart rate is 80/min, blood pressure 120/80 mm Hg. Lung and heart examinations are normal. An EKG shows normal sinus rhythm, a QRS axis of –60 degrees, a right bundle-branch block and left anterior fascicular block with minor ST-T wave changes, and an occasional PVC. An EKG performed 2 months ago was normal. Serum creatine phosphokinase (CPK) and troponin are normal. Of the choices below, your most appropriate choice is to:**

    a. Administer a fibrinolytic agent.

    b. Insert a transvenous pacemaker.

    c. Administer an antacid with viscous lidocaine; if the pain is relieved then discharge home with follow-up by a gastroenterologist.

    d. Administer 100 mg of intravenous lidocaine followed by a 2 mg/min drip and a repeat of 50 mg bolus 20 minutes later.

    e. Start a prophylactic amiodarone intravenous drip.

    The answer is b. A new conduction abnormality such as the bifascicular block in this patient with associated chest discomfort is highly suggestive of acute myocardial infarction (AMI). The risk of developing complete heart block in this setting is as high as 30–40% and is an indication for prophylactic insertion of a pacemaker. You should avoid lidocaine until the pacemaker is in place, as it can suppress ventricular escape rhythms. The utility of fibrinolytic therapy is limited to patients with acute ST elevation or a new left bundle-branch block presenting within 12 hours after the onset of symptoms. CPK values may not rise for at least 6–8 hours after the onset of symptoms and a normal value cannot be used to rule out AMI.

18. **A 25-year-old man complains of swelling and pain in right arm following a tennis match yesterday. There is generalized pitting edema of his entire right arm. His past history is unremarkable. Doppler ultrasound confirms thrombosis of the axillary and subclavian veins:**

    a. The thrombosis is probably not related to his athletic activity.

    b. He requires stat echocardiography to rule out atrial thrombus.

    c. Arterial flow and pulses are normally well preserved.

    d. The risk of pulmonary embolism from this site is 1–5%.

    e. Chronic edema and pain are common long-term complaints.

    The answer is e. Deep vein thrombosis of the subclavian and axillary veins is usually caused by placement of a subclavian catheter, but effort thrombosis is also seen in young people. The risk of pulmonary embolism is as high as 15%. The postphlebitic syndrome is common with anticoagulation, but fibrinolytic agents may reduce the symptoms.

19. **The most important factor in determining the natural history and prognosis of coronary artery disease is:**

    a. Left ventricular function.

    b. The number of prior heart attacks.

    c. The severity of ventricular dysrhythmia during the first 24–48 hours post-MI.

    d. Tobacco pack-years.

    e. The location of atherosclerotic narrowing as determined by coronary artery angiography.

    The answer is a. Left ventricular function and the extent of coronary artery obstruction are the two most important factors determining the natural history of coronary artery disease. Although left main coronary artery disease carries a poorer prognosis, it is the number of diseased vessels rather than the location of lesions that is more important. Ventricular arrhythmias during the first 48 hours of infarction are usually from irritability and are not independently prognostic. The number of infarctions is less significant than the degree of left ventricular function impairment.

20. **Of all cardiac enzymes and serum markers readily available, the one which will be present in the serum earliest and is most sensitive during the early hours after an acute event is:**

    a. Mass CK-MB.

    b. Troponin I.

    c. Troponin T.

    d. Myoglobin.

    e. Lactate dehydrogenase-1.

    The answer is d. Myoglobin levels are elevated in the serum within 1–2 hours after symptom onset, peaking 4–5 hours after acute myocardial infarction. Sensitivity improves from 62% on ED arrival to 100% 3 hours later, compared with 50% and 95% respectively for CK-MB. Specificity, however, is only 80% compared with 94% for CK-MB.

21. **By holding a magnet over a patient's pacemaker, you:**

    a. Turn it off.

    b. Inhibit its electrical conduction.

    c. Convert the pacemaker to an asynchronous or fixed-rate pacing mode.

    d. Recharge the battery.

    e. Convert it to a defibrillator.

The answer is c. A magnet placed externally over the pulse generator of a pacemaker does not inhibit or turn off a pacemaker. Rather it results in closure of a reed switch within the pacemaker circuitry, converting it to an asynchronous or fixed-rate pacer mode so the pacemaker is no longer inhibited by the patient's intrinsic electrical activity. This is helpful when the patient's intrinsic heart rate exceeds the pacemaker's set rate and pacemaker function is inhibited. Magnet application then allows pacing to occur, and pacing rate and the presence of capture can be determined.

22. **Concerning congestive heart failure:**

    a. Nitrates decrease afterload.

    b. Hydralazine decreases preload.

    c. Beta-blockers are to be avoided because of negative inotropic and chronotropic effects.

    d. Nitroprusside increases preload.

    e. ACE inhibitors have pure arterial effects.

    The answer is c. Beta-blockers are generally not used in patients with CHF, but some patients appear to benefit from their use because of reduced sympathetic activity. Vasodilators are a mainstay in the treatment of CHF, and evidence suggests that certain combinations of vasodilators and diuretics may improve the dismal long-term prognosis. Nitrates are preload reducers. Hydralazine is an arteriolar dilator and afterload reducer.

23. **A 65-year-old man complains of 12 hours of progressive dyspnea at rest. His past history is significant for a heart attack 5 years ago. Vital signs: respiratory rate 32/min; heart rate 120/min; blood pressure 95/60 mm Hg. You see jugular venous distention and pulsations, and you hear rales two-thirds up from both bases. You also hear a loud S3 and S4 gallop, and the point of maximal impulse (PMI) is displaced laterally. He is alert and oriented, with good peripheral pulses; his skin is warm and dry. EKG shows sinus tachycardia, Q waves in II, III, and AVF, and 4 mm ST elevation in leads V1 through V4. While in the ED he suffers ventricular fibrillation and you promptly defibrillate him to a sinus tachycardia with a BP of 100/60 mm Hg. On the basis of this information, what would be this patient's in-hospital mortality?**

    a. 5%.

    b. 20%.

    c. 40%.

    d. 60%.

    e. 80%.

    The answer is c. This patient has pulmonary edema in the setting of acute myocardial infarction. He is not in cardiogenic shock as his systolic BP is greater than 90 mm Hg. This patient would be in Killip-Kimball class III, which carries 40% mortality. The mortality doubles in class IV (cardiogenic shock). Arrhythmias occurring in the first 24–48 hours of AMI are usually from transient myocardial irritability and do not necessarily impart a worse prognosis. Keep in mind that arrhythmias are the most common cause of prehospital mortality in AMI.

24. **An inverted T wave is most likely caused by:**

    a. Ventricular repolarization occurring from endocardium to epicardium.

    b. Ventricular repolarization occurring from epicardium to endocardium.

    c. Ventricular depolarization occurring from endocardium to epicardium.

    d. Ventricular depolarization occurring from epicardium to endocardium.

    e. Abnormal delay in AV nodal reconduction.

    The answer is a. Since the normal direction for the repolarization wave is from epicardium to endocardium, reversing this sequence from endocardium to epicardium will produce an inverted T wave. A delay in AV nodal conduction will not affect the normal sequence of events in the ventricles.

25. **At a heart rate of 70/min, coronary artery blood flow is greatest immediately after the:**

a. Second heart sound.

b. Mitral valve has closed.

c. Aortic valve has closed.

d. Tricuspid valve has opened.

e. Pulmonic valve has opened.

The answer is a. When the ventricle starts to relax and ventricular pressure falls below arterial pressure, coronary artery blood flow reaches its peak value. During systole, flow to the left ventricle is depressed by the contracting muscle.

26. **At rest, a patient with mild right-sided heart failure will have:**

a. Low blood pressure.

b. Increased central venous pressure.

c. Reduced cardiac output.

d. Increased cardiac reserve.

e. Increased left atrial pressure.

The answer is b. A patient at rest with mild right-sided heart failure will most likely have a normal arterial blood pressure and cardiac output. His cardiac reserve, however, is diminished. Central venous pressure (and right atrial pressure) will be elevated since the right ventricle cannot generate a normal cardiac output at normal filling pressures. Since cardiac output at rest is normal, there is no reason for left atrial filling pressure to be elevated.

27. **A 26-year-old man with a bicuspid aortic valve presents with a fever of 39.4°C (103°F). He appears acutely ill, and has a bounding peripheral pulse of 110/min with a blood pressure of 100/30 mm Hg. His lungs are clear. Cardiac examination reveals an S4 gallop, a grade 2/6 crescendo–decrescendo systolic murmur and a 2/6 diastolic murmur present at the left sternal border. Soon after arrival, the cardiac monitor shows complete heart block with a rate of 30. Intravenous atropine restores a sinus rhythm, and you successfully insert a temporary pacemaker. The most likely cause of this patient's dysrhythmia is:**

a. Tricuspid valve endocarditis.

b. Acute aortic valve insufficiency.

c. Mitral valve endocarditis and aortic valve insufficiency.

d. Cocaine toxicity from intravenous use.

e. Burrowing abscess.

The answer is e. Sudden complete heart block developing in a patient with aortic insufficiency and aortic valve endocarditis indicates an abscess formation extending into the interventricular septum. Aortic insufficiency, tricuspid endocarditis, and mitral endocarditis are not likely to cause this problem. Cocaine toxicity is usually associated with tachyarrhythmias. IV drug abuse is a risk factor for endocarditis, particularly involving the tricuspid valve, but a structurally abnormal valve is a sufficient risk factor to explain endocarditis.

28. **During myocardial ischemia, echocardiography can detect wall-motion abnormalities:**

a. Within a few heartbeats.

b. In 5–10 minutes.

c. In 30 minutes.

d. In approximately 1 hour.

e. No sooner than 2–4 hours.

The answer is a. Soon after the onset of myocardial ischemia, muscle contraction is impaired. This may manifest on echocardiography as a wall-motion abnormality. Experimentally, hypokinesis, akinesis, or dyskinesis can be seen within a few heartbeats after coronary occlusion.

29. **Choose the true statement regarding patients with hypertrophic cardiomyopathy (HCM):**

    a. A vigorous exercise regimen is recommended for these patients as strict conditioning improves myocardial oxygen supply and demand ratios and thus cardiac performance.

    b. Bedside diagnostic interventions that increase left ventricular filling (such as the Valsalva maneuver or standing) or decrease myocardial contractility (such as intravenous isoproterenol) will accentuate the systolic ejection murmur.

    c. The mainstay of medical therapy for HCM is ACE inhibitors.

    d. The onset of paroxysmal or sustained atrial arrhythmias often results in a deterioration of functional status.

    e. Since there is no valvular pathology involved, prophylactic antibiotics are not needed prior to invasive procedures.

    The answer is d. HCM, an autosomal dominant disorder, is characterized by asymmetric septal hypertrophy and myocardial fiber disarray. Dyspnea on exertion is the most frequent presenting complaint, but palpitations, chest pain, and postexertional syncope are other manifestations. Symptoms worsen with age. Atrial and ventricular tachyarrhythmias are common. The systolic ejection murmur of HCM is decreased by actions that increase LV filling, such as isometric handgrip and squatting. EKG findings in "pure" HCM include left ventricular hypertrophy and left atrial enlargement and a "pseudoinfarction" pattern of Q waves without T-wave inversion. Sudden cardiac death occurs in 4% of patients per year and not uncommonly follows vigorous exercise. The severity of symptoms does not correlate with the risk of death. In symptomatic patients who fail to respond to beta-blockers, calcium channel blockers are used. Surgical therapy has not been conclusively shown to be beneficial. These patients should receive antibiotic prophylaxis for endocarditis.

30. **Choose the true statement about aortic dissection and aneurysms:**

    a. A dissecting thoracic aorta beginning proximal to the origin of the brachiocephalic trunk is classified as a type III DeBakey.

    b. The most common presentation of an aortic dissection is an incidental finding on routine chest radiograph.

    c. Severe chest pain radiating to the legs or abdomen is the most common presenting complaint of aortic dissection.

    d. Aortic aneurysms outnumber aortic dissections by at least 3 to 1.

    e. Unlike aortic aneurysm, emergency surgery is not indicated for most patients with dissection.

    The answer is e. Dissection is the most common acute disease to affect the aorta, outnumbering ruptured abdominal aortic aneurysms by a ratio of 2:1. Eighty percent of patients present with severe, tearing chest pain. Pain radiating to the back or abdomen is considered to be the classic presentation but is uncommon. Medial necrosis of the aortic wall can occur during pregnancy and with Marfan syndrome. Type I involves the ascending aorta and part of the distal aorta; type II involves the ascending aorta only; and type III involves the descending aorta, usually beginning distal to the left subclavian artery. Emergent surgery may be required, especially in types I and II, which may be complicated by aortic valvular insufficiency or pericardial tamponade. However, most patients (60%) present with type III dissections and are managed with medical therapy. The mainstay of medical therapy is control of hypertension.

31.   A 34-year-old woman complains of a red, painful left leg. You find tenderness and erythema running along the course of the greater saphenous vein all the way up to the groin, but her leg is not swollen. Her temperature is 37.8°C (100.1°F). Her white blood cell count is normal. Her history is significant only for taking oral contraceptives:

a. She requires admission and intravenous anticoagulation.

b. Treatment of choice may be an aminoglycoside antibiotic.

c. Phlebitis can easily be distinguished from lymphangitis.

d. Ice, elevation, and compressive dressing will probably be curative.

e. The risk of thrombotic episodes in women on oral contraceptives increases after age 30.

The answer is e. Superficial thrombophlebitis requires conservative treatment. Definitive diagnosis of phlebitis versus lymphangitis may require diagnostic studies in addition to clinical examination. If thrombosis of the greater saphenous vein extends into the iliofemoral system at the junction with the femoral vein, then systemic anticoagulant therapy is necessary to prevent PE and other complications. Massive iliofemoral thrombosis may cause Phlegmasia alba dolens (milk leg) in which the leg is swollen and painful but there is no arterial compromise. Phlegmasia cerulea dolens results if the process continues with thrombosis of most of the venous collaterals. Retrograde thrombosis of the arterial system eventually occurs. This venous gangrene results in a painful blue and swollen leg. Fasciotomy or amputation may be necessary.

32.   Choose the most likely scenario in the setting of mesenteric ischemia:

a. Patient with atrial fibrillation → dusky bowel extending from the ligament of Treitz to the splenic flexure.

b. Patient with CHF on digitalis → bowel dilated but of normal color; pseudoischemic pain from the effects of venous engorgement of CHF.

c. Patient with abdominal aortic aneurysm and hypotension → dusky sigmoid colon with remainder of bowel spared.

d. Patient with polycythemia vera and dehydration → bowel dilated but of normal color.

e. Patient with atherosclerosis and an episode of hypotension → dusky bowel extending from the ligament of Treitz to the splenic flexure.

The answer is a. Bowel infarction is a commonly misdiagnosed entity. Elderly patients with underlying cardiovascular disease are at great risk. Physical examination may be deceptive. The hallmark clue is abdominal pain out of proportion to the physical findings. Acute occlusion may be secondary to embolic disease, valvular heart disease and atrial fibrillation. Complete occlusion of the SMA would be expected to account for the pattern in patient **a**. Digitalis causes constriction of the splanchnic circulation and results in nonocclusive mesenteric infarction. Other causes of nonocclusive infarction are low cardiac output states and hypovolemia. Mesenteric venous thrombosis is a rare diagnosis, but might be expected in a patient with dehydration and a hypercoagulable state. The rest of the patterns are explained on the basis of the vascular anatomy of the colon.

33.   Concerning mitral valve pathology:

a. Stenosis usually takes years of progressive damage before symptoms develop.

b. Regurgitation tends to produce more medical complications than does mitral stenosis.

c. The most common clinical presentation of all mitral valve disease is hemoptysis.

d. The earliest radiographic evidence of mitral stenosis is cardiomegaly.

e. Mitral stenosis is almost always a consequence of ischemic coronary disease.

The answer is a. Mitral stenosis tends to produce more complications than does mitral regurgitation, in which the clinical course may be relatively benign. The mitral stenosis murmur usually occurs between age 20 and 40, and symptoms often do not develop for another 10–15 years. Exertion, infection, anemia, tachycardia, or pregnancy may precipitate dyspnea (the most common early symptom).

34. **Choose the true statement about hypertension:**

    a. Because of cerebral autoregulation, a BP of 140/90 mm Hg cannot cause hypertensive encephalopathy.

    b. A chronically hypertensive patient who presents with a BP of 250/135 mm Hg and encephalopathy would be appropriately treated if his pressure were reduced to 140/80.

    c. The presence of proteinuria, hematuria, and red cell casts with an elevated BUN and creatinine is evidence of target organ dysfunction even if the blood pressure is normal.

    d. Pulmonary edema and angina in a patient with a BP of 175/100 mm Hg is considered a hypertensive urgency.

    e. An asymptomatic patient presenting with a BP of 170/115 mm Hg should not be discharged until his pressure has been normalized.

    The answer is d. Hypertension accompanied by end-organ dysfunction defines a hypertensive emergency. Cerebral autoregulation (constant cerebral blood flow over a spectrum of pressures) resets to a higher range with chronic HTN and a lower range during pregnancy. In eclampsia, a blood pressure of 140/90 may cause hypertensive encephalopathy. In a chronic hypertensive patient, cerebral blood flow may decline precipitously if the lower limit of the autoregulatory mechanism (approximately 120 mm Hg mean arterial pressure) is reached. The goal of therapy is to achieve a reduction of 20–30% in the mean arterial pressure in 30 minutes. In the patient with hypertension (>115 mm Hg diastolic) and no signs of end-organ dysfunction, the treatment goal is to reduce BP within 24–48 hours.

35. **Choose the true statement about pericarditis:**

    a. The most common symptom is precordial or retrosternal chest pain aggravated by sitting up and improved by moving to the supine position.

    b. Hospital admission is generally advised because the most common cause, viral pericarditis, is often life-threatening.

    c. Pericarditis can be reliably diagnosed from the pattern of ST elevation on a standard EKG.

    d. Conventional posteroanterior lateral chest x-rays are of limited value in the diagnosis of acute pericarditis.

    e. A pericardial friction rub is not uncommon in the general population (5–7% incidence) and is thus of limited value in the diagnosis of acute pericarditis.

    The answer is d. Sharp, stabbing chest pain, intensified by inspiration or recumbence and relieved by sitting forward is characteristic of pericardial pain. Another feature is left trapezial ridge pain from diaphragmatic irritation. The friction rub, characteristically triphasic, is best heard with the patient sitting forward and may be intermittent. There are four stages of EKG changes. In stage one (acute), ST-segment elevation in the precordial leads and lead I is seen, often with PR-segment depression in II, AVF, and V4 to V6. The ST-T wave changes present in pericarditis can be difficult to differentiate from normal variants with early repolarization. In stage two, ST segments become isoelectric and T-wave amplitude decreases. In stage three, T-wave inversion occurs in leads that showed ST elevation. In stage four, there is resolution of the repolarization abnormalities. CXR is of limited value, although some patients will have effusions.

36.   **A 50-year-old woman complains of acute chest pain and shortness of breath. She describes the pain as sharp and "much worse than childbirth." Heart rate 100/min; blood pressure 190/110 mm Hg. You hear bibasilar rales and a grade 3/6 systolic murmur with a short diastolic component. Chest radiograph shows a left pleural effusion, mild mediastinal widening, and mild pulmonary vascular congestion. EKG shows 2 mm of ST depression in the lateral leads and voltage criteria for LVH. Her history is remarkable for hypertension, for she has refused therapy. Which statement about her diagnosis is true?**

   a. Treatment with a fibrinolytic agent within an hour of presentation significantly prolongs survival.

   b. A ventilation–perfusion scan will probably show mismatched defects.

   c. CPK isoenzymes and troponin levels will be positive.

   d. Emergency angiogram or transesophageal echocardiography is indicated.

   e. The mean 1-year survival of untreated patients is 50%.

   The answer is d. Acute, severe chest pain, aortic insufficiency, hypertension, ischemic EKG changes, and a left pleural effusion with mediastinal widening are consistent with acute aortic dissection. Ninety percent of these patients present with EKG changes, but MI patterns are rare. Unlike the case in acute MI, the chest radiograph is usually abnormal. An aortic knob with an abnormal amount of soft tissue density projecting beyond the aortic calcification may be seen. Emergency aortography (or in some centers contrast enhanced CT scan) confirms the process. Patients may also present with stroke or paraplegia from involvement of the carotid arteries. The diagnosis should be entertained in patients presenting with chest pain and neurologic findings. Differences in extremity blood pressure should be sought. Untreated aortic dissection has a mortality of 28% at 24 hours and 90% at 3 months.

37.   **A 21-year-old woman in her 16th week of pregnancy complains of 2 days of right chest pain approximately 1 week after she underwent a successful appendectomy. Vital signs: temperature 37.8°C (100.1°F); heart rate 100/min; respiratory rate 35/min. She appears mildly anxious. You can hear a few wheezes at the right lung base. She has a well-healing scar on her abdomen. The remainder of the examination is negative. A chest radiograph (with her abdomen appropriately shielded) shows subsegmental atelectasis of the right lower lobe with elevation of the right hemidiaphragm. Complete blood count and basic metabolic panel are unremarkable, and quantitative beta-HCG is appropriate to her pregnancy. Your next step is to:**

   a. Prescribe an albuterol inhaler and incentive spirometer with assurances that the lung effects of general anesthesia (atelectasis) will resolve soon.

   b. Obtain lower extremity duplex ultrasonography to rule out deep vein thrombosis (DVT).

   c. Obtain a ventilation–perfusion scan to rule out pulmonary emboli.

   d. Prescribe ibuprofen for the chest pain and refer to gynecology for follow-up.

   e. Presume venous thromboembolic disease and begin warfarin therapy.

   The answer is c. The diagnosis of exclusion is pulmonary embolism. This patient has risk factors for DVT, and presents with chest pain, subsegmental lung atelectasis, and tachypnea. Appropriate radiologic investigations should not be withheld from pregnant patients. A ventilation–perfusion lung scan or a pulmonary angiogram is an appropriate choice. Negative venograms occur in up to 30% of documented cases of pulmonary embolism. Warfarin is contraindicated during pregnancy, as it crosses the placental barrier.

38.   **Choose the appropriate statement about alcohol ingestion and heart disease:**

   a. Chronic alcohol ingestion can lead to a restrictive cardiomyopathy.

   b. If heart failure does develop, discontinuing alcohol will not change the prognosis.

   c. High-output congestive heart failure may be due to a thiamine deficiency.

   d. If a patient with alcoholic cardiomyopathy continues to drink, mortality rate is greater than 70% over the next 3 years.

   e. The most common dysrhythmia associated with a drinking binge is ventricular tachycardia.

The answer is d. Chronic alcoholics may develop a clinical picture identical to that of dilated cardiomyopathy. Stopping the consumption of alcohol can halt the progression of disease. With continued alcohol use, mortality rate approaches 75% within the next 3 years. While beriberi heart disease leads to a high-output congestive heart failure, alcoholic cardiomyopathy is associated with a low-output state. Binge drinking, or "holiday heart syndrome," causes atrial fibrillation more than any other dysrhythmia.

39. **Choose the true statement regarding the progression to complete atrioventricular block (AVB) in the setting of myocardial infarction:**

    a. The risk of complete AVB is the same regardless of the region of myocardium involved in the infarction.

    b. Mobitz I second-degree block is an indication for prophylactic insertion of a pacemaker.

    c. Mobitz II second-degree block infrequently progresses to complete AVB, and if it does, a stable infranodal pacemaker with an adequate rate is usually maintained.

    d. A first-degree AVB with a new left bundle-branch block (LBBB) is an indication for prophylactic insertion of a pacemaker.

    e. Infarctions that cause Mobitz II blocks are usually small and patients do well regardless of therapy.

    The answer is d. The risk of complete AVB in an AMI depends on the site of infarction and the appearance of new conduction disturbances. Patients with AMI are at risk for profound bradycardia if complete AVB develops because the ventricular escape pacemaker is often slow and unreliable. Increased vagal tone impairing AV conduction is often seen in inferior wall MI with first-degree AVB or Mobitz I (Wenckebach) second-degree AVB and usually requires no treatment. Symptomatic patients usually respond to simple measures such as administration of atropine.

40. **Choose the correct statement regarding acute myocardial infarction:**

    a. Elderly patients are more likely to present with nonspecific symptoms than younger ones.

    b. An S4 is rare and is probably the result of increased ventricular compliance.

    c. Inferior infarctions frequently cause tachycardia.

    d. A new systolic murmur usually represents tricuspid regurgitation.

    e. Acute fever precludes the diagnosis of myocardial infarction.

    The answer is a. New systolic murmurs in acute myocardial infarction require careful investigation. The most likely causes are acute papillary muscle dysfunction/rupture with mitral regurgitation or ventricular septal rupture. Mild fever in AMI is common. Elderly patients may present with symptoms related to decreased cardiac output, such as confusion or shortness of breath.

41. **Captopril:**

    a. Decreases plasma renin activity.

    b. Increases degradation of circulating bradykinin.

    c. Increases formation of angiotensin II.

    d. Cannot be safely used in combination with a beta-blocking agent.

    e. Is contraindicated in patients with bilateral renal artery stenosis.

    The answer is e. Captopril is an inhibitor of angiotensin converting enzyme and impairs production of angiotensin II, which is a potent vasoconstrictor. Through removal of the feedback mechanism, renin secretion is increased. There are additional antihypertensive effects from reduction of bradykinin degradation and stimulation of vasodilating prostaglandin production. Converting enzyme inhibitors such as captopril can be added to beta-adrenergic blockade therapy to achieve additional antihypertensive effects. Captopril is contraindicated in patients with bilateral renal artery stenosis, since a reduction in systemic arterial pressure may lead to progressive renal hypoperfusion.

42.   **The most important effect of digitalis therapy in heart failure is:**

   a. Controlling the ventricular response of atrial fibrillation.

   b. Controlling paroxysmal atrial tachycardia with block or accelerated junctional rhythms.

   c. Improving myocardial contractility, thus attenuating symptoms of congestive heart failure.

   d. Improving myocardial contractility to improve survival.

   e. Improving myocardial contractility and slowing the heart rate in high-output heart failure.

   The answer is a. Digitalis has been used for years to treat chronic CHF. Digitalis enhances contractility, reduces the heart's sympathetic response and controls the ventricular response (improving diastolic filling time) to atrial fibrillation. Paroxysmal atrial tachycardia and accelerated junctional rhythms are common arrhythmias seen in digitalis toxicity.

43.   **A 60-year-old man describes the onset of palpitations 8 hours ago that woke him from sleep. He has a history of hypertension and paroxysmal atrial fibrillation (AF). On presentation, he is noted to have a heart rate in the 140s with blood pressure of 110/60 mm Hg. Pertinent physical findings include mild basilar crackles in his lungs, an irregularly irregular rhythm, and a nondisplaced point of maximal intensity. His medications include aspirin and an ACE inhibitor. ECG confirms the presence of AF. Your next step is to:**

   a. Perform synchronized cardioversion immediately.

   b. Start metoprolol at 5 mg intravenously until the heart rate is 100/min, and follow this with oral metoprolol at 50 mg twice daily.

   c. Begin heparin drip and cardiovert.

   d. Perform transesophageal echocardiography to rule out thrombus, then cardiovert with 360 J synchronized to the R wave.

   e. Start oral dofetilide, intravenous heparin, and admit for anticoagulation with warfarin.

   The answer is b. While the other answers can be part of the clinical options to restore sinus rhythm, the most important immediate step is to control the ventricular response and prevent possible hemodynamic compromise. Starting a type I-C agent without an atrioventricular nodal blocking agent can lead to an even faster ventricular response. If sinus rhythm can be restored within 48 hours of the onset of atrial fibrillation, then most patients do not need transesophageal echocardiography or heparinization prior to cardioversion; however, if concern exists about the duration of AF and its frequency, start rate control and anticoagulation. The patient can be treated conservatively and cardioverted after 4 weeks of therapeutic International Normalized Ratio (INR) or have a transesophageal echo and cardioversion immediately. In both circumstances, anticoagulate the patient for 3–4 weeks after conversion to sinus rhythm.

44.   **Three drugs which have been shown to decrease mortality in patients suffering an acute myocardial infarction with ST-segment elevation are:**

   a. Calcium channel blockers, aspirin, and heparin.

   b. Fibrinolytic agents, beta-blockers, and heparin.

   c. Fibrinolytic agents, nitrates, and beta-blockers.

   d. Fibrinolytic agents, aspirin, and ACE inhibitors.

   e. Nitrates, aspirin, and heparin.

The answer is d. Calcium channel blockers have no role in the treatment of acute MI with ST elevation and actually may be harmful in this setting. Fibrinolytics, aspirin, and ACE inhibitors have been shown to reduce mortality rates. Beta-blockers reduce mortality in patients with ventricular dysrhythmias or anterior wall MI, but actually increase cardiogenic shock and death in patients who are hypotensive or have inferior wall ischemia. Nitrates are useful for symptomatic relief and preload reduction, but have not been shown to affect mortality. Heparin offers theoretical benefit, but does not affect mortality rates.

45. **The best choice for treatment of ventricular fibrillation in a patient with hypothermia is:**

   a. Procainamide.

   b. Lidocaine.

   c. Amiodarone.

   d. Atropine.

   e. Adenosine.

The answer is c. Procainamide is arrhythmogenic for patients with hypothermia and should not be used. Lidocaine is less effective in patients with hypothermia, and atropine is indicated for bradyarrhythmias. Adenosine is indicated for the treatment of supraventricular arrhythmias, but not ventricular fibrillation in hypothermia. Amiodarone is the drug of choice.

46. **An EKG finding that suggests a pacemaker abnormality is:**

   a. Pacer spike smaller than 5 mm.

   b. Lack of P wave.

   c. Right bundle-branch block.

   d. Left bundle-branch block.

   e. Paced QRS complexes independent of intrinsic atrial depolarization.

The answer is c. The pacer spike is a narrow deflection that is usually less than 5 mm in amplitude with a bipolar lead configuration and usually 20 mm or more in amplitude with a unipolar lead. A wide QRS complex appears immediately after the stimulus artifact. Depolarization begins in the right ventricular apex, and the spread of excitation does not follow normal conduction pathways. Characteristically, a left bundle-branch block conduction pattern is seen. A right bundle-branch pattern is abnormal and suggests lead displacement. In VVI pacing, the paced QRS complexes are independent of intrinsic atrial depolarization if present (AV dissociation).

47. **Choose the correct statement about the patient with a transplanted heart:**

   a. Heart rate does not increase with stress or exercise.

   b. The electrocardiogram frequently shows two P waves.

   c. Exogenous vasopressors do not work in a transplanted heart.

   d. Most antihypertensive agents are ineffective in a transplanted heart.

   e. Atropine is very effective in treating an atrioventricular block.

The answer is b. The transplanted heart maintains a rate of 100–110/min without vagal parasympathetic tone. The electrocardiogram typically demonstrates two P waves, with one wave from the native sinus node in the posterior right atrium, which is left in place with its vena caval connections during surgery, and the second from the donor sinoatrial node, which should conduct to the ventricles as usual with a normal PR interval. The heart rate can increase with exercise or stress through the effects of endogenous catecholamines, up to 70% of maximum for age. Exogenous pressor drugs work well in the transplanted heart. Antihypertensive agents can be used to treat hypertension, even of crisis proportions, as in the nontransplant patient. Atropine is ineffective at increasing the sinus node rate or relieving atrioventricular block.

CHAPTER 4

Cutaneous Emergencies

Stephanie Barbetta, MD

1. **In examining a patient suspected of being infested with body lice:**

   a. Eggs and lice are usually limited to the patient's body and are unlikely to be found on clothing or possessions.

   b. Egg casings are often found attached to the hairs of the arms and legs.

   c. Lice infestation is a superficial problem and should not cause adenopathy or fevers.

   d. Small pruritic erythematous spots on the skin are often found.

   e. Furrows are pathognomonic.

   The answer is d. Body lice and eggs are typically found on the inner surfaces of clothes in contact with the skin. The bites are small pruritic erythematous spots. Scratch marks may aid the diagnosis. Systemic reactions to lice feces and saliva, as well as pyogenic infections may lead to fever and regional lymphadenopathy. Egg casings are eccentrically located and firmly bound to terminal (thick) hair shafts. It is unusual to find lice on the fine (vellus) hair of the body. Furrows are characteristic of infestation by scabies mites.

2. **A 23-year-old woman complains of dysuria and her urine is dipstick positive for leukocyte esterase. She also has symptoms of a mild upper respiratory infection, but is otherwise healthy and has no known allergies. You give her a prescription for ampicillin, but she returns 2 days later with a diffuse, nonpruritic rash over her abdomen and trunk. She is otherwise asymptomatic. You should now:**

   a. Advise her to continue the antibiotic because the rash does not itch.

   b. Advise her to take diphenhydramine, 25 mg every 6 hours, and continue the ampicillin.

   c. Inform her that ampicillin interacts with viral URIs, and to continue the ampicillin.

   d. Discontinue the ampicillin and prescribe trimethoprim-sulfamethoxazole.

   e. Discontinue the ampicillin and prescribe cefaclor.

   The answer is d. Many drug eruptions can appear like viral exanthems. Ampicillin can cause skin rashes, particularly in patients with infectious mononucleosis. If a rash develops when taking a drug, the drug should be stopped and an appropriate alternative prescribed because continued administration can lead to erythroderma or exfoliative dermatitis. Although cefaclor is not contraindicated in this setting, it is expensive. Trimethoprim-sulfamethoxazole would be the best choice with the understanding that cutaneous reactions with this medication are not uncommon.

3. **In patients with suspected Stevens-Johnson syndrome:**

   a. Oral lesions are common but rarely become secondarily infected.

   b. Ocular involvement is exceedingly rare.

   c. It often is complicated by thrombophlebitis.

   d. Women may complain of vulvovaginitis.

   e. Discomfort may be severe but fatalities are virtually unheard of.

   The answer is d. The Stevens-Johnson syndrome is a severe form of erythema multiforme characterized by generalized bullae that involve the skin and mucous membranes, including the mouth, vagina, eyes, and esophagus. Dehydration results from painful stomatitis and weeping skin surfaces. Secondary infections of the denuded epithelium are common, as are severe ocular complications, including corneal ulcers and blindness. Thrombophlebitis is not particularly associated with the disease. Steroids provide symptomatic relief. The overall mortality is 5–10%.

4. **A 4-year-old girl has had an exudative, encrusting skin eruption on her upper lip and both cheeks for more than a week. Her mother has applied a 0.5% hydrocortisone cream twice daily, but says the rash is getting worse. The most likely diagnosis and best treatment is:**

   a. Acne vulgaris → treat with tetracycline, 25 mg/kg every 6 hours for 7 days.

   b. Impetigo contagiosa → treat with benzathine penicillin.

   c. Bullous impetigo → treat with dicloxacillin, 50 mg/kg every 6 hours for 10 days.

   d. Herpes zoster → treat with oral acyclovir and initiate immunodeficiency workup.

   e. Nummular eczema → treat with warm compresses and a more potent topical steroid lotion, such as fluocinolone acetonide cream.

   The answer is b. Acne does not occur in prepubescents, and tetracycline is contraindicated in children younger than 8 years. The two types of impetigo require different treatment. Impetigo contagiosa is caused by group A, beta-hemolytic *Streptococcus* and progresses from a small red papule to larger, honey-colored crusted lesions. Treatment should be the same as for a streptococcal infection of the throat, since some strains are nephrotoxic. Bullous impetigo is caused by phage group II staphylococci and the lesions appear as 0.5–3 cm pustular bullae without erythema. Presumptive treatment with oral antibiotics based on the clinical diagnosis is usually sufficient. Wound cleansing and topical antibiotics are also indicated in both types of impetigo. Eczema may become secondarily infected ("impetiginized"), and may be distinguished by the distribution of lesions and clinical history. Herpes zoster (shingles) is a vesicular eruption following a dermatomal pattern and does not cross the midline.

5. **The most common manifestation of Lyme disease is:**

   a. Erythema migrans.

   b. Meningitis.

   c. Cognitive impairment.

   d. Recurrent arthritis.

   e. Heart block

   The answer is a. Lyme disease is caused by the spirochete *Borrelia burgdorferi*. After *B. burgdorferi* is introduced into the skin, it spreads locally. The local spread leads to erythema migrans (EM), a rash that is found in approximately two-thirds of patients. Keep in mind that a rash may not be present in up to 20% of cases and even if present may be mild, nonspecific, and easily missed by the patient, family, caregivers, and/or the initial treating physicians.

6. **In evaluating the skin lesions of patients with AIDS:**

    a. Kaposi sarcoma is common but seldom more than a cosmetic problem.

    b. Candidiasis may occur but is easily treated with standard medications.

    c. Tinea corporis is no more likely in these patients than in the general population.

    d. Lichen planus of the oral mucosa is associated with the disease.

    e. Seborrheic dermatitis-like eruptions are frequently found.

    The answer is e. A virulent form of Kaposi sarcoma occurs in patients with AIDS. Recurrent, relatively refractory infections such as candidiasis and tinea corporis reflect the immunodeficiency state of AIDS. A seborrheic dermatitis-like eruption has been described in patients with AIDS and is characterized by abrupt onset of a symmetric, scaling erythematous rash primarily involving the face and chest. Lichen planus is a white lesion of the oral mucosa with no particular predominance in patients with AIDS (Tintinalli et al., 2003:932).

7. **Two weeks ago, a 54-year-old man developed a cold sore, which resolved uneventfully. He now complains of a nonpruritic skin rash. Examination reveals raised red lesions resembling hives, some with clear fluid bullae. They are located on his hands, including the palms, and his forearms and anterior tibia. The best way to confirm your suspected diagnosis is by:**

    a. Viral culture of blister fluid.

    b. Smear of blister fluid for Gram stain.

    c. Tzanck preparation of blister fluid to look for multinucleate giant cells.

    d. Full thickness skin biopsy of involved area.

    e. Wood's light examination of involved areas.

    The answer is d. Herpes simplex infection may precede erythema multiforme (EM). Affected patients may have recurrent bouts of the disease with each episode of herpes. The virus is not found in the blisters of EM, nor are fungi or bacteria. Immunofluorescent studies of a skin biopsy showing Ig-complement deposits at the dermoepidermal junction confirm the diagnosis. In mild cases, clinical diagnosis and outpatient treatment with topical steroids and close follow-up are sufficient. Other causes, such as drugs and malignancy, should be considered. Severe cases require hospitalization.

8. **Scabies infestations usually spare the:**

    a. Intertriginous spaces of the hands and feet.

    b. Areolar area in females.

    c. Penile shaft in males.

    d. Pubic area.

    e. Scalp.

    The answer is e. While scabies infestation may resemble lice infestation, the characteristic distribution of lesions aids in the differential diagnosis. Scabies bites are usually concentrated about the web spaces of the hands and feet. In adults, the nipple in females and the penis in males are frequent sites of involvement. Scabies rarely occurs above the neck in adults, who should be treated from the neck down with topical medications (permethrin, lindane, crotamiton, or in pregnant women, 5% sulfur ointment). Reapplication may be considered 1 week after initial treatment. The characteristic burrow of the female mite, a jagged white line with a gray dot at the end and overlying vesicles, is pathognomonic, but it is often obscured by the effects of scratching and may resemble dermatitis. Pruritus may persist after treatment and should not be interpreted as a treatment failure; antipruritic medications are indicated for symptomatic relief. Antibiotics may be indicated for secondary infections.

9. **A mother brings her twin 5-year-olds, who are scratching at their feet and rubbing their hands. You note lightning-shaped red lines on the dorsum of their feet, but no signs of cellulitis. The mother tells you that her family physician diagnosed scabies and prescribed 1% lindane, which she used as directed 4 days ago. She is insistent that the treatment must have failed and something more be done. Her physician is out of town. You should:**

   a. Prescribe lindane to be applied when necessary for 1 week.

   b. Prescribe lindane to be applied one additional time from the neck down in each child.

   c. Prescribe lindane to be applied to the scalp and below the neck one additional time, since reinfestation from the scalp is common.

   d. Reassure the mother, have her trim her children's nails, and prescribe calamine lotion and acetaminophen with codeine elixir as needed.

   e. Prescribe erythromycin, 200 mg every 6 hours for at least 7 days, and topical calamine lotion for itching.

   The answer is d. The lesions and itching of scabies often persist after successful treatment. Reapplication of scabicidal medications should not be considered until 1 week after initial treatment. Antipruritic agents and analgesics should be used as needed in the interim for relief. Lindane (gamma benzene hexachloride) is absorbed through intact skin, and neurotoxicity with seizures has been reported after its use. The drug itself can also result in a dermatitis. Alternative scabicidal agents (5% sulfur ointment) should be used in children and pregnant women. Antibiotics are used only if secondary infection is present.

10. **An avid 65-year-old male golfer presents with a 1-week history of a progressive eczematous skin rash. It is diffuse, symmetrical and involves the face, ears, and left forearm. He wears a golf glove on his right hand. Past medical history is positive for hypertension, which is controlled by a "water pill." Based on this information, he probably has:**

    a. Toxic epidermal necrolysis.

    b. Erythema nodosum.

    c. Erythema multiforme.

    d. Fixed drug eruption.

    e. Photoallergic dermatitis.

    The answer is e. Photoallergic dermatitis is an eczematous skin rash involving the sun-exposed surfaces of the body and may occur with the use of many drugs. This patient's right forearm was spared because of his use of a golf glove. Toxic epidermal necrolysis is a generalized blistering disease that involves the mucous membranes. Erythema nodosum has multiple, bilateral, tender nodules that occur on the lower legs. Erythema multiforme is a disease of evolving skin lesions, which begin as nonpruritic plaques that develop dusky centers ("target lesions"). Fixed drug eruptions are idiosyncratic reactions, typically a single, 2–3 cm, red lesion that develops in the same site every time the drug (tetracycline, barbiturates) is ingested.

11. **Choose the true statement concerning toxicodendron dermatitis:**

    a. Systemic corticosteroids are rarely effective in the treatment of poison ivy.

    b. In severe bullous toxicodendron dermatitis, care must be taken to avoid spreading the eruption by contact with allergens in the blister fluid.

    c. Patients sensitive to poison ivy react to poison oak but not poison sumac.

    d. The allergen of toxicodendron dermatitis is rapidly destroyed by alcohol, resulting in an inactive product called urushiol.

    e. The allergen of toxicodendron dermatitis is rapidly inactivated by household soap and water.

The answer is e. The characteristic rash of poison ivy develops 24–72 hours following exposure. Systemic corticosteroids are used to treat moderate-to-severe cases. Prednisone, 40–60 mg/day tapered over 2–3 weeks, should be prescribed; shorter treatment may result in a rebound dermatitis. Blister fluid is a plasma derivative, does not contain the active allergen and cannot spread the dermatitis. Urushiol is the allergen-containing plant resin and cannot be inactivated by alcohol. The allergens of the three plants (poison ivy, poison oak, and poison sumac) cross-react immunologically; an individual sensitive to one is sensitive to all. Soap and water rapidly inactivate the allergen.

12. **The most important initial therapy for a patient with toxic epidermal necrolysis (TEN) is:**

    a. Corticosteroids.
    b. Antibiotics.
    c. Anticoagulants.
    d. Analgesics.
    e. Crystalloids.

    The answer is e. Hydration is the single most important intervention. A patient with TEN is in acute skin failure. Because the most important function of the skin is to store water, loss of this barrier results in possible dehydration. Dehydration can result in acute renal failure and subsequent shock. Even with aggressive treatment; however, morbidity and mortality are high with this condition.

13. **A 45-year-old man presents with a nontender, 0.5 cm erosion at the base of the anterior aspect of the glans penis. After gently abrading the lesion, a sample is collected and immediate dark-field examination reveals spirochetes. Your next step is to:**

    a. Obtain a culture of the lesion and treat with procaine penicillin 4.8 million units IM, half in each buttock.
    b. Treat empirically with 4.8 million units of benzathine penicillin IM, report the case to the health department, and inform the patient he needs to notify his sexual partners.
    c. Treat empirically with 2.4 million units benzathine penicillin IM, obtain tests for VDRL and HIV antibody, and initiate case–control follow-up.
    d. Treat empirically with 4.8 million units procaine penicillin plus probenecid, 1 g po, and prescribe doxycycline 100 mg po bid for 10–14 days; initiate case–control follow-up and obtain urethral culture and serum VDRL.
    e. Treat empirically with 4.8 million units procaine penicillin plus probenecid, 1 g po, and prescribe doxycycline 100 mg po bid for 7 days; initiate case–control follow-up, obtain urethral, rectal, and oropharyngeal cultures, plus VDRL and FTA-ABS tests.

    The answer is c. This patient has primary syphilis. Adequate treatment is provided by choice c; however, since there is a high incidence of coexisting sexually transmitted diseases, many physicians might empirically treat with a regimen effective against gonorrhea and chlamydia. A baseline quantitative VDRL should be obtained. Whether to test for HIV antibody is controversial, but the patient should be questioned about risk factors. A urethral swab for gonorrhea would be appropriate, but in the absence of any suggestive findings rectal and pharyngeal cultures would not. Most states require notification of the health department of positive results. The patient should be counseled to notify his sexual partners. Follow-up is required to confirm successful treatment.

14.   **The condition that characteristically results in recurrent axillary and groin abscesses is:**

a. Regional enteritis.

b. Diabetes mellitus.

c. Ulcerative colitis.

d. Hidradenitis suppurativa.

e. Acne conglobata.

The answer is d. Hidradenitis suppurativa is characterized by recurrent infections of the apocrine glands. These glands are located in the axillary, anal, groin, and mammary areas. Carbuncles on the back of the neck and perianal abscesses are typical sites of infection in diabetic patients. Regional enteritis may lead to perianal fistulas, abscess formation; however, it would not involve the axilla. Ulcerative colitis is associated with pyoderma gangrenosum and erythema nodosum. Acne conglobata is a severe form of acne vulgaris and primarily involves sebaceous glands of the face and back.

15.   **A 22-year-old man is concerned about patches of skin on his arms and shoulders that do not tan like the surrounding skin. A likely diagnosis is:**

a. Tinea versicolor.

b. Vitiligo.

c. Pityriasis.

d. Acne vulgaris.

e. Piebald albinism.

The answer is a. Tinea versicolor, a yeast infection resulting in patches on the chest and trunk and occasionally the head and extremities. The lesions have a fine scaly appearance and appear hypopigmented.

16.   **A 20-year-old man complains of a rash on his back for 1 week. It is mildly pruritic. You note numerous oval, 1.5 cm slightly scaly lesions. One lesion on his left flank measures 3.5 cm and occurred several days before the other lesions. You recommend:**

a. Oral antifungal therapy.

b. Topical steroids.

c. High-dose IM penicillin for the patient and all sexual contacts.

d. Patience and antipruritics; the problem is self-limited.

e. Hepatic function panel.

The answer is d. Pityriasis rosea is a mild, self-limited skin eruption whose cause is unknown. It occurs primarily in children and young adults. Oval lesions occur in a Christmas tree-like pattern on the trunk. A larger "Herald patch" precedes the eruption in roughly half the cases. It resolves spontaneously in 2–3 months.

17. **Erythema nodosum may occur in patients with tuberculosis, sarcoid, ulcerative colitis, histoplasmosis, coccidiomycosis, or infections with *Streptococcus*, *Chlamydia*, and *Yersinia enterocolitica*. It can also be drug related, with the most common culprit being:**

    a. Penicillin.

    b. Sulfa drugs.

    c. Oral contraceptives.

    d. Cephalosporins.

    e. Erythromycin.

    The answer is c. Oral contraceptives are the medications most commonly associated with erythema nodosum. Pregnancy has also been noted to have an association with erythema nodosum.

CHAPTER 5

Endocrine and Metabolic Emergencies

Joseph Lex, MD, FACEP, FAAEM

1. **The two most common reasons that adult patients present to emergency departments with hypoglycemia are:**

   a. Diabetes and alcohol use.
   b. Diabetes and liver failure.
   c. Diabetes and sepsis.
   d. Liver failure and sepsis.
   e. Liver failure and alcohol use.

   The answer is a. The two most common causes of hypoglycemia are secondary to insulin treatment and alcohol use. Hypoglycemia can be classified into two main groups: spontaneous or induced. The blood glucose level at which symptoms occur is usually less than 50 mg/dL.

2. **You would expect a patient who is poorly compliant with his/her therapy for Graves disease to complain of:**

   a. Cold intolerance.
   b. Weight gain.
   c. A painful thyroid gland.
   d. Pretibial edema.
   e. Difficulty swallowing.

   The answer is d. Graves disease is an autoimmune disease. The resulting hyperthyroidism and goiter causes exophthalmos and a *peau d'orange* induration of the skin that usually is localized over the tibia, which differentiates it from the more generalized, dry, doughy skin of hypothyroidism. An elevated erythrocyte sedimentation rate (ESR), painful thyroid enlargement, and thyrotoxicosis are diagnostic of subacute (DeQuervain's) thyroiditis. In this disease, a viral infection is thought to cause inflammation and abnormal release of thyroid hormone from the gland. Patients with multinodular goiter may develop thyrotoxicosis if excess iodine is ingested or injected, such as that contained in iodinated radiologic contrast media. In patients with goiter who require such contrast, pretreatment with thyroid blocking drugs such as propylthiouracil should be considered.

3.   **A helpful clue to differentiate diabetic ketoacidosis (DKA) from hyperosmolar nonketotic hyperglycemia (HONK) is:**

   a. Serum glucose of 500 mg/dL is most consistent with the diagnosis of HONK.

   b. Fluid deficits are typically greater in DKA.

   c. Most patients who develop HONK have a prior history of complications of their IDDM.

   d. HONK most commonly presents as an acute event with illness developing over several hours, and coma is required to make the diagnosis.

   e. Focal neurologic symptoms occur more frequently in HONK.

   The answer is e. HONK and DKA have similar features: hyperglycemia (patients with HONK usually have a serum glucose >800 mg/dL), hyperosmolality, and dehydration; however, no ketoacidosis. HONK most commonly occurs in patients with non–insulin-dependent diabetes, usually the elderly. Precipitating illnesses include myocardial infarction, stroke, upper GI bleeding, sepsis, and renal failure. Some drugs that can cause HONK include thiazide diuretics, calcium channel blockers, phenytoin, and propranolol. There are no specific signs on physical examination, although neurologic pathology is most prominent and may present as hemisensory or hemiparesis, altered mental status, and focal motor seizures. Treatment for HONK includes correction of hypovolemia—the average fluid deficit is between 8 and 12 L—and hyperglycemia.

4.   **Choose the correct statement about diabetic ketoacidosis (DKA):**

   a. The most common cause of an episode of DKA is idiopathic.

   b. The level of consciousness of the patient correlates well with the severity of the acidosis and hyperglycemia.

   c. For every 180 mg/dL rise in the serum glucose, the measured serum sodium decreases by approximately 5 mEq/mL.

   d. Glucagon and other hormones probably have no importance in the genesis of DKA.

   e. Normothermic patients do not require evaluation of infection.

   The answer is c. Infection is the most common cause of diabetic ketoacidosis, yet most patients with diabetic ketoacidosis and infection have a normal body temperature. While other stresses (pregnancy, surgery, and myocardial infarction) can precipitate DKA, infection must be presumed regardless of the patient's temperature. The level of consciousness has no correlation with the severity of any biochemical abnormality except the serum osmolality. Altered mental status is likely to be present with osmolality >340 mOsm/kg. Nausea, abdominal pain, and other gastrointestinal complaints are commonly seen in patients with DKA and serve as a source of confusion when evaluating for signs of precipitating infection or illness. In general, abdominal symptoms that are a result of the DKA resolve as treatment progresses. A dilutional effect in serum sodium occurs with hyperglycemia. However, significant hypokalemia, hypomagnesemia, and hypochloremia are frequent findings in DKA.

5.   **Choose the true statement about lactic acidosis:**

   a. The absolute level of lactic acid in the blood correlates well with the observed clinical findings in all types of lactic acidosis.

   b. The most common type of lactic acidosis is associated with normal tissue perfusion.

   c. The mortality of patients with lactic acidosis of any cause is at least 50%.

   d. Pyruvate metabolism is not associated with the fate of lactic acid in the body.

   e. Most lactic acid is cleared by the kidneys.

The answer is c. Lactic acidosis is the most common metabolic acidosis. The classification of acidosis is based on the presence (type A) or the absence (type B) of tissue anoxia. Lactic acid is produced from pyruvate by anaerobic glycolysis. It is reconverted into pyruvate by the liver and kidneys. The liver is the most important organ in respect to removal of lactate. High levels of lactate are not deleterious per se, since runners, patients who have had seizures, and patients with certain chronic diseases can develop and tolerate relatively high levels of lactate. The disorder should be suspected in patients with elevated anion gap acidosis. The mortality in patients with lactic acidosis is up to 80%.

6. **The laboratory diagnostic test of choice to confirm thyroid storm is:**

    a. Serum T3 and T4 levels.
    b. Radionuclide thyroid scan.
    c. TSH level.
    d. TRH stimulation test.
    e. None of the above.

    The answer is e. Thyroid storm is usually due to inadequate treatment of hyperthyroidism. It is often precipitated by stress, and the disorder may be clinically difficult to differentiate from sepsis or transfusion reactions. Symptoms include fever, delirium, seizures, tachycardia, vomiting, and diarrhea. Although the serum levels of T3 and T4 are elevated in hyperthyroidism, thyroid storm is a clinical diagnosis.

7. **The most sensitive study to detect diabetic nephropathy in the emergency department is:**

    a. Serum creatinine level.
    b. Serum BUN.
    c. Urine albumin.
    d. Protein tolerance test.
    e. Renal ultrasound.

    The answer is c. Diabetic nephropathy can be clinically silent for 10–15 years after the development of disease. Clinically detectable nephropathy begins with the development of microalbuminuria, even though the glomerular filtration rate may be elevated at this time. Only when the protein level reaches 0.5 g/L will it be detectable on a urine dipstick test. Once proteinuria is detected by urine dipstick, there is a decline in renal function at an average of 1 mL/mo. Azotemia begins an average of 12 years after the diagnosis of diabetes.

8. **Choose the correct statement about treating an emergency department patient who presents with diabetic ketoacidosis (DKA):**

    a. The average fluid deficit in DKA is 4–6 L.

    b. Initial IV fluid replacement is best done with hypotonic fluids.

    c. A negative test for serum ketones in the ED does not exclude the diagnosis of DKA.

    d. Because of severe hemoconcentration, most patients with DKA have a dangerously high serum potassium level.

    e. Intravenous bicarbonate will rapidly and safely correct the severe metabolic acidosis.

    The answer is c. The most pressing problem in DKA is hypovolemia, with an average fluid loss of 5–10 L. Isotonic fluids are used for initial volume replacement. Probably half of the total estimated body fluid deficit should be replaced in the first 4 hours. Acidosis, ketonemia, and hyperglycemia will respond to fluid resuscitation. Bicarbonate is not recommended because of the danger of producing a paradoxical central nervous system acidosis. Insulin can be given as a continuous IV infusion or in frequent small IV or IM doses. Each IV bolus dose produces an effect for approximately 30 minutes; each IM dose produces an effect for approximately 2 hours. Avoid subcutaneous insulin. Begin potassium replacement (KCl or K_2PO_4) as soon as urine output is established. Despite apparently normal or high initial serum levels, the total body potassium is massively depleted. Acetoacetate and beta-hydroxybutyrate are the two major serum ketones in DKA. Nitroprusside-based tests do not detect beta-hydroxybutyrate and will underestimate the severity of the ketoacidosis.

9. **Choose the true statement about hypoadrenal crisis:**

    a. The most common cause is the abrupt discontinuation of long-term corticosteroids.

    b. Patients on short courses (less than a week) of high-dose corticosteroid therapy are at risk of developing the subacute adrenal crisis syndrome.

    c. Hypervolemia is a common finding.

    d. Rapid infusion of hypertonic saline can be a lifesaver.

    e. Mineralocorticoids must be added to glucocorticoid therapy.

    The answer is a. Chronic treatment with corticosteroids is necessary for the development of adrenal crisis from acute corticosteroid withdrawal. There is no such syndrome as subacute adrenal crisis. Other less frequent causes of adrenal crisis include bilateral gland hemorrhage and necrosis from meningococcal or other fulminant infections, or stress of a person with a low adrenal reserve, as in those patients with metastatic involvement of the adrenal from cancer. Patients who present with persistent hypotension unresponsive to the usual measures may have occult adrenal insufficiency. Patients with adrenal insufficiency have chronic volume depletion with a total body deficit that may reach 20%. Treatment of adrenal crisis includes volume resuscitation and intravenous administration of corticosteroids. Hydrocortisone or other steroids provide sufficient mineralocorticoid activity. Unresponsive hypotension can be treated with dopamine. Other important metabolic abnormalities include hyperkalemia and hypoglycemia. The major causes of death are hyperkalemia-induced cardiac arrhythmias and cardiovascular collapse.

10. **In evaluating patients with alcoholic ketoacidosis (AKA) it is important to remember that:**

    a. Serum glucose is usually elevated, making differentiation from DKA difficult.

    b. If serum and urine ketones are low and the anion gap is elevated in an alcoholic with a history of decreased food intake and vomiting, lactic acidosis is more likely than diabetic ketoacidosis.

    c. Patients with DKA are likely to have a low serum bicarbonate, in contrast to the near-normal or elevated levels of bicarbonate seen in patients with AKA.

    d. Glycosuria is a common finding in both DKA and AKA.

    e. Treatment of patients with AKA includes isotonic saline, glucose, and low-dose insulin therapy, and serial estimations of serum or urine ketones.

The answer is c. Alcoholic ketoacidosis develops in patients with heavy alcohol intake, decreased food intake, and vomiting. As a result of the vomiting, hypochloremic alkalosis is superimposed on a metabolic acidosis. Beta-hydroxybutyrate is preferentially produced, and the serum or urine ketone test may be falsely low or negative. Unlike the case in diabetic ketoacidosis, serum glucose in alcoholic ketoacidosis is near normal. Treatment of alcoholic ketoacidosis includes IV thiamine (to prevent precipitating Wernicke's encephalopathy) followed by isotonic saline and glucose.

11. **A 59-year-old man is brought to the ED by his son. The patient is disheveled and cannot walk without assistance. He appears apathetic and does not respond to questions. His son reports that the patient drinks alcohol daily and had complained of double vision. First-line therapy must include:**

    a. Glucose-containing intravenous fluid.
    b. Intravenous thiamine followed by intravenous fluids.
    c. Intravenous magnesium.
    d. Ophthalmology consultation.
    e. Neurology consultation.

    The answer is b. The patient described is a daily user of alcohol who is presenting with vision abnormalities, ataxia, and apathy. A high index of suspicion for Wernicke-Korsakoff syndrome should prompt initial treatment with intravenous thiamine, particularly before any glucose-containing fluids are administered. Glucose may deplete any existing stores of thiamine and result in worsening of the current condition. Although the patient is likely to require magnesium replenishment, this is not first-line therapy. Ophthalmology referral is not indicated in the acute setting. Keep in mind that Wernicke's (ataxia, ophthalmoplegia) syndrome can usually be reversed by thiamine but the Korsakoff's (behavioral and memory changes, confabulation) syndrome is more chronic and usually not reversed by thiamine.

12. **Choose the correct statement about thyroid disease:**

    a. The most common cause of hypothyroidism is chemical or surgical ablation for Graves disease.
    b. With treatment, the mortality of myxedema coma is less than 20%.
    c. Most hypothyroid patients present with myxedema coma during the summer heat waves.
    d. Approximately half of the patients ultimately diagnosed with myxedema coma first present for treatment in a stuporous or comatose condition.
    e. Hypernatremia, bradycardia, and diarrhea are common presenting signs in patients with significant hypothyroidism.

    The answer is a. Primary thyroid failure, usually in patients treated for Graves disease, is the most common reason for hypothyroidism; autoimmune hypothyroidism is the second most common cause. Women are more commonly affected than men. Mild hypothyroidism is accompanied by fatigue, cold intolerance, and skin changes. Hypothyroidism should be considered in patients with chronic constipation, bradycardia, or cardiomegaly. Myxedema coma is a rare but lethal stage of severe hypothyroidism most commonly occurring in patients older than 55 years. Cold exposure is a common precipitating event for the development of hypothyroidism. Although only a small percentage of hypothermic patients have hypothyroidism, 80% of patients with myxedema coma are hypothermic. Physical signs include respiratory failure, abdominal distention, seizures, psychosis, and sinus bradycardia. Laboratory findings include hypercholesterolemia, hypoglycemia, and elevated CSF protein, as well as low serum T3 and T4 levels. Treatment includes intravenous administration of thyroxine and corticosteroids because many of these patients may have adrenal insufficiency. Even with aggressive therapy, the mortality rate is close to 50%.

13. **A 46-year-old woman with a history of Graves disease is brought to the ED several hours after outpatient plastic facial surgery. She is delirious and agitated. Vital signs: temperature, 39.2°C; BP, 140/60 mm Hg, respiratory rate, 35/min; physical examination is otherwise unremarkable. Medications include propylthiouracil and a diuretic. A WBC is 10,000 with no left shift. Findings from other examinations, including CXR and urinalysis, are negative. Treatment at this time should include:**

   a. Aspirin, rather than acetaminophen, to treat hyperpyrexia.

   b. Calcium gluconate infusion to prevent rebound hypocalcemia.

   c. Propranolol 1–2 mg slow IV push.

   d. Ice baths.

   e. Gentamicin 100 mg and ampicillin 1 g IV.

   The answer is c. Thyroid storm may be precipitated in stressed hyperthyroid patients. Recent surgery and infection are two common causes. A major side effect of antithyroid drugs is leukopenia, but the white count is normal in this case. Mental status changes, hyperpyrexia, tachycardia, and diarrhea are the most typical manifestations; however, patients may present with lethargy, coma, and muscle weakness without the usual hyperdynamic symptoms (apathetic thyrotoxicosis) or unremitting atrial fibrillation and CHF. Thyroid storm is a clinical diagnosis. IV fluids for dehydration and supplemental oxygen should be given. Dexamethasone blocks peripheral conversion of T4 to T3. Propylthiouracil blocks the synthesis of thyroid hormone. Iodine is given 1 hour after antithyroid medication to inhibit thyroid hormone release. Propranolol blocks the sympathetic manifestations and blocks the peripheral conversion of T4 to T3. The mortality of untreated thyroid storm is virtually 100%. Aspirin should be avoided, as it can displace thyroid hormone from its binding sites and worsen the thyroid storm.

14. **A 67-year-old woman with a history of chronic obstructive pulmonary disease (COPD) and diabetes mellitus complains of 5 days of shortness of breath, weakness, and diarrhea. On examination, she has orthostatic hypotension, tachycardia, and expiratory wheezing. Initial laboratory results: sodium, 137 mEq/L; potassium, 2.0 mEq/L; chloride, 111 mEq/L; total CO$_2$, 15 mEq/L; glucose, 359 mg/dL. Urinalysis shows pH 5.0; there are no ketones. Her metabolic acidosis is probably due to:**

   a. Diabetic ketoacidosis.

   b. GI fluid losses.

   c. Proximal (type 2) renal tubular acidosis.

   d. Distal (type 1) renal tubular acidosis.

   e. Type 4 renal tubular acidosis.

   The answer is b. The patient has metabolic acidosis with a normal anion gap (i.e., hyperchloremic acidosis). The most common etiologies for this are gastrointestinal loss of HCO_3^- and renal tubular acidosis. The diarrhea is the likely source of her HCO_3^- and K$^+$ loss. Diabetic ketoacidosis is very unlikely with a normal anion gap and the absence of ketones in the urine. With type 1 RTA, the urine pH would be greater than 5.5; type 4 RTA typically is associated with hyperkalemia.

15. **A 50-year-old woman with a history of hypertension complains of 2 weeks of numbness and tingling in her extremities associated with progressive weakness. She takes amlodipine for blood pressure control. Laboratory results: sodium, 144 mEq/L; potassium, 1.9 mEq/L; bicarbonate, 15 mEq/L; chloride, 107 mEq/L; BUN, 17 mEq/L; creatinine, 0.6 mg/dL. Urinalysis shows: pH, 6.7, with no blood or ketones. The most likely associated symptom in this setting is:**

   a. Hypoaldosteronism.

   b. Fanconi syndrome.

   c. Nephrocalcinosis.

   d. Laxative abuse.

   e. Furosemide abuse.

The answer is c: This patient also has a metabolic acidosis with a normal anion gap. There is no history of gastrointestinal symptoms. The high urine pH, low serum potassium, and normal renal function exclude type 4 renal tubular acidosis (RTA). Proximal RTA is unlikely because of the high urine pH. The most likely diagnosis in this setting is distal RTA, which is associated with nephrocalcinosis. Laxative abuse would produce a picture of extrarenal HCO_3^- loss, and furosemide use would produce metabolic alkalosis rather than acidosis.

16. **Severe magnesium deficiency can lead directly to:**

    a. Hypercalcemia.
    b. Hypophosphatemia.
    c. Hypokalemia.
    d. Hyponatremia.
    e. Hyperchloremia.

    The answer is c. Approximately half of the patients who experience hypomagnesemia become hypokalemic. The mechanism is unclear, but probably involves secondary hypoaldosteronism, along with losses secondary to vomiting. Hypocalcemia is also common, and the combined loss of anions can lead to dangerous dysrhythmias.

17. **You would expect to find high circulating glucagon levels in a patient with:**

    a. Decreased plasma amino acid concentration.
    b. Increased somatostatin secretion.
    c. Plasma glucose concentrations above 100 mg/dL.
    d. Decreased plasma insulin levels.
    e. High levels of insulin in the absence of insulin resistance.

    The answer is e. The primary stimulus for glucagon release is low glucose, generally less than 70 mg/dL. An increase in plasma amino acids causes a stimulus for glucagon secretion. Somatostatin secretion inhibits glucagon and insulin secretion. High levels of insulin in the absence of insulin resistance will lead to a fall in plasma glucose, thus an increase in glucagon secretion.

18. **A patient in diabetic ketoacidosis has Kussmaul respirations because:**

    a. High blood glucose stimulates central respiratory centers.
    b. Serum acidification stimulates peripheral chemoreceptors.
    c. Increased plasma hydrogen ion concentration stimulates central respiratory receptors.
    d. Decreased extracellular volume enhances bicarbonate reabsorption.
    e. Insulin directly inhibits the respiratory center.

    The answer is c. The low pH of metabolic acidosis is a direct stimulus on the central respiratory center, leading to hyperventilation. Neither blood glucose nor insulin affect respiratory centers. While decreased extracellular volume does enhance bicarbonate resorption, it has nothing to do with respirations.

19.   **Choose the correct statement about these laboratory results: sodium, 136 mEq/L; potassium, 4.1 mEq/L; chloride, 108 mEq/L; sodium bicarbonate, 12 mEq/L; glucose, 600 mg/dL; venous pH, 7.10:**

    a. The anion gap is 26.

    b. The corrected potassium is 2.3 mEq/L.

    c. The corrected potassium is 5.9 mEq/L.

    d. The corrected sodium is 126 mEq/L.

    e. The corrected sodium is 152 mEq/L.

The answer is b. The reported serum sodium is often misleading in DKA. The true value of sodium may be approximated by adding 1.6 mEq/L to the reported value for every 100 mg/dL of glucose over the norm. Acidosis and dehydration contribute to high measured serum potassium despite total body deficits. Correction for acidosis can be made by subtracting 0.6 mEq/L from the laboratory value for every 0.1 decrease in pH below 7.4.

20.   **The most common cause of metabolic acidosis in children is:**

    a. Cystic fibrosis.

    b. Diabetes.

    c. Febrile seizure.

    d. Nephrotic syndrome.

    e. Prolonged diarrhea.

The answer is e. Metabolic acidosis can be caused by one of three mechanisms: (1) increased production of acids, (2) decreased renal excretion of acids, or (3) loss of alkali. The etiologies of metabolic acidosis can be clinically divided into those that create an elevation in anion gap and those that do not. In the pediatric age group, dehydration from prolonged diarrhea is the most common cause of metabolic acidosis.

21.   **It is well known that vomiting leads to hypokalemia. The reason for this is:**

    a. Direct loss of potassium from stomach contents.

    b. Hypovolemia from volume loss leads to increases in aldosterone secretion, causing the kidney to preserve sodium and bicarbonate in exchange for potassium, resulting in alkalosis, which causes potassium to shift into cells in exchange for hydrogen ions.

    c. Vomiting causes hyperventilation, leading to respiratory alkalosis and compensatory extracellular to intracellular potassium shifts.

    d. With the loss of hydrogen ions after a first episode of vomiting, the gastric parietal cells stop secreting potassium, so secretion cannot keep up with losses.

    e. Unknown.

The answer is b. The hypokalemia associated with vomiting has very little to do with the actual potassium lost in the vomitus and much more to do with the metabolic alkalosis that follows. The hypovolemia from volume loss leads to increases in aldosterone secretion, which acts on the kidney to preserve Na^+ and bicarbonate in exchange for K^+. The resultant alkalosis also causes K^+ to shift into cells in exchange for H^+.

22. **You are treating a patient in thyroid storm. You have given propranolol intravenously. An appropriate follow-up regimen would be:**

    a. Intravenous methimazole followed by rapid intravenous sodium iodide.

    b. Intravenous propylthiouracil (PTU) followed by slow intravenous sodium iodide.

    c. Oral propylthiouracil followed by slow intravenous sodium iodide.

    d. Oral sodium iodide followed by intravenous methimazole.

    e. Oral sodium iodide followed by intravenous propylthiouracil.

    The answer is c. Thioamides, including propylthiouracil (PTU) and methimazole, inhibit thyroidal peroxidase, thereby preventing hormone synthesis. PTU is generally preferred over methimazole because it has the additional minor effect of inhibiting peripheral conversion of T4 to T3. PTU is given by mouth (PO) or by nasogastric (NG) tube every 4–6 hours. Further organification of iodine will be blocked within 1 hour of PTU administration, but the drug should be continued for several weeks while the hyperthyroidism is brought under control. Because preformed T4 and T3 are stored in the thyroid colloid, release of hormone can occur for weeks despite synthesis inhibition. Thus prevention of colloid hormone release is the second goal of therapy. Both iodine and lithium can inhibit thyroid hormone release. Lithium is not generally used because it can be difficult to titrate the dose, and toxic effects are common. Thioamides should be given at least 1 hour before iodine therapy to prevent organification of the iodine. Lugol's iodine solution, PO or by NG tube; potassium iodide (SSKI), PO or by NG tube; or sodium iodide, intravenous (IV) drip is acceptable.

23. **Common laboratory findings in a patient with adrenal insufficiency include:**

    a. High sodium, high potassium, high glucose.

    b. High sodium, low potassium, low glucose.

    c. Low sodium, high potassium, low glucose.

    d. Low sodium, low potassium, high glucose.

    e. Low sodium, low potassium, low glucose.

    The correct answer is c. The usual laboratory findings in patients with primary adrenal insufficiency include hyponatremia, hyperkalemia, hypoglycemia, and azotemia. Hyponatremia is present in 88% of cases and is usually mild to moderate; severe hyponatremia (<120 mEq/L) is rare. Hyperkalemia is present in 64% of cases, usually mild; the potassium level rarely exceeds 7 mEq/L. Two-thirds of patients with adrenal failure have hypoglycemia and the glucose levels less than 45 mg/dL; the pathophysiology is decreased gluconeogenesis and increased peripheral glucose use secondary to lipolysis.

24. **The most important blood protein buffer is:**

    a. Albumin.

    b. Fibrinogen.

    c. Glucose-6 phosphatase.

    d. Hemoglobin.

    e. Myoglobin.

    The answer is d. Many protein buffers in blood are effective in maintaining acid–base homeostasis. The most important is hemoglobin, which can buffer large amounts of H^+, preventing significant changes in the pH. If hemoglobin did not exist, venous blood would be 800 times more acidic than arterial blood, circulating at a pH of 4.5 instead of the normal venous pH of 7.37.

25. **In patients with symptomatic chronic hyponatremia, correction must take place in a controlled fashion. Overaggressive saline administration can lead to:**

    a. Acute renal failure.

    b. ARDS.

    c. Coma and quadriplegia.

    d. Fulminant hepatic failure.

    e. Life-threatening cardiac dysrhythmias.

    The answer is c. Acute hyponatremia may be corrected at rates of up to 1–2 mEq/L/h, and chronic hyponatremia should be corrected at a rate not greater than 0.5 mEq/L/h. In general, the serum sodium should not be corrected to above 120 mEq/L or increased by more than 10 mEq/L in a 24-hour period. Hypertonic saline should be administered through a controlled intravenous (IV) infusion, with careful attention to fluid input and output and frequent assessment of serum electrolytes. The approximate required dose of hypertonic saline can be calculated with the following formula:

    $$(\text{desired } [Na^+] - \text{measured } [Na^+]) \times (0.6) \, (\text{weight in kg}) = mEq \, [Na^+] \text{ administered.}$$

    Overaggressive correction of the serum sodium may have serious consequences. Central pontine myelinolysis (CPM), also known as cerebral demyelination, involves the destruction of myelin in the pons and is thought to result from rapid elevation of the serum sodium. Patients may develop cranial nerve palsies, quadriplegia, or coma. CPM is more likely to occur in patients with chronic hyponatremia than in those with acute hyponatremia.

26. **A 68-year-old alcoholic with cirrhosis is highly agitated, disoriented, and diaphoretic. Vital signs: temperature 38.0°C; heart rate 132/min; respiratory rate 24/min; blood pressure 160/100 mm Hg. Initial pharmacotherapy should include:**

    a. Diazepam (Valium).

    b. Lorazepam (Ativan).

    c. Pentobarbital (Nembutal).

    d. Ethanol drip.

    e. Valproic acid (Depakote).

    The answer is b. This patient's history and clinical picture is consistent with delirium tremens (DTs). Initial drug treatment should be with a benzodiazepine. Considering this patient's age (>60 years) and history of cirrhosis, lorazepam would be the appropriate choice because this drug does not produce active metabolites, which can lead to toxicity. Fluid and electrolyte deficits should be corrected, and thiamine should be administered. In addition, searching for other etiologies of altered mental status, fever, and tachycardia is important. It must be remembered that DTs are life threatening and are a more severe form of alcohol withdrawal.

27. **Urine dipstick for ketones uses a nitroprusside reaction, which measures:**

    a. Acetoacetate.

    b. Beta-hydroxybutyrate.

    c. Insulin levels.

    d. Ketones.

    e. Lactic acids.

The answer is a. Urine ketone dipsticks use the nitroprusside reaction, which is a good test for acetoacetate but does not measure beta-hydroxybutyrate. Although the usual acetoacetate–beta-hydroxybutyrate ratio in diabetic ketoacidosis is 1:2.8, it may be as high as 1:30, in which case the urine dipstick does not reflect the true level of ketosis. When ketones are in the form of beta-hydroxybutyrate, the urine ketone dipsticks may infrequently yield negative reactions in patients with significant ketosis.

28. **The laboratory values most consistent with a diagnosis of DKA are:**

    a. Glucose >350 mg/dL, bicarbonate >20 mEq/L, arterial pH <7.3, severe ketonuria.
    b. Glucose >250 mg/dL, bicarbonate >15 mEq/L, arterial pH >7.3, moderate ketonemia.
    c. Glucose >250 mg/dL, bicarbonate <20 mEq/L, arterial pH <7.0, moderate ketonuria.
    d. Glucose >350 mg/dL, bicarbonate <15 mEq/L, arterial pH <7.3, moderate ketonemia.
    e. Glucose >700 mg/dL, bicarbonate >15 mEq/L, arterial pH >7.3, moderate ketonuria.

    The answer is d. Athough the exact definition of DKA is variable, most experts agree that a blood glucose greater than 350 mg/dL, bicarbonate level less than 15 mEq/L, and an arterial pH of less than 7.3 with moderate ketonemia constitute the disease.

29. **The single most important initial treatment for the patient in diabetic ketoacidosis is:**

    a. Oxygen therapy.
    b. Rapid bicarbonate administration.
    c. Rapid fluid administration.
    d. Rapid insulin administration.
    e. Rapid potassium replacement.

    The answer is c. Rapid fluid administration is the single most important initial step in the treatment of diabetic ketoacidosis. Fluid helps restore intravascular volume and normal tonicity, perfuse vital organs, improve glomerular filtration rate, and lower serum glucose and ketones. The average adult patient has a water deficit of 100 mL/kg (5–10 L) and a sodium deficit of 7–10 mEq/kg. Normal saline is the most frequently recommended fluid for initial rehydration even though the extracellular fluid of the patient is initially hypertonic.

30. **A 62-year-old man has classic symptoms of hypothyroidism—mild hypothermia, bradycardia, hoarse voice, and bilateral carpal tunnel syndrome. You find no signs of infection. He has an extensive cardiac history, including an automatic internal defibrillator, and is on a waiting list for heart transplant. He takes many medications, but the one you suspect is probably causing his thyroid malfunction is:**

    a. Amiodarone (Cordarone).
    b. Bumetinide (Bumex).
    c. Enalapril maleate/felodipine (Lexxel).
    d. Lovastatin (Mevacor).
    e. Sotalol (Betapace).

    The answer is a: The many complex effects of iodine-rich amiodarone on thyroid physiology may lead to asymptomatic abnormalities of thyroid hormone levels, including an elevated TSH, as well as clinically relevant hypofunction of the thyroid gland. Hypothyroidism has been estimated to occur in 1–32% of patients taking amiodarone, which is 37% iodine by molecular weight.

31.   **In a patient with diabetes insipidus:**

    a. Fluid restriction is essential.

    b. Hypernatremia is the rule.

    c. Intranasal vasopressin may be helpful.

    d. There is an osmolar gap.

    e. Urine specific gravity is high.

The answer is c. Diabetes insipidus (DI) results in loss of large amounts of dilute urine because of the loss of concentrating ability in the distal nephrons. DI can be central (lack of ADH secretion from the pituitary) or nephrogenic (lack of responsiveness to circulating ADH). Patients are usually able to maintain near-normal serum levels as long as access to water is maintained. Patients will have a low urine-specific gravity (<1.005) and low urine osmolality. Patients with central DI require administration of parenteral or intranasal vasopressin.

32.   **You are treating a pregnant woman for preeclampsia while awaiting emergent delivery. She shows signs of iatrogenic hypermagnesmeia. After infusing isotonic saline and giving a loop diuretic, you can reverse her respiratory depression and hypotension by giving:**

    a. 20 mL of 10% calcium chloride IV bolus.

    b. 25 mL of intravenous potassium phosphate.

    c. 40 mEq potassium chloride intravenously over 2 hours.

    d. 50–100 mEq IV sodium bicarbonate.

    e. intravenous methotrexate.

The answer is a. Patients with severe hypermagnesemia should receive intravenous calcium, which directly antagonizes the membrane effects of hypermagnesemia and reverses respiratory depression, hypotension, and cardiac dysrhythmias. For life-threatening manifestations of hypermagnesemia, 100–200 mg of calcium, as either 10% calcium gluconate (93 mg calcium per ampule) or 10% calcium chloride (360 mg calcium per ampule), is a reasonable dose.

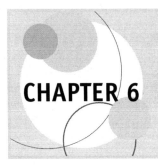

Manish Garg, MD, FAAEM

CHAPTER 6

Environmental Emergencies

1. **A 32-year-old worker is brought by ambulance from a silver recovery plant complaining of weakness and dizziness after being overcome by fumes from the recovery tanks. Shortly after arrival, he becomes unconscious. You are concerned about toxic exposure, so you remove the patient's clothing, intubate him, and administer 100% oxygen and:**

   a. Crush a pearl of amyl nitrite and hold it in the intake valve of the Ambu bag.

   b. Administer methylene blue.

   c. Begin chelation therapy.

   d. Consult hyperbarics.

   e. Consult nephrology for possible hemodialysis.

   The answer is a. Cyanide poisoning must be treated if suspected. Burning polyurethane or nylon, electroplating and silver recovery plants, and pest fumigation are some of the most common sources. Detecting the presence of a bitter almond odor is helpful, but 40% of the population cannot smell this. Initial treatment is to remove contaminated clothing and begin 100% oxygen. Amyl nitrite is used initially, followed by sodium nitrite. Both of these agents form methemoglobin, which acts to remove cyanide from the cytochrome oxidase system and form cyanomethemoglobin. Thiosulfate complexes form thiocyanate, which is excreted in the urine. Laboratory tests are obtained after treatment is started. Sodium nitrite may cause hypotension, which should be treated with fluid and pressors as needed.

2. **A 24-year-old woman complains of an itching, burning skin rash over her upper trunk that started about halfway through her flight back from a scuba-diving vacation in the Caribbean. Physical examination reveals a mottled rash over her upper arms and anterior trunk with some induration. She has no other findings and denies allergies or other medical problems. She wore a wet-suit top while diving. The most likely cause of these findings is:**

    a. The "bends" (decompression sickness).

    b. Angioedema.

    c. Sulfite anaphylaxis.

    d. Allergic reaction to neoprene rubber.

    e. Envenomation by a marine organism.

    The answer is a. Decompression sickness (DS) occurs as nitrogen gas bubbles out of solution when ambient air pressure is decreased too rapidly after diving or breathing pressurized air. Even scuba divers adhering to proper diving techniques may "get bent" because of the decreased air pressure at altitude that occurs even in pressurized commercial jets. The bubbles exert their effects directly by mechanical obstruction of vessels and indirectly by activating Hageman factor (factor XII) and the clotting, kinin, and complement systems. Cutaneous symptoms may be the only manifestation of decompression sickness or a harbinger of more severe involvement. Many cases of "skin bends" are probably overlooked or attributed to other causes. Musculoskeletal DS is the most commonly recognized. Typically, deep periarticular pain most commonly of the elbows and shoulders occurs. CNS involvement is a more serious type of DS. Most commonly the lumbar and thoracic spinal cord is affected, resulting in back or abdominal pain, paresthesias of the legs, weakness or paralysis, and urinary retention. Vertigo may occur from involvement of the inner ear ("the staggers"). The most life-threatening type is pulmonary DS, known among divers as "the chokes." Cough, dyspnea, and chest pain may be followed by circulatory collapse and death in pulmonary DS. Treatment of all but the most minor cases is by chamber decompression. Immediate management includes intravenous fluids, 100% high-flow oxygen by mask, and parenteral corticosteroids.

3. **Choose the true statement about Hymenoptera envenomation:**

    a. The formation of cataracts has been described after a sting to a site remote from the eye.

    b. With true anaphylaxis 0.3 mL of a 1:1000 epinephrine solution should be given intravenously.

    c. Killer bees contain an extremely potent toxin, which can result in death after one sting.

    d. Serum sickness may develop 2 or 3 days following the sting.

    e. Treatment of significant reactions to Hymenoptera stings may include epinephrine, antihistamines, and steroids just like any anaphylactic reaction.

    The answer is e. The acute local complications of a Hymenoptera sting include swelling and pain. Stings into the eye globe can cause perforation, cataracts, and other long-term complications. A neuropathy can develop if the stinger injects into a peripheral nerve. Killer bees are venomous but the venom has the same potency of other Hymenoptera. Killer bees are fierce and attack in numbers, so death is secondary to the enormous load of toxin delivered by a swarm of bees rather than the potency of the toxin. Systemic anaphylactic reactions can occur in sensitized persons after one sting, but direct toxic reactions can develop in nonsensitized people after multiple stings and include vomiting, syncope, and convulsions. Anaphylaxis is treated with epinephrine, antihistamines, and steroids. In the patient with severe anaphylaxis 1 mL of 1:10,000 epinephrine may be given intravenously. The 1:1000 dilution is reserved for subcutaneous administration. A serum sickness-type illness may develop with fever, arthralgias, and malaise 10 days to 2 weeks following stings.

4. **Choose the true statement concerning treatment of snakebite:**

   a. Snakebites should be treated prophylactically with an antibiotic selected for its Gram-positive activity, particularly against staphylococcal species.

   b. The amount of antivenin given is based on the severity of the symptoms and laboratory data.

   c. The dose of antivenin given to children is weight based.

   d. Of the calculated dose of antivenin, 25–50% should be infiltrated into the local wound of the bite and the rest given intravenously.

   e. Copperhead bites always require antivenin administration.

   The answer is b. Snakebites generally do not get infected; therefore, prophylactic antibiotics are not warranted. The amount of antivenin given is primarily a function of the severity of the envenomation. Children (or small adults) should be given proportionately more antivenin because they receive a proportionately greater amount of venom per kilogram of body weight than an adult. Antivenin is given intravenously and never injected into the area of the local wound. The venom of the copperhead is mild and in general no antivenin is needed. However, antivenin is indicated regardless of sensitivity if any symptoms occur after the bite of a coral snake.

5. **You are evaluating a 70-kg woman who suffered 55% total body surface area second-degree burn in a kitchen fire. She arrives within less than 20 minutes after the injury occurred. Using the Parkland formula, you calculate the estimated total fluid requirements for the next 24 hours and the type and rate of fluid administration (round to the nearest 10 mL) to be:**

   a. Ringer lactate, 960 mL/h in the first 8 hours, then 480 mL/h for the next 16 hours.

   b. Ringer lactate, 640 mL/h for the next 24 hours.

   c. Normal saline, 480 mL/h in the first 8 hours, then 960 mL/h for the next 16 hours.

   d. Normal saline, 540 mL/h for the next 24 hours.

   e. None of the above.

   The answer is a. Several formulas for fluid replacement in burns are available. The Parkland formula calls for 4 mL of lactated Ringer solution to be given per kilogram of body weight times the percentage burn. Half of this amount is given in the first 8 hours and the rest given over the next 16 hours. Thus, $4 \times 70 \times 55 = 15,400$ mL/24 h. In the first 8 hours after the burn, 7700 mL is given at approximately 960 mL/h, and the remainder over the next 16 hours at approximately 480 mL/h. An important gauge of fluid replacement is the urine output, and the rate of fluid administration should be modified to maintain a urine output of 30–50 mL/h in adults, and 1 mL/kg/h in children.

6. **A 17-year-old man is pulled from the bottom of a neighbor's swimming pool where he was submerged for an unknown period. Although initially pulseless and in respiratory arrest, his vital signs are now: heart rate 110/min; blood pressure 134/88 mm Hg; respiratory rate 4/min. His Glasgow Coma Score is eyes, 1; verbal, 1 (intubated); motor, 2. His pupils are fixed and dilated. You know that:**

    a. Aspirated water significantly interferes with successful ventilation from mechanical obstruction of airways.

    b. Injuries of the cervical spine are uncommon.

    c. A normal chest x-ray excludes significant lung abnormalities.

    d. Application of the Heimlich maneuver will help evacuate his lungs of excess fluid.

    e. Twenty percent of near-drowning patients who are comatose and flaccid with fixed and dilated pupils on arrival in the ED fully recover.

    The answer is e. The appearance of a patient after a near-drowning accident cannot reliably predict the outcome. In particular, hypothermic near-drowning patients cannot be declared dead until their body temperature is at least 32.2°C (90°F). Not all patients require admission, but observation is indicated if there is any evidence of significant immersion or breathing abnormalities. Pulmonary complications may take several hours to evolve, and initial normal chest x-rays do not exclude the development of pulmonary edema or hypoxia. These delayed complications may account for past reports of a postimmersion syndrome and death following successful resuscitation. Cervical spine injuries should be suspected in every near-drowning patient. Burst fractures of C1 and injuries of the midcervical spine are common in diving accidents. Aspiration of large quantities of water is uncommon and no special efforts should be made to "pump out" excess water. However, aspiration of water and water-borne contaminants, with secondary loss of surfactant, inflammation, and neurogenic pulmonary edema, contributes to the respiratory insufficiency seen in near-drowning patients. Resuscitative efforts follow standard guidelines in near-drowning patients, with consideration of possible hypothermia and occult cervical trauma or intoxication.

7. **An 87-year-old woman is brought to the ED by fire rescue when her neighbors realized they had not seen her for a few days. It is mid-August and the daily temperature has not gone below 87°F for more than a week. The paramedics report that her apartment was "unbearably hot" and apparently cooled only by a small revolving fan. The patient is comatose with a core temperature of 109.3°F and a blood pressure palpable at 60 mm Hg. You institute therapy, knowing that:**

    a. Coagulation studies usually stay normal even after severe heatstroke.

    b. Shivering that occurs during treatment must not be suppressed with chlorpromazine.

    c. Sedation, paralysis and intubation reduce temperature by inhibiting muscular activity.

    d. The presence of sweating excludes the diagnosis of heatstroke.

    e. Heatstroke and heat exhaustion are differentiated by the height of fever.

    The answer is c. Sweating can be present in early heatstroke, but later in the syndrome most patients develop hot, dry skin and do not sweat. The most common reason for impaired sweating is use of drugs with anticholinergic properties. Although exercise in hot weather is classically associated with its development, the disorder can occur, especially in older patients, even at rest. The earliest clinical abnormality is a change in central neurologic function, usually of the mental status; mental status changes are what differentiate heatstroke from the less severe heat exhaustion. Focal neurologic findings suggesting a mass lesion may be seen. Tachycardia and fever are usually present, but a sort of high-output cardiac failure can develop leading to pulmonary edema and cardiovascular collapse. Purpura, thrombocytopenia, and clinically significant bleeding can occur, sometimes progressing to DIC. Patients with clinically significant bleeding may require plasma and platelet replacement. The object of treatment is to lower the temperature. Ice water baths, hypothermia blankets, and iced saline lavage all have their proponents, but there is no clearly superior method of cooling. Paralysis is employed to decrease temperature through the inhibition of muscular activity. Shivering can and should be suppressed using a phenothiazine or benzodiazepine. Chlorpromazine can be used for this and will not contribute to the hyperpyrexia under these circumstances. Oxygen should be given and urine output measured, with central venous pressure measurements often helpful in determining fluid requirements.

8. **The NBA (National Bombers Association) is having its annual convention in your town. While one of the exhibitors is demonstrating the safety features of a homemade bomb to a large audience, there is an explosion. Several people are brought to your ED for treatment. You see no penetrating injuries and it appears most complaints are related to the blast wave. While evaluating and treating these patients, you keep in mind that:**

   a. Significant injuries are almost always immediately recognized clinically.

   b. The lungs are usually spared from injury.

   c. Injury to solid organs is far more common than injury to air filled organs.

   d. Air embolism to the CNS is treated with hyperbaric therapy.

   e. Ossicular injuries without tympanic membrane involvement are more common than tympanic membrane perforations.

   The answer is d. Blast injuries occur as a result of the pressure wave, flying debris, flying victims, and such effects as burns and exposure to toxic gases. The ears are most often injured. Disruption of the ossicles or perilymphatic fistulas can occur with intact tympanic membranes, but tympanic perforations are the most common ear injury. Blast patients should be observed for 6–12 hours for delayed injuries to appear. A perforated eardrum is a clue to significant overpressurization. The lungs are usually the most severely affected organ by blast waves, and injuries range from pulmonary contusion to hemorrhage, edema, air embolism, and the pulmonary overpressurization syndrome. Hyperbaric oxygen is the treatment for air embolism. Blast waves are most likely to damage air-filled organs; the large bowel is the most commonly ruptured. Solid-organ injuries are somewhat less common in air, but in underwater explosions, the solid abdominal viscera are at greater risk. Musculoskeletal injuries are obviously not rare. CNS injuries include concussion, bleeding, and air embolism with stroke.

9. **You are evaluating a 47-year-old man who suffered more than 75% total body surface area burns in an explosion at a local glass-etching factory. You must evacuate him by helicopter to the burn center, which is located more than 150 miles away. You know that:**

   a. Nasogastric suction is not necessary in burn patients when transferring by helicopter or ambulance if they have not eaten within the last 6 hours or if they are otherwise alert and the gag reflex is intact.

   b. Sheets soaked in sterile ice water or iced saline should be used to cover all large burn areas to prevent further tissue injury and reduce pain.

   c. If the burns are from hydrofluoric acid, subcutaneous calcium chloride injected until the pain stops is the treatment of choice.

   d. Escharotomies of the chest and limbs are performed by infiltrating the site to be cut with 1% lidocaine and making an incision roughly one-fourth of an inch deep extending to uninvolved tissue.

   e. Burn patients should not receive morphine sulfate intramuscularly or subcutaneously for pain.

   The answer is e. Only intravenous pain medication should be given in burn patients because of erratic absorption of medication from the subcutaneous and intramuscular routes. Ice should not be directly applied to wounds, and while cold compresses are helpful in small burns, hypothermia can result if they are applied to larger burns. Clean sheets are sufficient covering. Oxygen should be provided, blood gases and COHb levels checked, and in patients with evidence of severe heat injury to the face, stridor, or evidence of significant upper airway burns, early intubation should be considered before swelling makes this impossible. Patients with burns of greater than 20% of the body surface should all probably get an NG tube since ileus and gastric distension are common. Gastric rupture is a possibility in patients with distension and who are to be transported by helicopter. Third-degree burns are painless by definition and no local anesthesia is needed for escharotomy. The cut is made deep enough so the subcutaneous fat bulges through the incision and through the entire length of the eschar. Burns from hydrofluoric acid are extremely painful and destructive. Treatment includes subcutaneous or intra-arterial injection of calcium gluconate (not calcium chloride) solution until the pain stops.

10.   **While scaling Mt. McKinley, a 34-year-old woman triathlete develops headache, anorexia, nausea, vomiting, and fatigue. The base camp physician will know that:**

a. Cerebral edema is a possible consequence secondary to hypocapnia or hypoxia.

b. These symptoms will likely resolve without treatment as she ascends higher.

c. This condition is best treated with acetazolamide.

d. Prior physical conditioning should have been effective in preventing this illness.

e. Because of the estrogen-protective effect, this patient will have less severe symptoms than her male counterpart.

The answer is a. Although physical exercise may improve climbing skills, there is no relationship between the development of acute mountain sickness (AMS) and prior physical conditioning or gender. Headache is attributed to cerebral edema or spasm of cerebral blood vessels secondary to hypocapnia or hypoxia. Symptoms of AMS usually develop within 4–6 hours of reaching a high altitude and peak within 24–48 hours, resolving after 3–4 days. Acetazolamide may prevent or ameliorate AMS. Dexamethasone may be effective in preventing AMS in sedentary people, but not in athletes. The treatment of choice is descent to a lower altitude.

11.   **As you are driving to the ED to begin your midday shift, you hear that a hijacked jet has just crashed into the local nuclear power plant and survivors are being transported to your hospital as recovery occurs. You realize that you will arrive to a chaotic scene and start reviewing in your mind the effects of radiation. You recall that:**

a. The median lethal dose (LD_{50}) in humans is 400 rem.

b. The presence of early signs and symptoms does not influence the prognosis.

c. Symptomatology is rare in the patient exposed to 200 rem or less.

d. Nausea and vomiting early after exposure is common and therefore an unreliable predictor of exposure.

e. The lymphocyte count at 24 hours is a good prognostic indicator for survival.

The answer is a. Doses less than 100 rem are associated with minimal toxicity (anorexia, vomiting, transient WBC depression). Doses of 200 rem are associated with significant symptoms, including transient disability, and lymphocyte depression. The LD_{50} in humans is 400 rem, and at 600 rem the mortality is nearly 100%. The emergency once-in-a-lifetime exposure is officially 100 rem. The absolute lymphocyte count at 48 hours is a good predictor of hematopoietic involvement. If the absolute lymphocyte count is greater than 1200, it is unlikely that the patient has received a fatal radiation dose. If the absolute lymphocyte count falls between 300 and 1200 at 48 hours then a lethal dose is suspected. Decontamination and supportive care are the mainstays of therapy, but chelation therapy is available for specific agents and can significantly reduce whole-body half-life. Stem cell transplantation and cytokine are new advances that may raise the LD_{50}. Nausea and vomiting developing within 2 hours of exposure implies a dose of greater than 400 rem.

12.   **Select the correct pairing of toxins and symptoms or treatment:**

a. Inhalation of ammonia → lower airway symptoms.

b. Inhalation of phosgene → upper airway symptoms.

c. Inhalation of hydrogen sulfide → methylene blue therapy.

d. Chlorosulfonic acid → water irrigation.

e. Inhalation of metal fumes → headache, cough, fever, chills, and myalgia.

The answer is e. Water solubility of inhaled toxic agents determines the predominant respiratory symptoms. Ammonia is very soluble and results in upper airway irritation. Because phosgene is insoluble, it is deposited deep in the tracheobronchial tree and causes pulmonary edema. Hydrogen sulfide poisons the cytochrome oxidase system and is treated with sodium nitrite to form methemoglobin. The cyanosis produced by methemoglobin, sulfhemoglobin, and cyanide does not respond to administration of oxygen, but the absence of cyanosis does not exclude the diagnosis of any of these. Metal fume fever occurs in foundry workers and may mimic the flu. In general, chemical splashes are washed off with water, but certain chemicals are either insoluble in water (phosphorus) or react violently with water (calcium oxide, titanium tetrachloride, chlorosulfonic acid) and should be removed by blotting.

13.   **You are evaluating a 3-year-old girl who bit into an electrical cord. She is crying and you note blisters on the lips and a small charred lesion at the lip angles. The most frequent serious complication which must concern you is:**

   a. Delayed oral swelling and airway compromise.

   b. Fracture of the mandible or teeth.

   c. Cardiac dysrhythmias.

   d. Bleeding.

   e. Cataracts.

The answer is d. Delayed hemorrhage from the labial arteries 3–5 days later is a frequent complication of this type of injury. Injuries from alternating current are often more extensive than is apparent on first examination. Tetanic muscle contraction and deep muscle injury may cause myoglobinuria, and x-rays of bone and the cervical spine are indicated to exclude occult fractures. A full physical examination is mandatory, since the current may have flowed anywhere through the body through the path of least resistance to ground. An EKG and cardiac monitoring are routinely performed. Admission to the hospital for observation is indicated although some authorities say children can be followed as outpatients when they leave reliable caregivers. Cataracts are a frequent complication of lightning strikes but are uncommon in injuries of this type.

14.   **Choose the true statement about the physiology or diagnosis of diving accidents:**

a. A diver who surfaced and lost consciousness within 10 minutes is probably suffering from decompression sickness.

b. The risk of air embolism is greatest at shallow depths (i.e., less than 33 ft).

c. The onset of tinnitus, vertigo, and sensorineural hearing loss during a diving descent not associated with rupture of the tympanic membrane is most likely due to middle-ear overpressurization; a return to diving is acceptable when symptoms abate.

d. A diver who surfaced and developed dyspnea and subcutaneous emphysema of the neck is most likely experiencing pulmonary decompression illness; emergency recompression should be carried out in the water.

e. A patient with mild otitis externa who wants to scuba dive should be advised to wear earplugs to protect the ear from water and keep pressure equalized to prevent imbalances of middle-ear pressure and vertigo.

The answer is b. Rupture of the tympanic membrane, air embolism, sinus squeeze, and other injuries caused by the expansion or compression of gas collections are most likely to happen when the diver is at depths less than 33 ft, because it is at these relatively shallow depths that the greatest pressure changes occur. A diver who loses consciousness or develops neurologic dysfunction immediately or within 10 minutes of surfacing is most likely to have an air embolism. Rupture of the lung may result in benign pneumomediastinum or pneumothorax, which is prone to become a tension pneumothorax as the diver ascends and continues to breathe pressurized air. Breath holding during ascent is the most common cause of these air-embolism/lung-rupture injuries. Rupture of the tympanic membrane is associated with vertigo and a conductive hearing loss. Diving should not be allowed until the rupture is fully healed. Under no circumstances should a diver use earplugs, since they will create a closed air cavity and prevent pressure equalization. Rupture of the round window will result in acute vertigo, tinnitus, and a sensorineural hearing loss. The result is a perilymphatic fistula, a contraindication to further diving. Injury to the tympanic membrane is common with this but not always present. Divers with decompression or barotrauma-related injuries should never be treated by attempted recompression in the water.

15.   **A 7-year-old boy is brought to the ED with scratch marks on his forearm and minor bleeding. The parents say that they found the boy playing with a raccoon, which apparently scratched him. The animal ran off, but the parents did not notice anything strange and actually brought him to the ED for antitetanus immunization. You inform the family that rabies has been reported in raccoons in your state. You must now:**

a. Scrub the child's scratches with soap and water, then apply tincture of iodine to the wounds; discharge home on prophylactic antibiotics.

b. Scrub the child's scratches with soap and water, then apply tincture of iodine to the wounds; discharge home on prophylactic antibiotics, and advise follow-up the next day with family physician for possible rabies immune prophylaxis.

c. Clean the patient's scratches with soap and water, avoiding further tissue injury by not scrubbing; administer tetanus prophylaxis and discharge home after advising parents to contact animal control and the local health department regarding need for immunization.

d. Initiate human rabies immune globulin (HRIG) by infiltrating one-half the dose in the area of the deepest scratches and give the other half IM; start rabies human diploid cell vaccine (HDCV) immunizations, preferably in the limb with the maximum exposure.

e. Scrub the child's wounds with soap and water; immunize with HRIG using as much as possible in the area of the wound and the rest IM if necessary; begin immunizations with HDCV in the deltoid muscle.

The answer is e. Although animal bites are the most common form of exposure for consideration for rabies prophylaxis, other exposures should be considered. Animals may lick their paws and the wounds may become contaminated with saliva. Skunks, bats, raccoons, and foxes are common animal vectors, but with the exception of rodent bites, any animal bite is suspect, including those of horses and cattle. The decision to treat should not be delayed. If the animal cannot be observed or examined, and rabies is endemic in the area, then prophylaxis is indicated. The incidence of severe complications from HRIG and HDCV is low. After mechanical cleansing of the wound with soap and water, as much as possible of the calculated HRIG dose should be infiltrated into the wound area and the rest given intramuscularly. HDCV is given in the deltoid muscle in five doses over 28 days (days 0, 3, 7, 14, 28). Tetanus prophylaxis and antibiotics are given if indicated.

16. **A 24-year-old woman was struck by lightning while playing golf. She was initially in respiratory arrest but was easily intubated by the ACLS unit prior to arrival. Her pupils are fixed and dilated, and she has no spontaneous respirations. Her blood pressure is 112/65 mm Hg. She is 8 months pregnant. Her tearful husband asks about the prognosis:**

   a. The mortality from lightning strikes exceeds 80%.

   b. Morbidity and permanent sequelae occur in less than 20% of survivors.

   c. The patient will almost certainly have serious internal injuries as a result of the lightning, including massive muscle injury.

   d. Fixed and dilated pupils cannot be used as evidence of brain death.

   e. The chances that she will bear a living, healthy baby are nearly nonexistent.

The answer is d. Because ocular autonomic disturbances may cause dilated unresponsive pupils, this presentation cannot be used to determine brain death. Cataracts are a common ophthalmologic complication and occur at any time up to 2 years later. Lightning accounts for 150–300 deaths a year in the United States, and the overall mortality of lightning strikes is 20–30%. Burns are usually superficial and deep tissue injury with rhabdomyolysis, while it should be excluded, is not common, unlike the case with injury from alternating current. Two-thirds of patients present with lower extremity paralysis and one-third with upper extremity paralysis. The extremities may appear lifeless from vascular spasm. Resolution of these findings over the succeeding hours is the rule rather than the exception, but spinal cord injury should be excluded. Some patients are left with permanent limb paralysis or paresthesias. Patients who present in a coma following lightning strikes may have a correctable intracranial lesion such as a hematoma from an acute skull fracture, and CT scan is imperative before postulating hypoxic brain injury. Amnesia, personality changes, and neuralgias are among the other long-term CNS complications.

17.   **A 25-year-old man was drinking an excessive amount of alcohol and apparently fell asleep in the park on a February night. On arrival at the ED, he is unresponsive with a core temperature of 27.8°C (82°F) and a pulse of 40/min. You know that:**

a. Continuous CPR must be performed until the patient is rewarmed.

b. A large positive deflection at the end of the QRS complex indicates a poor prognosis.

c. Bradycardia should be treated with intravenous pacemaker placement.

d. Cardiopulmonary bypass therapy is useless in the hypothermic patient without a pulse.

e. Hypothermic patients are usually volume depleted.

The answer is e. Hypothermic patients are volume-depleted for a variety of reasons, including alcohol, cold-induced diuresis, and third spacing of intravascular volume. The hypothermic kidney loses its ability to concentrate urine, rendering urine output and specific gravity inaccurate as a sole guide to intravascular volume. Controversy exists about the indications for CPR in hypothermic patients. It may be difficult to monitor cardiac activity in these patients. If no pulse is detected after a minute in the hypothermic patient, or if obvious ventricular fibrillation or asystole is present, CPR is clearly indicated. A variety of EKG changes are often seen in hypothermia, including the Osborn (J) wave, a positive deflection at the end of the QRS complex. The Osborn wave has no bearing on prognosis and resolves with rewarming. Dysrhythmosis are common, especially with a core temperature below 30°C (86°F), and are generally best treated with rewarming rather than pharmacologic therapy. The cold myocardium is both susceptible to ventricular fibrillation (which may be precipitated by rough handing of the patient or intracardiac devices) and refractory to defibrillation. If one or two attempts to defibrillate the hypothermic patient are unsuccessful, CPR is carried out simultaneously with rewarming efforts and defibrillation attempted after each few degrees increase in core temperature. Cardiopulmonary bypass therapy is extremely beneficial in the pulseless, hypothermic patient.

18.   **You are marooned on a large desert island with several other people after the grounding and wreck of your tour boat. Fortunately you have a good store of supplies and agree to provide the correct medical services to your compatriots as long as they can bring you food. Which of the following remedies is correctly paired with the injuries?**

a. A 23-year-old actress was stung on the thigh by a Portuguese man-of-war and tentacles are still present → tentacle removal using surgical gloves and irrigation with fresh water.

b. A 42-year-old college professor with rash on his arms from handling sponges → apply dilute baking soda soaks tid.

c. An obese 50-year-old captain with a wound to his calf from a stingray tail → remove retained fragments and soak leg in 46.1°C (115°F) water for 90 minutes.

d. A 62-year-old millionaire and his slightly younger wife who have puncture wounds to their hands and arms from sea urchin spines → remove foreign bodies and inject 2% lidocaine with epinephrine at the puncture sites, avoiding use in the fingers.

e. A 21-year-old first mate with a puncture wound of the arm from a catfish spine → apply ice packs to the area tid and remove foreign body.

The answer is c. Direct identification of the organism may not be possible, so it is acceptable to treat wounds by unidentified marine organisms in a similar fashion. The toxins found in many spines, including the tail of the stingray, catfish, and stone fish, are heat labile; therefore, the affected part should be immersed in water as hot as the patient can comfortably withstand (not over 45°C [113°F]) for 30–90 minutes depending on the size of the wound and the organism, if known. Ice treatment for these acute puncture wounds should not be used. Local anesthetics without epinephrine and systemic analgesics may be needed. The stings of the Portuguese man-of-war in particular can cause severe systemic reactions. The tentacles should be picked off with forceps and not with gloved hands. A weak vinegar solution may be used to inactivate the nematocysts, or salt water used to wash off the skin. In general, most coelenterate (some coral, anemones, and jellyfish) stings should not be treated with basic solutions or exposed to fresh water as this causes the nematocysts to discharge. The same applies to acute stings from handling sponges. General measures include antihistamines for itching, topical steroids for dermatitis, debridement and wound treatment, and tetanus prophylaxis. Certain envenomations (sea snake, sea wasp) may require antitoxin treatment.

19. **Choose the true statement about carbon monoxide poisoning:**

    a. Cherry-red skin and mucous membranes are sensitive findings commonly seen.
    b. Nausea, vomiting, and diarrhea are the most common early complaints confusing the diagnosis with gastroenteritis.
    c. COHb (carboxyhemoglobin) levels of 10–20% are found in daily smokers.
    d. Red retinal veins are not a sensitive or early finding.
    e. The COHb level at the scene correlates best with the clinical presentation.

    The answer is e. Patients with CO poisoning usually have pale or cyanotic, not cherry-red skin. However, red retinal veins are a sensitive early finding. Headache is the most common complaint, followed by dizziness and weakness. A high index of suspicion must be maintained for CO poisoning in the winter months to avoid misdiagnosis of CO poisoning as the flu. With higher blood levels of COHb, visual disturbances, dyspnea, confusion, and finally coma and respiratory failure occur. Patients exposed to high levels of CO may collapse without progressing through this sequence. CO not only combines with hemoglobin more avidly than oxygen, but it shifts the oxygen–hemoglobin dissociation curve to the left and prevents any remaining oxygen from being released in the tissues. CO combines with other heme-structure molecules, including cytochromes and myoglobin. Considerable debate over the relative importance of each of these sites of poisoning exists, but the effect can be important clinically, since rebound increases in the blood CO may occur as these tissue stores are mobilized and cause confusion in interpreting COHb results. The COHb level at the scene correlates best with the clinical presentation. Administering 100% oxygen can lead to underestimating the degree of toxicity; however is necessary as this is the treatment. Cigarette smokers have COHb levels of 5–10%.

20. **Choose the true statement about spider bites or scorpion stings:**

a. Although local symptoms predominate, Loxosceles (brown recluse) spider bites can cause systemic symptoms, including seizures and myocarditis.

b. If a severe bite by the brown recluse is suspected, brown recluse antivenin should be given, with 50% of the dose infiltrated locally around the bite.

c. Abdominal pain and rebound tenderness with board-like rigidity of the abdomen may be prominent physical findings in patients bitten by the black widow spider.

d. Intravenous magnesium chloride provides prompt relief of the painful symptoms caused by black widow spider bites.

e. Absence of a local reaction at the site of a scorpion sting is not uncommon in envenomations by potentially fatal species.

The answer is e. Scorpion stings are most likely to be fatal in children or the elderly. Most scorpion stings produce a local reaction similar to a bee sting, but some lethal species have a sting that produces no local findings. Toxicity is manifested by local paresthesias spreading to the entire extremity, followed by an excited state (from catecholamine release) that may progress to seizures and coma. Treatment for minor envenomations is symptomatic; severe stings require administration of antivenin. Beta-blockers for the hypercatecholamine state and diazepam for anxiety and seizures may be needed. The bite of the black widow spider causes muscle contractions involving the muscles of the trunk proximal to the site of the bite. Since the buttocks and genitalia are most often bitten, board-like abdominal rigidity is a common presenting sign. Although the symptoms may suggest intra-abdominal catastrophe, the coexistent muscle cramps of the extremities and lack of peritoneal signs should help distinguish it. Horse antivenin is used in children and patients with coexistent medical problems. The brown recluse spider, which now ranges from the Midwest to southern portions of the United States, can cause a severe local tissue necrosis with its bite that may require skin excision and grafting. No clearly effective treatment exists. Systemic toxicity is uncommon, but hemolysis and renal failure may occur.

21. **A 25-year-old man presents after claiming to have been bitten by a snake, which he was unable to identify. You realize that:**

a. In the presence of apparent fang marks that are oozing blood, venomous snakebite is unlikely.

b. If psychosis, muscle weakness or fasciculations, and slurred speech with minimal swelling of the affected area are associated with a snakebite, presumptive administration of coral snake rather than pit viper antivenin is justified.

c. Pit vipers produce a coagulopathic state similar to disseminated intravascular (DIC) coagulation with a prolonged PT and PTT, thrombocytopenia, hypofibrinogenemia, increased fibrin split products, bleeding, and clot formation.

d. The use of crotalid polyvalent immune Fab fragments (CroFab) has resulted in the same incidence of serum sickness as the equine derived polyvalent crotalid antivenom.

e. The bite of a snake at the end of summer is usually more severe than the bite of a snake after winter.

The answer is b. The venom of the coral snake is primarily neurotoxic. Antivenin must be given when there are any signs of envenomation. Symptoms are often delayed for several hours but progress rapidly and can lead to death in less than 24 hours from respiratory paralysis. Coral snakes do not have the same type of fangs as pit vipers, and the bite may appear surprisingly innocuous. Pit vipers produce a coagulopathic state (increased PT and PTT, thrombocytopenia, hypofibrinogenemia, increased fibrin split products, and bleeding) similar to DIC; but unlike DIC, clot formation does not occur. In a true bite with envenomation the fang marks should be oozing blood. Fang marks greater than 1.5 cm apart indicate a bite by a large snake. Bites in the spring after hibernation are often more serious. The location of the bite is important; the most toxicity results from truncal or facial bites or those on the proximal upper limbs. Lower extremity bites may produce delayed symptoms. The bite of a copperhead does not require antivenin in every instance, but the bite of any other pit viper with signs of envenomation probably needs antivenin. The equine derived polyvalent crotalid antivenom has largely been replaced with the ovine derived crotalid polyvalent Fab fragments (CroFab). Anaphylactoid reactions and serum sickness have decreased with the use of CroFab.

22. **A 42-year-old, 70-kg man attempts suicide by drenching himself in gasoline and setting himself on fire. He presents screaming in pain with extensive burns to the head and neck, anterior and posterior torso, entire right upper and lower extremity, and the genitals. Using the rule of nines, estimate the total percentage burn:**

   a. 37%.
   b. 55%.
   c. 64%.
   d. 73%.
   e. 82%.

The answer is d. The rule of nine in adults is as follows: head and neck 9%; torso 18% anterior, 18% posterior; each arm 9%; each leg 18%; and genitals 1%. Children have a relatively larger head, and for infants the head is 18% of the total body surface. Charts are available for estimating burns at various ages.

23. **An unconscious patient who is 32 weeks pregnant presents with probable carbon monoxide (CO) poisoning. Choose the true statement:**

   a. Because fetal hemoglobin does not bind CO as readily as adult hemoglobin does, significant fetal toxicity is rare.
   b. The maternal PaO_2 is usually depressed in CO poisoning.
   c. Oxygen treatment of CO poisoning in the pregnant woman should be extended 5 times longer than is needed to complete the maternal course of treatment.
   d. If the patient requires intubation, establishing a normal PCO_2 will result in a normal pH.
   e. Carboxygen (95% oxygen, 5% carbon dioxide) and hypothermia are useful adjuncts for treatment in severe CO poisoning.

The answer is c. CO crosses the placenta and efficiently binds to fetal hemoglobin. The uptake of CO by the fetus lags behind that by the mother as does elimination, and prolonged therapy is recommended to eliminate CO from the fetus. Neurologic impairment may occur in 60% of neonates born to mothers with CO poisoning. ABG results can be deceiving in CO poisoning. Low levels of COHb do not exclude the diagnosis of poisoning. The PaO_2 will be normal in most patients with CO poisoning, and if the hemoglobin saturation is based on a calculation from the measured PaO_2, it will be falsely high. Direct oximetric measurement will reveal the true, lower hemoglobin saturation. A metabolic acidosis from anaerobic metabolism is common in significant poisoning. This is not necessarily deleterious since it shifts the oxygen–hemoglobin dissociation curve to the right and facilitates tissue oxygenation (whereas CO poisoning shifts the oxygen–hemoglobin dissociation curve to the left). Alkalosis should be avoided. The delivery of 100% oxygen by a close-fitting high-flow mask with a reservoir is the initial treatment of choice in CO poisoning and is continued until the COHb level is below 10% and the patient is asymptomatic. Hyperbaric oxygen therapy, which considerably shortens the time required for treatment, should be considered in severe cases.

24. **Choose the true statement concerning hyperpyrexia:**

   a. The definition of heat exhaustion includes a temperature greater than 102°F (38.9°C).

   b. Intracerebral hemorrhage presents more commonly with hypothermia rather than hyperthermia.

   c. Both the neuroleptic malignant syndrome and malignant hyperthermia are successfully treated with nondepolarizing paralytics.

   d. Both the neuroleptic malignant syndrome and malignant hyperthermia are successfully treated with dantrolene.

   e. Neuroleptic malignant syndrome is a genetically inherited disorder.

   The answer is d. A mildly increased temperature may accompany heat exhaustion, but significant elevations do not occur. In addition to heatstroke, other causes of hyperpyrexia include infection, intracerebral hemorrhage, stroke, and various drugs. Phenothiazines, antidepressants, and anticholinergics are drugs that increase susceptibility to heatstroke. The neuroleptic malignant syndrome is associated with the use of phenothiazines and causes hyperpyrexia independent of the ambient temperature; the disorder is not inherited. Malignant hyperthermia occurs most often in patients with a genetic predisposition and given anesthesia with succinylcholine and inhalational anesthetics. Patients suffering from the neuroleptic malignant syndrome can be successfully paralyzed with nondepolarizing paralytics. Patients with malignant hyperthermia are resistant to the nondepolarizing paralytics. In malignant hyperthermia calcium is released from the sarcoplasmic reticulum resulting in muscular rigidity. Blocking the acetylcholine receptor on the cell surface with paralytics will not influence muscular contraction. Dantrolene sodium inhibits calcium release from the sarcoplasmic reticulum and may be used to treat both disorders.

25. **A 6-year-old boy complains of nausea, vomiting, and abdominal pain. His physical examination is unremarkable and you diagnose gastroenteritis. On his way out the door, you notice that he drops a small brown object into the garbage. You inspect the trashcan and recover a small brown mushroom. You know that:**

   a. Cortinarius species contain the toxin orelline that produces renal failure.

   b. Amanita phalloides produces a peripheral zonal liver necrosis similar to acetaminophen.

   c. If more than 6 hours has elapsed between the time of ingestion and the onset of symptoms, the likelihood of a fatal or severe poisoning is minimal.

   d. Poisoning by Gyromitra species causes seizures controlled with benzodiazepines.

   e. Toxic mushrooms, with few exceptions, produce initial symptoms of fever, nausea, vomiting, diarrhea, and abdominal cramps.

   The answer is a. With few exceptions gastrointestinal symptoms are the first manifestation of mushroom poisoning. Fever is not a manifestation of poisoning. If more than 6 hours has elapsed between ingestion and the onset of symptoms, one should suspect poisoning with a potentially fatal species such as Amanita species (cyclopeptide) which causes hepatic necrosis, a Gyromitra species (monomethylhydrazine) which causes seizures, methemoglobinemia, and hemolytic anemia, or Cortinarius species (orelline and orellanine) which produce renal failure. Amanita phalloides produces a centrilobular necrosis of the liver similar to acetaminophen toxicity. Monomethylhydrazine and isoniazid inhibit the enzyme pyridoxine phosphokinase that converts pyridoxine to the active metabolite pyridoxal 5'-phosphate. Pyridoxal 5'-phosphate is a cofactor used by the enzyme glutamic acid decarboxylase that converts glutamic acid to GABA. Both poisoning by monomethylhydrazine and isoniazid require the antidote pyridoxine. Benzodiazepines will not be effective without GABA. Patients who have ingested potentially toxic mushrooms should receive activated charcoal and be admitted for observation.

26. **The best way to rewarm a frozen extremity is to:**

    a. Do a slow thaw, starting with ice water and increasing the temperature through a series of baths.

    b. Use a forced-air warming device, such as a Bair Hugger.

    c. Perform direct tissue massage.

    d. Immerse directly in a warm water bath kept at 40–42°C.

    e. Directly expose to open flame.

    The answer is d. Although there is some controversy about the exact temperature required, experts agree that immersion in a closely monitored warm water bath is the preferred method of rewarming a frozen or partially frozen extremity. Indicators of successful thawing include increased flexibility, redness, and hyperemia. This can be intensely painful, and patients may need parenteral opioids. Field rewarming is discouraged due to the risk of refreezing, which causes even worse tissue loss.

27. **Which statement concerning the physiology of electrical injuries is true?**

    a. Direct current exposure to the same voltage tends to be 3 times more dangerous than alternating current.

    b. The thorax is the most common site of contact with an AC electric source.

    c. The higher the resistance of a tissue to the flow of current, the less likely is transformation of electrical energy to thermal energy.

    d. Tissue resistance remains constant throughout length of exposure to current.

    e. Tetany occurs when muscle fibers are stimulated at 40–110 cycles/s.

    The answer is e. Alternating current exposure to the same voltage tends to be 3 times more dangerous than direct current. Continuous muscle contraction, or tetany, can occur when the muscle fibers are stimulated at between 40 and 110 times per second. Electrical transmission frequency used in the United States is 60 cycles/sec. The hand is the most common site of contact via a tool that is in contact with an AC electric source. The higher the resistance of a tissue to the flow of current, the greater the potential for transformation of electrical energy to thermal energy at any given current. As the tissue breaks down under the energy of the current flow, its resistance may change markedly, making it difficult to predict the amperage for any given electrical injury.

28. **Lightning is:**

    a. Direct current.

    b. Alternating current.

    c. A combination of both direct and alternating current.

    d. Neither direct nor alternating current, but a unidirectional current impulse.

    e. A voltage phenomenon.

    The answer is d. Lightning is neither a direct current nor an alternating current. At best, it is a unidirectional massive current impulse. Therefore, lightning is classed as a current phenomenon rather than a voltage phenomenon.

29.   A "kissing burn" occurs:

a. At extensor surfaces in electrical exposure when the current causes flexion at a joint, protecting that area but leaving the exposed extensor surfaces at greater risk for damage.

b. At flexor surfaces in electrical exposure when the current causes flexion at a joint, and the moisture in the flexor crease leads to an arc burn and extensive deep tissue damage.

c. When a child "sucks" an electrical outlet.

d. When a child bites an electric cord.

e. When lightning "kisses" the skin, leaving a typical fernlike pattern.

The answer is b. A peculiar type of burn associated with electrical injury is the kissing burn, which occurs at the flexor creases. As the current causes flexion of the extremity, the skin of the flexor surfaces at the joints touches. Combined with the moist environment that often occurs at the flexor areas, the electric current may arc across the flexor crease, causing arc burns on both flexor surfaces and extensive underlying tissue damage.

30.   The most common medical complaint of scuba divers is:

a. Inner ear squeeze.

b. Middle ear squeeze.

c. Nitrogen narcosis.

d. Swimmer's ear.

e. The bends.

The answer is b. Middle ear barotrauma (barotitis or "ear squeeze,") is the most common complaint of scuba divers, experienced by 30% of novice scuba divers and 10% of experienced divers. The middle ear is an air-filled space with solid bony walls except for the tympanic membrane. The Eustachian tube is the only anatomic passage to the external environment. As the diver descends, each foot of water exerts an additional 23 mm Hg pressure against the intact tympanic membrane. Ear squeeze occurs when a negative differential pressure is created within the middle ear because the diver could not "equalize" to ambient pressure, leading to pain. If equilibration of middle ear pressure does not occur, the floppy medial third of the Eustachian tube collapses shut, making any further attempts at equalization futile. Further pressure increases can cause the TM to rupture.

CHAPTER 7

Head, Eye, Ear, Nose, and Throat Emergencies

Stephanie Barbetta, MD, and
Scott H. Plantz, MD, FAAEM

1. **A 78-year-old woman complains of a new rash on the left side of her face. The dermatomal distribution is consistent with herpes zoster ophthalmicus (HZO). You should:**

   a. Prescribe the oral antiviral acyclovir 800 mg 5 times/d for 7 days.

   b. Prescribe oral antiviral acyclovir 800 mg 5 times/d for 7 days, and desipramine 25 mg, taper up to 75 mg at bedtime for several weeks.

   c. Treat with oral antiviral famciclovir 500 mg tid, valacyclovir 1 g tid, or acyclovir 800 mg 5 times/d for 7 days; nortriptyline or desipramine 25 mg, taper up to 75 mg at bedtime for several weeks (if needed) to inhibit acute and prolonged postherpetic neuralgia.

   d. Document all external lesions and ocular findings. Proceed with treatment protocol for acute herpes zoster ophthalmicus. Prescribe oral antiviral (famciclovir 500 mg tid, valacyclovir 1 g tid, or acyclovir 800 mg 5 times/d for 7 days); prescribe tricyclic antidepressant (nortriptyline or desipramine 25 mg, taper up to 75 mg at bedtime for several weeks if needed) to inhibit acute and prolonged postherpetic neuralgia. Prescribe additional topical steroids, antibiotics, dilators, antivirals, and glaucoma medications as necessary for keratitis, iritis, or glaucoma. Advise the patient of disease prognosis, and prepare the patient for the possibility of postherpetic neuralgia. Consult an ophthalmologist.

   e. Document all external lesions and ocular findings. Proceed with treatment protocol for acute herpes zoster ophthalmicus. Prescribe oral antiviral (famciclovir 500 mg tid, valacyclovir 1 g tid, or acyclovir 800 mg 5 times/d for 7 days); prescribe tricyclic antidepressant (nortriptyline or desipramine 25 mg, taper up to 75 mg at bedtime for several weeks if needed) to inhibit acute and prolonged postherpetic neuralgia. Prescribe additional topical steroids, antibiotics, dilators, antivirals, and glaucoma medications as necessary for keratitis, iritis, or glaucoma. Advise the patient of the disease prognosis, and prepare the patient for the possibility of postherpetic neuralgia. Set up an appointment with a neurologist.

   The answer is d. Prescribe oral antiviral (famciclovir 500 mg tid, valacyclovir 1 g tid, or acyclovir 800 mg 5 times/d for 7 days); prescribe tricyclic antidepressant (nortriptyline or desipramine 25 mg, taper up to 75 mg at bedtime for several weeks if needed) to inhibit acute and prolonged postherpetic neuralgia. Prescribe additional topical steroids, antibiotics, dilators, antivirals, and glaucoma medications as necessary for keratitis, iritis, or glaucoma. Advise the patient of disease prognosis, and prepare the patient for the possibility of postherpetic neuralgia. Consult an ophthalmologist.

2.   **Proper treatment for a hordeolum consists of:**

   a. Systemic antibiotic therapy.
   b. Topical antibiotic ointment.
   c. Daily warm compresses.
   d. Surgical incision and curettage.
   e. Observation.

   The answer is c. Frequent use of daily warm compresses is the mainstay in the treatment of this lesion. Warm compresses also are used in the prevention of new lesions in patients with blepharitis or meibomian gland dysfunction.

3.   **The canilicula are located:**

   a. In the nose.
   b. In the palpebral portion of the eyelid.
   c. Lateral to the puncta.
   d. Inferior to the puncta.
   e. In the superficial aspect of the medial eyelid.

   The answer is e. The canaliculi are located in the vulnerable medial aspect of the superior and inferior eyelid.

4.   **A 55-year-old woman complains of painful double vision. Examination shows her right pupil is 7 mm with sluggish reaction, her left pupil is 4 mm and briskly constricts. There is 3 mm ptosis of the right lid. She cannot adduct her right eye when asked to do so. You should now:**

   a. Tell the patient she has Horner syndrome and needs evaluation of her carotid artery.
   b. Arrange emergent evaluation for possible aneurysmal compression, as she has a pupil-involved third nerve palsy.
   c. Place pilocarpine drops in her right eye, as this is probably a pharmacologically dilated pupil.
   d. Administer a serotonergic (5HT) triptan, as this is almost certainly a migraine variant.
   e. Place a dilating drop in her eyes and perform direct ophthalmoscopy to confirm your suspicion of retinal tear involving the fovea.

   The answer is b. A painful, pupil-involved third nerve palsy demands emergent evaluation for possible aneurysmal compression. Approximately 25% of posterior communicating artery aneurysms produce a third nerve palsy. Aneurysms may affect the third nerve via enlargement, sentinel leak, or frank subarachnoid hemorrhage, which is a life-threatening event.

5.   **A 40-year-old man complains of right facial pain for 24 hours that started shortly after he was elbowed in the neck while playing football. His right pupil is 4 mm, his left is 5.5 mm, and both are reactive. He has approximately 1 mm ptosis of the right lid. This patient has:**

   a. Partial third nerve palsy which may represent uncal herniation; he requires an emergent CT scan.
   b. Partial third nerve palsy which may represent aneurysmal compression; he requires emergent angiography.
   c. Horner syndrome which likely represents carotid dissection; he requires emergent angiography.
   d. Physiologic anisocoria and requires no further workup.
   e. Traumatic iritis; he needs a careful slit lamp examination.

The answer is c. Painful Horner syndrome demands consideration for carotid dissection. Sympathetic fibers travel up the carotid to enter the orbit after traversing the cavernous sinus. The fibers are vulnerable to carotid disease within the neck. Dissections commonly produce ipsilateral neck, face, or periorbital pain. The clinical scenario of anisocoria greater in dark with normally reactive pupils only can result from physiologic anisocoria or Horner syndrome.

6. **The most common cause of branch retinal artery occlusion in patients older than 60 years is:**

    a. Vasculitis.

    b. Idiopathic.

    c. Embolism.

    d. Vasospasm.

    e. Blood dyscrasia.

    The answer is c. Embolic causes are the most common cause of branch retinal artery occlusion. In many cases, the emboli are visible on funduscopic examination.

7. **When confronted with a patient who suffered a chemical burn to the eye, your first step in evaluation or treatment is to:**

    a. Assess visual acuity (the "vital sign" of the eye).

    b. Determine how long ago the injury occurred.

    c. Determine how the patient treated the injury prior to visit.

    d. Copiously irrigate the affected eye.

    e. Perform fluorescein staining of the cornea to check for the presence of a corneal abrasion.

    The answer is d. Time is of the essence when dealing with chemical injuries, and the top priority should be to irrigate the eye, even if the patient says that the eye has been washed out. The eye should be irrigated again, and the pH must be determined to be neutral before continuing with the examination.

8. **A 22-year-old college student presents at 3 AM approximately 1 week after he was struck in the face with a fist during a fight with a fellow student. He complains of double vision in dim light. His visual acuity is 20/25 in the right eye, 20/20 in the left eye. You note resolving periorbital ecchymosis on the right. His globes are intact and intraocular pressure is 14 mm Hg in both. There is no afferent pupillary defect, and his extraocular movements are normal. His corneas are clear, and anterior chambers are deep and quiet. There is no angle recession in either eye. His right lens is slightly displaced inferonasally. The remainder of his examination is normal. Your ophthalmologist on call is not answering his pager. You should now:**

    a. Do nothing—this patient requires only observation.

    b. Begin a trial of miotic therapy in the right eye and arrange follow-up with an ophthalmologist in the morning.

    c. Admit for emergent eye surgery in the morning.

    d. Contact the partner of the ophthalmologist whom you cannot reach, as this patient needs immediate vitrectomy of his right eye.

    e. Place a protective eyeshield, keep the patient upright, and transfer to an eye specialty center.

    The answer is b. The patient's complaint is monocular diplopia and is secondary to lens subluxation in the right eye following blunt trauma. Miotic therapy may relieve his symptoms and prevent surgery in this case. If he cannot tolerate miotics or if they fail to alleviate his diplopia, lens extraction and intraocular lens implantation would be the next course of action. This evaluation can wait until morning.

9. A 40-year-old construction worker was inadvertently struck in his left eye 2 hours ago by a coworker carrying a wooden beam. His visual acuity is 20/20 in the right eye, and counting fingers at 3 ft in the left eye. His globes are intact. He has an afferent pupillary defect in his left eye, and there is a rosette-shaped lens opacity. Ophthalmoscopic examination shows an inferior vitreous hemorrhage of the left eye with a small inferotemporal retinal tear. Your most pressing concern is the:

   a. Vitreous hemorrhage.
   b. Traumatic cataract.
   c. Afferent pupillary defect.
   d. Abnormal visual acuity.
   e. Retinal tear.

   The answer is c. An afferent pupillary defect in this setting should alert you to the possibility of traumatic optic neuropathy. The patient should be started on a course of high-dose intravenous methylprednisolone and should be observed closely for progressive visual loss. Surgical intervention may be indicated if visual decline continues while on corticosteroid therapy. Other ocular injuries also should be addressed, but traumatic optic neuropathy should be the most pressing concern.

10. A 14-year-old girl complains of sudden fever, unilateral eyelid redness, and double vision. You find limitation of extraocular movement and pain when the patient tries to move her eyes. Your most important diagnostic study is:

   a. MRI.
   b. CT scan.
   c. Blood culture.
   d. Eyelid culture.
   e. White blood cell count.

   The answer is b. This patient's presentation is suspicious for orbital cellulitis. A CT scan will assess and stage orbital involvement, such as subperiosteal abscess or orbital abscess. It also can evaluate the paranasal sinuses. Blood culture and eyelid culture results tend to be negative; therefore, antibiotic choice is empiric. White blood cell counts cannot be used to differentiate between preseptal cellulitis and orbital cellulitis.

11. A 10-year-old patient complains of unilateral eyelid swelling and erythema. You suspect this is preseptal (periorbital) cellulitis because on physical examination you find:

   a. Limited ocular motility.
   b. An afferent pupillary defect (Marcus Gunn pupil).
   c. Tenderness and purulent reflux from the lacrimal sac.
   d. Resistance to retropulsion.
   e. Eye pain and photophobia.

   The answer is c. Pain and purulent reflux from the lacrimal sac is likely from dacryocystitis, which is a common predisposing condition for preseptal cellulitis. An afferent pupillary defect is caused by a lesion of the anterior visual pathway (i.e., optic nerve and tract), and it is suggestive of orbital cellulitis. Resistance to retropulsion is a physical finding in the presence of an orbital mass. Eye pain and photophobia has a large differential diagnosis and does not specifically point to preseptal cellulitis.

12. **A 33-year-old woman complains of red eyes with a watery discharge for 2 weeks despite treatment with gentamicin and bacitracin eyedrops. She denies genitourinary symptoms but is sexually active. Your next step is to:**

    a. Send conjunctival swab for routine bacterial culture and sensitivities.

    b. Change to a combination antibiotic–steroid eyedrop.

    c. Do conjunctival scraping for Gram stain and Giemsa stain.

    d. Change to a fluoroquinolone eyedrop.

    e. Begin empiric systemic therapy with doxycycline.

    The answer is c. Persistent conjunctivitis which does not improve with usual topical therapy may be caused by chlamydia infection. Chlamydial sexually transmitted disease is characteristically asymptomatic in females. Certainly culture and sensitivities will be useful if this is a resistant bacterial infection. However, the diagnosis of chlamydia will be missed on routine culture without special collection and processing. Conjunctival scraping will determine if bacteria predominate or if inclusion bodies diagnostic of chlamydia are present. Therefore, this is the best answer. Changing the antibiotic or adding steroid without further study would not be ideal.

13. **A 44-year-old man reports that he has been using neomycin eyedrops for 1 week to treat a red eye and discharge. The discharge has stopped, but his eye is still red and irritated. On slit lamp examination, you find injection of the small conjunctival vessels and a trace of punctate staining of the cornea. You should now:**

    a. Change to gentamicin eyedrops.

    b. Change to an antibiotic–steroid combination eyedrop.

    c. Perform conjunctival scraping for Gram stain and Giemsa stain.

    d. Discontinue the neomycin, and monitor the patient's progress.

    e. Add systemic doxycycline.

    The answer is d. Neomycin is known to cause irritation of the conjunctiva and the corneal epithelium. In this case, it is most reasonable to stop the suspected agent and monitor the patient without subjecting him to further tests. Empirically, changing the therapy is not ideal.

14. **Corneal abrasions can lead to infection because:**

    a. Human tears contain a large number of pathogens.

    b. Scarring occurs.

    c. A de-epithelialized cornea is susceptible to infection.

    d. The cornea is a "protected space," and white cells cannot migrate appropriately to aid in healing.

    e. Meibomian glands frequently harbor occult pathogens.

    The answer is c. A de-epithelialized cornea is more susceptible to infection. Such a cornea is vulnerable not only to pathogens contaminating the foreign body that produced the abrasion but also to potential pathogens that are present in the normal conjunctival flora. Prophylactic topical antibiotics are generally prescribed for corneal abrasions. The use of prophylactic periocular injections or systemic administration of antibiotics after corneal abrasions is controversial.

15. **A 47-year-old workman complains of severe left eye pain, which started 15 minutes ago while he was hammering a nail into a wall. Your first step is to:**

 a. Perform an x-ray of the orbits.

 b. Check visual acuity in each eye separately.

 c. Place a drop of proparacaine in the eye for the pain.

 d. Examine the eye with a slit lamp.

 e. Order a CT scan of the orbits.

The answer is b. Before proceeding with any extensive ocular examination or treatment, vision should be checked in each eye separately. Documenting the initial visual acuity of the patient, both for medical and medicolegal purposes, is important.

16. **In a patient with acute central retinal artery occlusion, sight can generally be retained if circulation is restored within:**

 a. 30 minutes.

 b. 60 minutes.

 c. 90 minutes.

 d. 120 minutes.

 e. 150 minutes.

The answer is c. Because acute retinal artery occlusion is an ophthalmic emergency, efforts should be directed toward restoring retinal circulation as soon as possible. It has been proven that restoration of vision is minimal beyond 90 minutes. Nonetheless, all attempts should be made within the first 24 hours.

17. **A 62-year-old woman complains of sudden, painless, vision loss in her right eye. Your funduscopic examination shows a diffuse retinal hemorrhage, including marked tortuosity and dilatation of all the retinal veins. You tell your ophthalmologist consultant that you suspect:**

 a. Acute angle-closure glaucoma.

 b. Acute central retinal artery occlusion.

 c. Nonischemic central retinal vein occlusion.

 d. Ischemic central retinal vein occlusion.

 e. Macular degeneration.

The answer is d. This is a classic presentation of retinal vein occlusion. Fundus examination is essential to differentiate artery occlusion from vein occlusion. Ischemic and nonischemic types present with visual loss; fundus examination shows dilatation and tortuosity of all retinal branch veins. Nonischemic forms have a few scattered retinal hemorrhages in the posterior pole; ischemic forms have diffuse retinal hemorrhages extending from the optic disc to the periphery of the fundus. Acute central retinal artery occlusion typically results in a pale retina and a small reddish dot near the fovea (Tintinalli et al., 2003:1461).

18. **A 56-year-old woman complains of nausea, headache, and a painful, red right eye. Her visual acuity is 20/200 in the right eye, 20/20 in the left eye. Her right pupil is 6 mm and does not react to light. Her left pupil is 3 mm and reactive. The right cornea looks cloudy. You should now:**

    a. Order emergent head MRI.

    b. Order emergent head CT.

    c. Dilate the pupils for funduscopic examination.

    d. Obtain intraocular pressures.

    e. Begin high-dose steroid therapy for optic neuritis.

    The answer is d. The patient must be evaluated for evidence of acute narrow-angle glaucoma; this is vision threatening. Glaucoma commonly presents with systemic signs of nausea, vomiting, or headache and must be considered in the differential of all patients with these complaints. Tonometry is essential in making the diagnosis. Signs include a middilated, poorly reactive pupil with corneal edema and a shallow anterior chamber. An inflammatory reaction is often present. These classic findings may not always be present early in the clinical course.

19. **A 38-year-old man without past medical history woke up this morning and noted a collection of blood in his left eye. His visual acuity is 20/20 in each eye. The blood is superficial and does not cross the limbus. He requires:**

    a. Blood coagulation studies.

    b. Emergent ophthalmology consult.

    c. Reassurance—send home without treatment.

    d. Drainage of the blood.

    e. Fluorescein angiography to determine vascular anomalies.

    The answer is c. This patient has a subconjunctival hemorrhage. These usually develop spontaneously or from trauma. Most patients can be sent home without further treatment. The hemorrhage should resolve within 2–3 weeks. More complicated cases may result from a large collection of blood (which prevents lid closure) or from an associated conjunctivitis.

20. **A 35-year-old man was struck in the left eye with a softball. He complains of blurred vision, vertical double vision, numbness of his cheek, and eye pain. The most important evaluation is:**

    a. Visual acuity and pupil evaluation.

    b. Orbital x-ray.

    c. Slit lamp evaluation.

    d. Orbital CT scan with 3-D reconstructions.

    e. Muscle balance evaluation.

    The answer is a. Traumatic optic neuropathy, ruptured globe, or an intraocular injury must be ruled out before any consideration should be given to an orbital floor fracture. Loss of vision and/or an afferent pupil must be investigated first.

21. **A 45-year-old man has watery discharge and erythema of his right eye. Visual acuity is normal. A tender, ipsilateral preauricular lymph node is present on examination. The sclera is diffusely erythematous. The cornea has small punctate opacities that stain poorly with fluorescein. His most likely diagnosis is:**

   a. Allergic conjunctivitis.

   b. Herpes zoster conjunctivitis.

   c. Blepharitis.

   d. Epidemic keratoconjunctivitis.

   e. Corneal abrasion.

   The answer is d. Erythema and eye irritation are characteristic of both viral and bacterial causes of conjunctivitis. A purulent discharge is more commonly seen in bacterial conjunctivitis. Empiric therapy for uncomplicated conjunctivitis includes systemic analgesics and topical antibiotics. Epidemic keratoconjunctivitis, caused by adenovirus, is a highly contagious eye infection associated with tender preauricular lymph nodes and a mild keratitis. It is self-limited condition.

22. **A 29-year-old man sustained blunt trauma to his right eye from a racquetball. He complains of eye pain only. Visual acuity is normal. Extraocular muscles are intact. The pupils are equal, the light reflexes are intact, and no photophobia is present. Funduscopic examination reveals a small inferior vitreous hemorrhage. The remainder of the ocular examination is unremarkable. An appropriate action is to:**

   a. Refer the patient for immediate ophthalmologic evaluation.

   b. Instruct the patient to return for reexamination in 24 hours or sooner if he notices blurry vision or eye pain.

   c. Advise the patient to use cool compresses as needed and see an ophthalmologist in 5–7 days for follow-up.

   d. Apply an eye patch, prescribe a topical cycloplegic and topical anesthetic, and instruct the patient to return in 24 hours.

   e. Administer a topical cycloplegic and topical steroid and refer the patient for follow-up.

   The answer is a. Posttraumatic vitreous hemorrhage suggests the possibility of a retinal tear. Peripheral traumatic tears may be difficult to visualize. Ultrasonography may be used to search for retinal injury and the need for operative repair. Treatment of vitreous hemorrhage includes elevating the head of the bed as well as avoiding platelet-inhibiting drugs and Valsalva maneuver. Vitrectomy is performed for vitreous hemorrhage with an associated retinal detachment. In the above case, there is no evidence of a traumatic iritis and therefore no indication for a topical cycloplegic or ophthalmic steroid preparation. Topical ocular anesthetics should never be prescribed for use by the patient. Other injuries associated with blunt eye trauma include traumatic lens dislocation, traumatic mydriasis, and orbital wall fractures.

23. **The bacterial organism most commonly associated with bullous myringitis is:**

   a. *Staphylococcus pyogenes.*

   b. *Staphylococcus aureus.*

   c. *Chlamydia trachomata.*

   d. *Mycoplasma pneumoniae.*

   e. *Pseudomonas aeruginosa.*

The answer is d. Bullous myringitis is a painful condition of the ear characterized by bulla formation on the tympanic membrane. The blisters occur between the highly innervated outer epithelium and the inner fibrous layer of the TM, explaining the severe otalgia. Opioid pain medication is often required. It is believed that most cases are viral in nature but *Mycoplasma* still remains the most frequent bacterial organism isolated. Treatment consists of warm compresses, analgesics, and systemic macrolide antibiotics. In severe cases, the patient should be referred to an ENT surgeon for therapeutic rupture of the bullae.

24. **A 4-year-old boy presents with high fever, anorexia, and drooling. He has mild inspiratory stridor and resists the nurse's efforts to assist him into the supine position. You should next:**
   a. Use a tongue blade to visualize the posterior oropharynx and rule out epiglottitis.
   b. Obtain a portable lateral soft tissue x-ray of the neck with the child in his mother's arms, while arranging airway management in the operating room.
   c. Perform immediate tracheostomy.
   d. Begin high-dose steroid therapy and arrange for a croup tent.
   e. Sedate the patient and place him supine, while starting beta-agonist therapy.

The answer is b. Although it remains one of the most feared childhood emergencies, pediatric epiglottitis has markedly declined in incidence in the last several years following the widespread use of the Haemophilus influenzae B (HIB) vaccine. Pediatric epiglottitis typically affects children between 3 and 7 years of age and occurs year round. Typically, there is an acute onset of a severe sore throat and high fever with drooling and dysphagia. The child often sits with the neck slightly extended and chin thrust out to open the airway. Air hunger and retractions are common, while coughing is absent. The child resists efforts to be placed supine, but otherwise sits quietly with all efforts directed toward breathing. The child with suspected epiglottitis should not be left unattended by the physician. A bag-valve mask with oxygen, endotracheal tube, laryngoscope, and a 14-gauge needle-catheter for needle cricothyrotomy should be kept close at hand. Attempts to visualize the epiglottis with a tongue blade should be avoided as they may precipitate airway occlusion and respiratory arrest. A lateral neck film in the ED may help confirm the diagnosis. Optimal treatment includes intubating the patient in the operating room under general anesthesia.

25. **A 16-year-old girl was struck in the mouth with a baseball. She complains of mild nasal tenderness and a sore tooth. Her left central incisor is chipped and blood is visible at the site. You must:**
   a. Place a calcium hydroxide dressing on the tooth and advise the patient to see a dentist within 24 hours.
   b. Administer a regional anesthetic block, smooth off the rough edge, and refer to the dentist for elective treatment.
   c. Apply oil of cloves for analgesia, administer antibiotics, and refer to a dentist within 24 hours.
   d. Arrange immediate dental referral.
   e. Debride the protruding pulpal tissue after dental nerve block, then cover with foil and refer to a dentist.

The answer is d. Management of dental fractures is determined by the Ellis classification. An Ellis class I fracture only involves the enamel. The patient should be referred to a dentist for elective cosmetic treatment. An Ellis class II fracture exposes the dentin. The patient will typically note extreme temperature sensitivity. If the patient is younger than 12 years or if the fracture involves a large portion of the tooth, a calcium hydroxide dressing covered with gauze or foil is applied and the patient is referred to a dentist within 24 hours. Older patients do not require the dressing but should see a dentist within the same time frame. An Ellis class III fracture exposes the pulp and therefore bleeds. This fracture is a dental emergency and requires immediate dental referral. If a dentist is not immediately available, moist cotton can be placed over the exposed pulp and covered with a piece of dry foil. Never debride the pulp. In cases of extreme pain a dental nerve block may be helpful. Topical analgesics should not be used, since they may cause additional damage or promote sterile abscess formation.

26. **A 65-year-old man complains of vertigo. For the past 2 weeks he has felt unsteady on his feet. He has an unremarkable past medical history. Neurologic examination reveals vertical nystagmus and a mild ataxic gait. The source of his symptoms is likely the:**

     a. Brainstem.

     b. Middle ear.

     c. Labyrinthine system.

     d. Eighth cranial nerve.

     e. Occipital lobe.

The answer is a. Vertigo is the illusion of motion. One must first establish that the patient has vertigo rather than presyncope or disequilibrium. Next, one must attempt to determine whether the vertigo is central (brainstem, cerebellum) or peripheral (eighth nerve, inner and middle ear) in origin. Peripheral vertigo usually presents with nausea, vomiting, hearing loss, tinnitus, and marked, almost violent rotational symptoms, with no associated neurologic abnormalities. Nausea, vomiting, hearing loss, and tinnitus are mild or rarely present in central vertigo. Vertical nystagmus is a finding highly suggestive of brainstem disease, as are associated ocular palsies, ataxia, dysarthria, and peripheral sensory deficits.

27. **The most frequent cause of epistaxis is:**

     a. Atherosclerosis of the nasal blood vessels.

     b. Coagulation disorders.

     c. Traumatic injury of the ethmoidal arteries.

     d. Erosion of the vessels of the anterior nasal septum.

     e. Erosion of the posterior sphenopalatine arteries.

The answer is d. Erosion of the vessels of anterior nasal septum (Kisselbach's plexus) either from trauma, dry air, infection, nasal irritants, or telangiectasias (Osler-Weber-Rendu syndrome), is the most common cause of epistaxis. Systemic disorders such as blood dyscrasias, liver disease, and atherosclerotic nasal arteries are important causes of posterior epistaxis. Anterior epistaxis, which accounts for 90% of all nosebleeds, usually responds to direct pressure or chemical cauterization with silver nitrate. Posterior epistaxis or severe anterior epistaxis require nasal packing or a balloon device for tamponade control. Patients with anterior nasal packs may be managed as outpatients. Patients with posterior bleeding should be admitted to the hospital. All patients with nasal packing require antibiotic prophylaxis, such as amoxicillin-clavulanate or a first-generation cephalosporin, to prevent toxic shock syndrome and sinusitis.

28. **A 3-year-old child apparently knocked out a tooth at play, but did not retrieve the tooth. You should now:**

     a. Obtain an x-ray of the tooth socket.

     b. Reassure the mother that the lost tooth will not make any difference.

     c. Obtain a chest x-ray.

     d. Send the mother home to look for the tooth so it can be reimplanted.

     e. None of the above

The answer is c. If a tooth or piece of a tooth cannot be found after trauma, a chest x-ray must be obtained to rule out possible aspiration. Avulsed primary teeth in the pediatric patient aged 6 months to 6 years should not be replaced in the socket. Reimplanted primary teeth ankylose or fuse to the alveolar bone and interfere with the eruption of the permanent teeth. These patients should however be referred to a dentist for possible space maintainers or cosmetic appliances. Avulsed permanent teeth should be reimplanted as soon as possible. Each minute that reimplantation is delayed equals a 1% decrease in the probability of the tooth's survival. The tooth should only be rinsed gently with saline, never scrubbed, since this will damage the periodontal ligaments. If the tooth cannot be immediately reimplanted, it can be kept moist in gauze, milk, or saliva. The best storage and transport medium is Hanks's solution ("Save-A-Tooth").

29. **The most valuable radiographic study in the initial evaluation of a patient with a potential midface fracture is the:**

    a. Lateral view.
    b. Waters view.
    c. Caldwell view.
    d. Submental vertex view.
    e. Towne view.

The answer is b. The standard plain film facial series usually consists of the Waters (occipitomental) view, the Caldwell (occipitofrontal or PA) view, and lateral view. The Waters view is the best study for the initial evaluation of the maxilla, maxillary sinuses, and orbital rims. An air–fluid level in the maxillary sinus is almost pathognomonic for a fracture in the setting of acute trauma. A soft tissue density seen within the maxillary sinus suggests an orbital blowout fracture. The Caldwell view best details the bones of the upper face and lateral orbits. The lateral view may demonstrate elongation of the face in LeFort injuries or disruption of the posterior sinus walls. The submental vertex view, commonly referred to as the "jug handle" view, is useful for evaluating the base of the skull and the zygomatic arches. The Towne view is useful for evaluating the mandibular rami and condyles.

30. **The eye disorder which will probably require the patient to be hospitalized is:**

    a. Corneal ulcer.
    b. Ultraviolet keratitis.
    c. Blepharitis.
    d. Hordeolum.
    e. Subconjunctival hemorrhage.

The answer is a. The differential diagnosis of a painful red eye includes, but is not limited to, acute glaucoma, foreign body, acute iritis, and corneal ulcer. The corneal ulcer appears as a white corneal opacity. Hypopyon, white cells in the anterior chamber, may be present. Extended-wear contact lens wearers are at risk for *Pseudomonas* infections.

31.   **Choose the most accurate statement concerning the treatment of acute angle-closure glaucoma:**

   a. Topical beta-blockers are used to decrease aqueous humor secretion.

   b. Topical alpha-blockers are used to decrease aqueous humor secretion.

   c. Topical steroids are used to decrease the volume of fluid in the eye.

   d. Topical cycloplegics are used to promote aqueous outflow.

   e. Topical miotics, by promoting aqueous outflow, provide immediate pain relief.

The answer is a. Acute angle-closure glaucoma occurs in patients with shallow anterior chamber angles. Acute narrowing of this angle produces a resistance to the normal flow of aqueous humor and an abrupt increase in intraocular pressure (IOP). This can be precipitated by stress, administration of topical cycloplegics, or by moving from daylight to a darkened room. Symptoms include ocular pain, blurred vision, and halos around lights. A red eye with a fixed, mid-dilated pupil and a hazy cornea is noted on examination. Intraocular pressures usually exceed 40 mm Hg. Treatment consists of the sequential administration of several different agents to decrease the intraocular pressure. Topical beta-blockers (e.g., timolol), topical alpha-agonists (e.g., apraclonidine), and carbonic anhydrase inhibitors (e.g., acetazolamide) are used initially to decrease the secretion of aqueous humor by the ciliary body. Topical steroids are used to reduce inflammation. Hyperosmotic agents (e.g., mannitol) are used to decrease the volume of fluid in the eye. Topical miotics (e.g., pilocarpine) are used to promote aqueous outflow but they do not usually have an effect until the IOP is < 40 mm Hg. Analgesics should be provided as needed. Immediate ophthalmologic consultation is required.

32.   **A 41-year-old woman is elbowed in the left eye. 5 hours later she has photophobia and decreased visual acuity (OS 20/60; OD 20/20). Ciliary flush is present. You would also expect to find:**

   a. Cell and flare in the anterior chamber.

   b. Pupillary constriction.

   c. Consensual photophobia.

   d. Improved symptoms with cycloplegic drops.

   e. All of the above.

The answer is e. The diagnosis is acute traumatic iritis. Ocular pain, decreased vision, and photophobia are characteristic symptoms of iritis. Ciliary flush and a constricted and sometimes irregular pupil are present on examination. Intraocular pressure is variable. Slit lamp examination may reveal cells (leukocytes) and flare (protein) in the anterior chamber. Initial treatment includes long acting cycloplegic agents. Topical steroids may be used in consultation with an ophthalmologist. If the pupil is not dilated properly, adhesions (synechiae) may form between the iris and anterior lens surface. These adhesions may produce permanent pupillary disfigurement and can lead to secondary glaucoma.

33.   **A 42-year-old diabetic woman presents with a history of severe right otalgia. She has a recent history of otitis externa and states that the acetic acid drops are now ineffective. Her other medications include nifedipine and insulin. Her temperature is 38.5°C (101.3°F). Her right external canal is erythematous, swollen, and tender, and her tympanic membrane is slightly erythematous, but there is no effusion present. Prudent management requires you to:**

   a. Obtain ear cultures, change eardrops, and reexamine in 1 week.

   b. Prescribe an oral cephalosporin for 10 days along with a systemic analgesic.

   c. Prescribe an oral cephalosporin, a topical antibiotic, an oral analgesic, and warm compresses 3 times daily.

   d. Prescribe an oral fluoroquinolone, a topical antibiotic, an oral analgesic, and warm compresses 3 times daily.

   e. None of the above.

The answer is e. Malignant otitis externa, or necrotizing external otitis, is an extremely aggressive form of otitis externa. It occurs primarily in adults with diabetes and should be suspected when otitis externa fails to respond to conventional therapy. Symptoms include pain, tenderness, swelling around the periauricular area, headache, and otorrhea. The examination finding most characteristic of the disease is granulation tissue in the floor of the ear canal at the bony cartilaginous junction. Although the infection begins in the external canal, involvement of the adjacent soft tissues and cartilage may quickly result in extension to the underlying bone. Complications include osteomyelitis, cranial nerve palsies, sigmoid sinus thrombosis, and meningitis. These patients require hospitalization for parenteral antibiotics and possible surgical debridement.

34. **Choose the correct statement about nasal fractures:**

    a. Nasal films should be obtained in all cases.
    b. Persistent epistaxis and CSF rhinorrhea are common complications.
    c. Immediate reduction of nasal fractures is required in the ED.
    d. Septal hematomas should be drained immediately in the ED.
    e. Immediate ENT consultation and hospitalization is recommended.

    The answer is d. The nose is the most common site of facial trauma. The diagnosis of a simple nasal fracture is primarily clinical. Suggestive findings include the presence of tenderness, swelling, ecchymosis, deformity, or crepitus. Epistaxis may occur but is usually transient. Nasal films are of little or no value in the initial management and need not be obtained in most cases. Although immediate reduction may be possible, it is generally deferred until the swelling has subsided. All patients with nasal trauma should be carefully evaluated for the presence of a septal hematoma. These hematomas should be drained immediately to prevent avascular necrosis of the nasal septum and/or septal abscess formation. All patients with suspected or confirmed nasal fractures should be referred for reevaluation in 5–7 days. Trauma to the bridge of the nose may cause a more complex nasoethmoid fracture. These fractures may be complicated fractures of the cribiform plate and CSF rhinorrhea. CT scanning, neurosurgical consultation, and admission are generally required.

35. **A 23-year-old male patient complains of facial swelling and epistaxis after sustaining a significant blow to the face. On examination, you are able to freely move the patient's maxilla and nasal bridge with gentle traction on the upper incisors. You suspect he has:**

    a. Nasal fracture.
    b. LeFort I fracture.
    c. LeFort II fracture.
    d. LeFort III fracture.
    e. Tripod fracture.

    The answer is c. Maxillary fractures result from massive, direct facial trauma. These fractures are often classified as LeFort I, II, or III fractures. A LeFort I fracture (palatal–facial disjunction) involves a horizontal fracture of the maxilla at the level of the nasal floor. It can be diagnosed by gently grasping the upper incisors and moving the maxilla back and forth. A LeFort II fracture (pyramidal disjunction) includes fractures through the maxilla, nasal bones, and infraorbital rim. Grasping the upper incisors and gently moving them back and forth will result in motion of the maxilla and the bridge of the nose. A LeFort III fracture (craniofacial disjunction) is similar to a LeFort II fracture, except that the fracture extends bilaterally across the frontozygomatic sutures, the lateral orbits, and through the bridge of the nose. The face is generally pushed inward. Gently moving the upper teeth results in movement of the midface and zygoma together. The LeFort III fracture has the highest incidence of CSF rhinorrhea. Of note, these fractures rarely occur in their pure form and usually present in combination. Plain films may demonstrate these fractures but CT imaging is generally needed to delineate the extent and number of fractures present. Treatment includes airway management, prophylactic antibiotics, and surgical evaluation. Tripod fractures generally result from a blow to the cheek and involve fractures at the zygomatic arch, zygomaticofrontal suture, and infraorbital rim.

36.   Regarding acute necrotizing ulcerative gingivitis (ANUG):

    a. Herpes virus is the most commonly implicated pathogen.

    b. Metallic taste and foul breath are common presenting complaints.

    c. Systemic symptoms, such as fever and malaise, are uncommon.

    d. Systemic antibiotics are generally not helpful.

    e. Dental follow-up is recommended on an as-needed basis.

The answer is b. Acute necrotizing ulcerative gingivitis (ANUG or "trench mouth") is a periodontal infection caused by fusobacteria and spirochetes. Patients present complaining of gingival pain, a metallic taste, and foul breath. Systemic symptoms such as fever, malaise, and regional lymphadenopathy are common. On examination, the gingiva is swollen and fiery red. The interdental papillae are ulcerated or "punched out" and covered with a grayish pseudomembrane. Treatment includes warm saline irrigation, antibiotics (PCN, erythromycin, or tetracycline), systemic analgesics, and local topical anesthetics. Antibiotics often provide dramatic relief within 24 hours. Dental follow-up is required because ANUG can be complicated by the destruction of underlying alveolar bone.

37.   A 32-year-old alcoholic man presents with facial pain and swelling. He reports difficulty swallowing as well as trouble opening his mouth. He sits with his lower jaw slightly thrust out and chin extended. His temperature is 38.9°C (102°F). There is marked submandibular swelling bilaterally and the tongue is slightly elevated. A periapical tooth abscess of the second right lower molar is noted on examination. Your next step is to:

    a. Prescribe oral penicillin, PRN analgesics, and discharge home.

    b. Administer a tetanus booster and tetanus immune globulin at two separate sites and consider admission to the ICU for prophylactic neuromuscular blockade.

    c. Perform local I&D of the periapical abscess and discharge home.

    d. Administer high-dose penicillin and metronidazole IV, obtain immediate ENT consultation, and admit to the ICU.

    e. Administer diphenhydramine and prednisolone IV and observe in the ED for 6 hours.

The answer is d. Ludwig's angina is a progressive cellulitis of the floor of the mouth involving the sublingual, submandibular, and submaxillary spaces bilaterally. It is a polymicrobial infection of mixed aerobic and anaerobic bacteria. The most commonly isolated organisms are streptococci, staphylococci, and *Bacteroides* sp. Signs and symptoms include fever, drooling, dysphagia, dysphonia, and trismus. The most common physical examination findings are bilateral submandibular swelling and elevation of the tongue. The swelling is often noted to be "brawny" or "woody" in nature. Since most of these infections are odontogenic in origin, it is not uncommon for an infected or recently extracted tooth to be present on examination.

38.   The usual complaint of a patient with optic neuritis is:

    a. Flashing lights and a visual field defect.

    b. Sudden, painless, diffuse monocular vision loss.

    c. Rapidly progressive loss of central vision.

    d. Gradual loss of peripheral vision.

    e. None of the above.

The answer is c. Optic neuritis is an inflammatory process of the optic nerve. It is often characterized by loss of central vision with preservation of peripheral vision. Visual loss ranges from mild to severe and is rapidly progressive over hours to days. Associated symptoms include painful extraocular movements and red vision desaturation. An afferent pupillary defect (Marcus-Gunn pupil) is almost universally present. The disc may be normal (retrobulbar optic neuritis) or swollen and hyperemic (anterior optic neuritis). Of note, approximately 30% of patients presenting with acute optic neuritis will develop multiple sclerosis within 5 years.

39. **After 2 days of URI symptoms, a 3-year-old girl has developed a barking cough and moderate stridor. The parents state that her condition is worse at night. Physical examination shows a low-grade fever of 38°C (100.4°F), pulse of 140, respirations of 40, and inspiratory stridor at rest. Following two treatments of racemic epinephrine the child's stridor has resolved. At this point you should:**

    a. Provide instructions to use a cool-mist humidifier and discharge home.

    b. Prescribe ampicillin and discharge home.

    c. Administer steroids and discharge home.

    d. Administer steroids and observe the patient for at least 3 hours.

    e. Obtain a lateral soft tissue x-ray of the neck and emergent ENT consultation.

    The answer is d. Croup, most commonly caused by parainfluenza virus, is usually a benign, self-limited disease characterized by edema and inflammation of the upper airway. It most often occurs in children 6 months to 3 years of age in the late fall and early winter. The typical history is 2–3 days of a URI with a gradually worsening cough, especially at night. Fever is absent or low grade and the child is nontoxic in appearance. Treatment may include cool-mist, oxygen, steroids, racemic epinephrine, and Heliox in severe cases. Steroids should be administered to any child with moderate to severe stridor and any child who receives racemic epinephrine. Racemic epinephrine is usually reserved for children with resting stridor and respiratory distress that does not respond to supportive measures. Children who respond to racemic epinephrine should be observed for at least 3 hours prior to final disposition.

40. **The Centor criteria for determining which patient with a sore throat should receive antibiotics:**

    a. Rarely leads to overtreatment.

    b. Are not valid in children.

    c. Determine which antibiotic will be most effective.

    d. Were developed in an attempt to reduce the occurrence of acute rheumatic fever.

    e. Includes both historical and anatomic findings.

    The answer is e. Centor criteria (presence of tonsillar exudates, tender anterior cervical adenopathy, fever by history, and absence of cough) combine both historical features and physical findings to help determine which patient has streptococcal pharyngitis and therefore may benefit from treatment with antibiotic. They are equally valid in adults and children; some experts recommend adding one point for patients younger than 15 years and subtracting one point for patients older than 45 years. The criteria do not determine which antibiotic should be used, only which patient should be treated with antibiotic. Even in patients with all four Centor criteria (high pretest probability), overtreatment will occur in approximately 50% of cases.

41. **The most sensitive test for determining maxillary sinusitis is:**

a. Sinus x-ray.

b. CT scan.

c. Percussive tenderness.

d. Transillumination.

e. Ultrasound.

The answer is b. Radiologic studies do not have a significant clinical role in the diagnosis of acute rhinosinusitis. Coronal CT scan of the sinuses is the most sensitive test. Transillumination is probably more useful (and practical) in the emergency department. None of these methods can determine whether the patient has a bacterial infection amenable to treatment with antibiotics.

CHAPTER 8

Hematologic and Oncologic Emergencies

Sachin J. Shah, MD, MBA, FAAEM

1. **In children with sickle cell disease presenting with osteomyelitis, the most common pathogen is:**

   a. *S. aureus.*

   b. *S. pneumoniae.*

   c. *E. coli.*

   d. *Salmonella* species.

   e. Enterococcal species.

   The answer is d. Up to two-thirds of cases of osteomyelitis in children with sickle cell disease involve *Salmonella*. It is unclear why these patients are susceptible to *Salmonella* specifically. Patients with sickle cell disease are at higher risk for infection with encapsulated organisms due to the impairment of macrophage function.

2. **In alcoholic patients, thrombocytopenia is due to:**

   a. Toxic effects on megakaryocytes.

   b. Liver sequestration.

   c. Bone marrow infarcts.

   d. Platelet lysis.

   e. Unknown.

   The answer is e. Apart from acquired immune deficiency syndrome (AIDS), alcoholism is probably the leading cause of thrombocytopenia. However patients generally do not exhibit manifestations of excessive bleeding. Alcohol-related thrombocytopenia is usually transient, and platelet counts generally return to normal within 1 week of abstinence. The exact mechanisms underlying alcohol-related thrombocytopenia remain unknown. Some researchers have suggested that alcohol intoxication itself, rather than alcohol-related nutritional deficiencies, causes the decrease in platelet numbers. This view is supported by findings that thrombocytopenia developed in healthy subjects who received a diet containing adequate protein and vitamin levels, including large doses of folic acid, and consumed the equivalent of 1.5 pints (i.e., 745 mL) of 86-proof whiskey for at least 10 days.

3. **A 19-year-old man was riding a motorcycle, which collided with a delivery truck. He complains of severe abdominal pain and is tachycardiac. He tells you that he has a history of von Willebrand disease. The product you should order to help control improve this patient's clotting ability is:**

    a. 4 units of whole blood.

    b. A 6 pack of platelets.

    c. Recombinant factor VIIa.

    d. Packed red cells.

    e. Factor VIII.

    The answer is e. Patients with von Willebrand disease have normal platelet counts and morphology but have diminished function due to lack of circulating von Willebrand factor. The ideal choice for this patient to help improve platelet aggregation would be Factor VIII. The initial dose would be 20–30 IU/kg every 12 hours. Fresh frozen plasma can be used as well in extreme conditions as desmopressin.

4. **A 13-year-old girl complains of heavy vaginal bleeding during her menstrual period. She has a history of menorrhagia. A urine pregnancy test is negative. A platelet count, PT, and PTT are normal. The laboratory test that might reveal a bleeding diathesis is:**

    a. Thrombin time.

    b. Factor VIII level.

    c. Fibrinogen level.

    d. Bleeding time.

    e. Ristocetin platelet aggregation.

    The answer is d. A bleeding disorder should be suspected in any patient with recurrent bleeding, as in this patient with menorrhagia. Type I von Willebrand disease, the most common inherited bleeding disorder, is an autosomal dominant trait in which an abnormality in a plasma glycoprotein (von Willebrand factor) results in abnormal platelet adhesion and a prolonged bleeding time. The PT and PTT are usually normal.

5. **A local ambulance company brings you a 25-year-old woman; her husband tells you "she's confused." Temperature 38.9°C (102°F); blood pressure 130/100 mm Hg. She has a diffuse petechial rash and generalized edema. She is oriented only to self and is delirious. Laboratory studies show: BUN, 29 mg/dL; creatinine, 2.7 mg/dL; platelet count, 27,000/mm³; and hematocrit, 30% with numerous schistocytes seen on the peripheral smear. WBC count is normal with no left shift. Which of the following statements is TRUE?**

    a. The patient requires urgent heparinization.

    b. A PT and PTT would probably be prolonged in this patient.

    c. Antibiotic coverage is indicated.

    d. Plasmaphoresis and treatment with fresh frozen plasma is needed.

    e. Intravenous steroids are not recommended.

    The answer is d. This patient has classic signs of thrombotic thrombocytopenic purpura (TTP) including anemia, thrombocytopenia, fever, neurologic, and renal dysfunction. Patients may present in coma. The PT and PTT are not prolonged in TTP. Heparinization is not routinely indicated for the initial treatment of TTP. Large doses of intravenous steroids are used if the diagnosis is suspected. Plasmaphoresis and transfusion with fresh frozen plasma may reverse the clinical and laboratory abnormalities.

6. **ABO matching of donor and recipient is unnecessary in the patient receiving:**

    a. Whole blood.

    b. Platelets.

    c. Packed red blood cells (PRBCs).

    d. Fresh frozen plasma.

    e. Leukocyte-poor red blood cells.

    The answer is b. Spontaneous bleeding is unusual when platelet counts are more than 20,000/mm^3. Platelet counts less than 10,000/mm^3 may cause spontaneous bleeding. HLA matching may be performed for platelets in special circumstances. ABO matching is unnecessary.

7. **A 20-year-old man with hemophilia A complains of a swollen right knee, which started after he played basketball. He says that his factor VIII level is generally measured at 7%. His knee is swollen and tense. Appropriate management for this patient is:**

    a. Immobilize his knee and insist on several days bed rest with aspirin therapy to reduce joint inflammation.

    b. Infuse with cryoprecipitate to raise factor VIII level to 30% and repeat infusions twice daily for 3 days.

    c. Continuously infuse with fresh frozen plasma to raise factor VIII level to 50–100%.

    d. Infuse with standard factor VIII concentrate to raise his factor VIII level to 90%.

    e. None of the above.

    The answer is e. Factor VIII levels of less than 1% predispose patients with Hemophilia A to frequent, severe bleeding episodes. Levels between 1% and 5% indicate moderate disease and levels above 5% indicate mild disease. Heat-treated factor VIII concentrate, monoclonal antibody purified factor VIII concentrate, and recombinant factor VIII concentrate cannot transmit HIV or hepatitis viruses. A small hemarthrosis or bleeding episode can be treated with a single infusion of factor VIII concentrate to achieve a plasma level of factor VIII of 15–20%. Each unit will raise the plasma level of factor VIII by 2% pcr kg of body weight. Alternatively, DDAVP (desmopressin acetate) will transiently increase levels of factor VIII. Factor VIII levels should be raised to 25–50% of normal for at least 3 days. Moderate bleeding episodes require twice-daily infusions as the half-life of factor VIII is 12 hours. Patients with severe trauma or intracranial bleeding should have factor VIII levels raised to 80–100%. Cryoprecipitate may also be given to raise levels of factor VIII. The risk of transmitting virus with this is low because cryoprecipitate is not prepared from pooled plasma sources. Fresh frozen plasma has very low factor VIII activity and requires much greater volume, which limits its use in hemophiliacs.

8. **A 52-year-old man arrives by ambulance complaining of several weeks of progressive lethargy. He is stuporous but arousable and complains of back pain and constipation. His vital signs are normal. Physical examination is remarkable for sausage-shaped retinal vessels and decreased consciousness. Neurologic examination reveals no focal findings. A chest x-ray shows a left pleural-based density with associated bony destruction. An abdominal series is remarkable for osteopenia of the pelvis. The hematology laboratory reports the machines keep clogging up. The hematocrit is 21%; RBCs are hypochromic and microcytic with marked rouleaux formation; WBC is 14,000/mm^3 with no left shift. Choose the correct statement:**

    a. The patient will probably have hypernatremia.

    b. The diagnostic test of choice is a CT or MRI scan of the head.

    c. Treatment includes fluid restriction.

    d. Hypocalcemia may be present.

    e. The radiographic findings are virtually diagnostic, but the diagnostic tests of choice include a serum viscosity determination.

    The answer is e. The hyperviscosity syndrome occurs when either abnormal amounts of serum protein are produced (multiple myeloma or Waldenström macroglobulinemia) or from the presence of massive numbers of white blood cells (chronic myelocytic leukemia [CML] and blast crisis). Vascular stasis and capillary sludging result in headache, fatigue, lethargy, seizures, and coma. Laboratory abnormalities in the paraproteinemias include RBC rouleaux formation, factitious hyponatremia, and abnormally high serum viscosity. Protein electrophoresis is diagnostic. Treatment of the hyperviscosity syndromes include hydration and plasmapheresis. Blast crisis and hyperviscosity in CML are treated with hydration and chemotherapy. Multiple myeloma is a common cause of destructive rib lesions and generalized osteopenia in patients older than 40 years. Additional clinical features include back pain (from lumbar vertebral fractures), constipation, and a decreased mental status (from hypercalcemia).

9. **A 65-year-old man whom you are treating for an acute upper GI bleeding inadvertently receives packed red cells intended for the patient with trauma in the next room. He develops a severe transfusion reaction before this error can be corrected. His urine turns dark and when you do a bedside hematocrit you notice that his serum is pink. You can help prevent renal complications by:**

    a. Infusing mannitol.

    b. Restricting fluid.

    c. Alkalinizing the urine.

    d. Performing emergent dialysis.

    e. Giving intravenous diphenhydramine and continuing the transfusion.

    The answer is c. Maintaining urine output of 0.5–1 mL/kg/h may prevent hemoglobin-induced acute tubular necrosis. Alkalinization of the urine prevents precipitation of hemoglobin in the renal tubules. Furosemide increases renal cortical blood flow and promotes diuresis. Osmotic diuresis with agents such as mannitol does not increase blood flow. Many physicians believe it should not be used in pigment-induced renal failure.

10. **Which statement about sickle cell disease is true?**

    a. Aplastic crisis can be diagnosed with a hematocrit less than 17% and a high reticulocyte count.

    b. Sequestration crisis is common in older patients.

    c. Hemolysis may cause icterus.

    d. Thrombotic (vasoocclusive) sickle cell crisis is a laboratory diagnosis.

    e. A urine specific gravity defines the hydration status.

The answer is c. Sickle cell patients have papillary necrosis of the kidneys and their urine becomes isosthenic. The inability to concentrate the urine contributes to dehydration and the thrombotic crisis. The painful thrombotic crisis is the most familiar crisis. Sickle cell disease is a hemolytic process and may cause an unconjugated hyperbilirubinemia. The reticulocyte count should be elevated. In aplastic crisis, bone marrow suppression secondary to folate deficiency or a viral (parvovirus) infection, the hematocrit declines and the reticulocyte count is low. The diagnosis of thrombotic crisis is clinical. Severe pain in the back, abdomen, or joints may be present. There is no specific laboratory test to diagnose a thrombotic crisis. Laboratory evaluation helps exclude infection or dehydration as contributing factors. In situ, thrombosis causes pulmonary infarction, autosplenectomy, and CNS disease. CNS vascular thrombosis may cause transient or permanent motor/sensory deficits or seizures.

11.   **A 70-year-old man with paroxysmal atrial fibrillation is on chronic warfarin therapy. The therapeutic goal for the patient's INR is:**

   a. <1.
   b. 1–1.5.
   c. 1.5–2.0.
   d. 3–4.
   e. None of the above.

The answer is c. For patients being anticoagulated for atrial fibrillation, the therapeutic goal for INR is between 1.5 and 2.0. For mechanical valves, the goal for INR can be as high as 2.5–3.5.

12.   **A 62-year-old woman complains of profound weakness and dyspnea on exertion for several weeks. Physical examination shows pallor, an unsteady gait, and guaiac-positive stool. She has been taking one pill a day for an "irregular heartbeat" and thyroxine. Laboratory studies include hemoglobin of 7.0 g/dL, hematocrit of 21%, leucopenia, and thrombocytopenia. A peripheral smear shows a macrocytic anemia with some hypochromic microcytic RBCs. Her probable diagnosis is:**

   a. Aplastic anemia.
   b. Myelofibrosis.
   c. Folate deficiency.
   d. Vitamin B_{12} deficiency.
   e. Drug-induced immune-mediated blood cell destruction.

The answer is d. The patient is pancytopenic and has signs of posterior column dysfunction. This presentation is very suggestive of pernicious anemia caused by vitamin B_{12} deficiency. Vitamin B_{12} deficiency is most commonly due to atrophic gastritis, which leads to the loss of production of intrinsic factor and malabsorption of the vitamin. There is a higher incidence of pernicious anemia in patients with a history of hypothyroidism and other immune-related endocrine disorders. Atrophic gastritis may be the result of an autoimmune reaction against gastric parietal cells. Patients with pernicious anemia have a higher risk of developing gastric carcinoma. Folate deficiency may cause a megaloblastic anemia; however, no neurologic abnormalities occur.

13.   **A patient with liver disease receives a transfusion of citrated blood. The rate of the transfusion is greater than 1 mL/kg/min. A complication you would expect is:**

   a. Decreased sensorium from ammonia build-up.

   b. Thrombocytopenia.

   c. Prolonged QT interval.

   d. Ventricular fibrillation.

   e. First-degree AV block.

   The answer is c. Citrate may chelate calcium and lower the serum's ionized levels. Hypocalcemia may be manifested as a prolonged QT interval. The liver metabolizes citrate to bicarbonate. Calcium supplementation should be reserved for patients who exhibit myocardial dysfunction.

14.   **Evaluation and treatment of a patient experiencing sickle cell vasoocclusive crisis should always include:**

   a. PRBC transfusion.

   b. Serial hematocrits and reticulocyte counts.

   c. Intravenous hydration.

   d. Analgesia.

   e. Supplemental oxygen.

   The answer is d. Transfusion of PRBCs should be avoided unless the patient is severely anemic (hematocrit <17–18%). Transfusion to a hematocrit above 30% may promote further sludging and vasoocclusion. The treatment of a vasoocclusive crisis includes analgesics, and possible oxygen, hydration. Evaluate for infection and the following crises: hemolytic, aplastic, and sequestration.

15.   **A patient with alcoholic cirrhosis and GI bleeding is most likely to have:**

   a. Increased bone marrow production of platelets.

   b. Normal absorption of vitamin K.

   c. Increased production of factor VII.

   d. Abnormal bleeding time.

   e. Congestive splenomegaly and thrombocytopenia.

   The answer is e. Vitamin K deficiency in patients with liver disease stems from malnutrition and malabsorption. The production of factors II, VII, IX, and X are vitamin K dependent. Thrombocytopenia is commonly due to hypersplenism (a consequence of portal hypertension) and bone marrow suppression. Alcohol directly suppresses bone marrow hematopoiesis.

16.   **A 45-year-old man complains of severe weakness and is found to have a hemoglobin level of 5 g/dL. Fragmented erythrocytes are present on the peripheral smear. The test which could help establish the diagnosis is:**

   a. Direct Coombs test.

   b. Indirect Coombs test.

   c. Serum B12.

   d. Serum folate.

   e. Urine for hemosiderin.

The answer is e. Fragmented erythrocytes suggest a microangiopathic hemolytic anemia. This form of anemia occurs in patients with cardiac valvular dysfunction or transfusion reactions. The only test that is helpful in this form of anemia is testing for urinary hemosiderin. The mechanism for a positive urine hemosiderin is that patients with this form of anemia can have hemoglobinemia and hemoglobinuria. The distal tubular renal cells reabsorb hemoglobin from the urine and convert it into hemosiderin. When the hemosiderin-laden renal tubules are sloughed, hemosiderin can be detected in the cellular component of the urinary sediment, and thus, urine is positive for hemosiderin. Fragmented RBCs do not suggest conditions in which a direct or indirect Coombs test would be positive or conditions in which the serum folate and vitamin B_{12} levels would be abnormal. A direct Coombs test is positive in autoimmune hemolytic anemia, and an indirect Coombs test is positive following transfusion reactions.

17. **The viral agent implicated in an aplastic crisis of patients with sickle cell disease is:**

    a. Bunyavirus.

    b. Atypical herpes simplex.

    c. Parvovirus.

    d. Coxsackie virus.

    e. HTLV-IV.

    The answer is c. Aplastic crises can be precipitated by viral infections (particularly parvovirus B19), folic acid deficiency, or the ingestion of bone marrow toxins such as phenylbutazone. Bone marrow erythropoiesis is slowed or stopped. The hematocrit falls to as low as 10%, and the reticulocyte count falls to as low as 0.5%. The white blood cell count and platelet counts usually remain stable.

18. **The laboratory study to differentiate poor RBC production from increased RBC destruction is the:**

    a. Sedimentation rate.

    b. C-reactive protein level.

    c. Schleptoglobin level.

    d. Total to direct bilirubin ratio.

    e. Reticulocyte count.

    The answer is e. The reticulocyte retains its ribosomal network for approximately 4 days, of which 3 are spent in the bone marrow and 1 in the peripheral circulation. The red blood cell matures as the reticulocyte loses its ribosomal network and circulates for 110–120 days. Under steady state conditions, the rate of red blood cell production equals the rate of destruction. Red blood cell mass remains constant as an equal number of reticulocytes replace the destroyed, senescent erythrocytes during the same period.

19. **By far, the most important way an emergency physician can treat DIC is to:**

    a. Stabilize the patient hemodynamically and treat the underlying disorder.

    b. Rapidly correct the thrombocytopenia.

    c. Aggressively resuscitate the patient with colloid solution.

    d. Arrange for emergent plasmapheresis.

    e. Arrange for emergent hemodialysis.

    The answer is a. The goals of emergency care in cases of DIC include initial suspicion, aggressive diagnostic pursuit, understanding of potential life-threatening complications, and only rarely, initiation of therapy.

20.   Heparin-induced thrombocytopenia:

a. Does not occur with low molecular weight heparins.

b. Requires a minimum number of units, so a heparin "flush" is always safe.

c. Can paradoxically cause thrombosis, ischemia, and amputation.

d. Never occurs during the first 24 hours of infusion.

e. Is easily treated with warfarin and fresh frozen plasma.

The answer is c. A number of drugs have been associated with thrombocytopenia of immunologic origin. Because of its relatively high frequency, heparin is an important cause of drug-induced thrombocytopenia in hospitalized patients. Platelets are activated by the formation of an IgG-heparin complex. Low–molecular-weight heparin may be associated with less thrombocytopenia than standard, unfractionated heparin; however, both forms of heparin have cross-reactivity. Heparin-induced thrombocytopenia can occasionally lead to the "white clot" syndrome, causing impaired peripheral circulation, gangrene, and amputation.

21.   Following antileukemic therapy, a 52-year-old man develops febrile neutropenia and receives broad-spectrum antibiotics intravenously at home for 4 days, yet he is persistently running a temperature of 102.6°F. His chest x-ray shows no infiltrates. Blood cultures are negative for growth of bacterial or fungal pathogens to date. His WBC count is 0.1/mm³, hemoglobin is 10.2, and platelet count is 22,000/mm³. Your most appropriate next step in the care of this patient is to:

a. Continue the same broad-spectrum antibiotics and admit to a respiratory isolation bed.

b. Initiate intravenous fluconazole therapy (200 mg/d).

c. Initiate intravenous amphotericin B therapy.

d. Administer rectal nonsteroidal anti-inflammatory agents to suppress the fever.

e. Give high-dose steroids intravenously.

The answer is c. Administer early empiric treatment with amphotericin B (e.g., conventional, other formulations) for patients who are persistently febrile, neutropenic, and already on broad-spectrum antibiotics for a few days, despite the absence of any documented evidence of fungal infection. The clinical scenario is suspicious for an acid-fast bacillus infection.

CHAPTER 9

Immunologic Emergencies

Sachin J. Shah, MD, MBA, FAAEM

1. **Which of the pairings of patients and drug regimens used to treat anaphylaxis is correct?**

   a. Mildly hypotensive adult patient → 5 mg epinephrine 1:10,000 IM, IV crystalloid infusion.

   b. Adult patient in cardiovascular collapse → 1 mg epinephrine (10 mL of a 1:10,000 dilution) via the cricothyroid membrane, IV fluids.

   c. 10-kg child in cardiovascular collapse → 10 mL/kg IV fluid bolus, 0.6 mg epinephrine 1:10,000 IV bolus.

   d. Normotensive adult patient → 2.5 mg SQ epinephrine 1:10,000.

   e. Normotensive 10-kg child → 1 mg SQ epinephrine 1:1000.

   The answer is b. Anaphylactic shock requires prompt administration of epinephrine. The intravenous or endotracheal route should be used in severe hypotension or cardiovascular collapse. Intramuscular or subcutaneous administration may be used for less severe reactions. Generally, epinephrine at a 1:10,000 dilution is used when given via the endotracheal or intravenous route. A 1:1000 solution is used for subcutaneous or intramuscular injection. The initial dose, whether given subcutaneously, intramuscularly, or via the trachea, is 0.01 mg/kg to a maximum of 0.3 mg in children, and 0.5–1.0 mg in adults (which may be repeated q 5–20 min). The intravenous infusion dose is 0.1 mg/kg/min. The usual initial intravenous bolus dose is 0.1 mg (1 mL of a 1:10,000 solution), but 0.5–1.0 mg IV may be needed in severe hypotension.

2. **Which of the following statements about anaphylaxis is true?**

   a. Anaphylactic reactions are less common in atopic individuals.

   b. Anaphylactic-type reactions from IV radiocontrast agents always occur less than 10 minutes postinfusion.

   c. Diphenhydramine blocks histamine release and reverses the physiologic effects of anaphylaxis.

   d. In a patient taking propranolol and exhibiting anaphylactic shock unresponsive to IV epinephrine, give 1 mg IV glucagon.

   e. Anaphylactic reactions do not recur after successful treatment with epinephrine and diphenhydramine.

   The answer is d. Anaphylactic reactions are IgE mediated. Reactions to certain drugs, foods, and intravenous radiocontrast resemble anaphylactic reactions but occur via a different mechanism. Reactions to intravenous contrast may be delayed for 10–20 minutes. Beta-blockers and calcium channel blockers contribute to myocardial depression and hypotension. Intravenous glucagon should be used in patients on beta-blockers unresponsive to epinephrine; MAST garments may be considered for unresponsive hypotension. Relapses from initial therapy may occur in people who have deposits of the allergen (e.g., intramuscular penicillin or bee stings). Patients should be observed for several hours after treatment of acute anaphylactic reactions. Diphenhydramine does not block histamine release or reverse the physiologic changes that have occurred in anaphylaxis, but it prevents further histamine binding.

3. **A 22-year-old man with asthma becomes acutely ill within 1 hour after ingesting tuna. He complains of facial flushing, weakness, diarrhea, and an itchy rash. The most likely cause of his symptoms is:**

    a. Scombroidosis.

    b. Sulfites in the salad.

    c. Ciguatera fish poisoning.

    d. Monosodium glutamate.

    e. Iodine allergy.

    The answer is b. Sulfites are used as preservatives in food, wines, and some medications. Ten percent of asthmatics may be sensitive to sulfites and exposure may cause life-threatening bronchospasm and hypotension. Monosodium glutamate (MSG) has been associated with reactions ranging from flushing and wheezing to nausea and vomiting. MSG reactions are not felt to be immune mediated. Scombroid poisoning is caused by ingesting a histamine-like compound found in certain spoiled fish (tuna, mackerel). Facial flushing, diarrhea, and urticaria are common manifestations. Ciguatera fish poisoning produces nausea, vomiting, diarrhea, and neurologic symptoms (myalgias, painful sensory paresthesias).
    The toxin is found in fish (grouper, snapper) that have fed on a particular marine dinoflagellate.

4. **A 63-year-old man presents with a history of several weeks of intermittent fevers, muscle weakness, arthralgias, and headaches. He also notes recent pain and tenderness on the side of his scalp when he puts on his glasses. On examination, his temperature is 38.3°C (101°F). He has mild proximal muscle weakness. There is marked tenderness to palpation over the right temporal area. A CPK is normal, CBC shows a mild normochromic normocytic anemia, and WBC is 10,000. The ESR is 110 mm/h. You know that:**

    a. Temporal artery biopsy may confirm the diagnosis.

    b. Treatment of choice is a third- or fourth-generation fluoroquinolone.

    c. This is a migraine headache.

    d. The underlying pathophysiology is a virus.

    e. Prognosis is poor despite treatment.

    The answer is a. Giant cell arteritis, of which temporal arteritis is the most common presentation, is a systemic vasculitis involving medium and large arteries. It often presents with fever, a markedly elevated ESR, anemia, myalgias, cephalgia, and temporal artery tenderness. The serum CPK levels are usually normal. Blindness may occur from involvement of the ophthalmic artery. The disease responds rapidly to systemic steroids and the prognosis is good if treated early. A positive biopsy of the temporal artery confirms the clinical diagnosis.

5. **Angioedema:**

    a. Appears as indurated patches of the periorbital and perioral tissue, hands, feet, and scrotum.

    b. Causes intensely pruritic lesions.

    c. When hereditary is caused by overproduction of C1 esterase, and may result in life-threatening laryngeal edema or intestinal colic.

    d. When hereditary almost always improves with epinephrine and steroids.

    e. Involves the superficial dermis, as opposed to urticaria.

    The answer is a. Alterations of vascular permeability cause urticaria and angioedema. Acute urticaria is IgE mediated and more common in adolescents. Chronic urticaria (>6 weeks duration) is nonallergic and more common in adults. Lung or colon cancer, pregnancy, hypothyroidism, viral infections (hepatitis), and drugs (oral contraceptives, ASA) have been associated with urticaria. Angioedema involves the deep dermis and subcutaneous tissues. Urticaria lesions are pruritic. Treatment for hereditary angioedema may include steroids and androgens to increase C1 esterase production. The treatment of acute urticaria may include removal of the offending agent and administering H1 and H2 antagonists, epinephrine, and corticosteroids.

6. **Of conditions listed, the one most frequently implicated in lower extremity pain is:**
   a. Reactive arthritis.
   b. Calcific tendonitis.
   c. Adhesive capsulitis.
   d. Rotator cuff injury.
   e. Pancoast tumor.

   The answer is a. Reactive arthritis (formerly Reiter's syndrome) generally involves the joints of the lower extremities. Calcific tendonitis or rupture of the rotator cuff are common causes of shoulder pain. Loss of abduction is not a specific finding for these and occurs in other disorders. Shoulder arthrography or MRI is necessary to diagnose rotator cuff tears. NSAIDs are the treatment of choice for tendonitis, but select cases may benefit from local steroid injection. Aseptic necrosis is more commonly seen in the hip, but can occur in the humeral head. Causes of aseptic necrosis include systemic corticosteroid therapy, repeated intra-articular steroid injections, sickle cell disease, alcoholism, and dysbaric injury. Adhesive capsulitis may occur following trauma and is characterized by pain and severe limitation of movement. The apex of the lung should always be inspected on shoulder films as a Pancoast tumor may produce shoulder pain.

7. **A common EKG finding in a patient with rheumatoid arthritis is:**
   a. Atrial bigeminy.
   b. Left anterior hemiblock.
   c. Prolonged PR interval.
   d. Right atrial hypertrophy.
   e. Shortened QT interval.

   The answer is c. ECG is indicated for patients with arthritis who have a history of chest pain or complaints that might be related to the heart, or physical examination findings of a new or changing heart murmur, evidence of congestive heart failure, or cardiomegaly. In carditis, prolongation of the P-R interval is the most common finding, and if pericarditis is present, acute diffuse ST segment elevations may be noted.

8. **The triad of fever, joint pain, and rash in a woman of childbearing age should suggest the diagnosis of systemic lupus. You also know that:**
   a. The most common cardiac manifestation is left bundle-branch block is, reported in 30% of patients.
   b. Exudative pleural effusions are relatively common.
   c. Persistent hematuria is seen in approximately 50% of patients.
   d. Neurologic presentations, such as seizures, stroke, psychosis, migraines, and peripheral neuropathies, are frequently the first signs of disease.
   e. Unlike rheumatoid arthritis, the inflammation of the hands is asymmetric.

   The answer is b. Pleural effusions, seen in 12% of SLE patients, are usually exudative in nature. Like rheumatoid arthritis, the inflammation of the hands, specifically the proximal interphalangeal and the metacarpophalangeal joints, is symmetric. Clinical nephritis, defined as persistent proteinuria, is seen in approximately 50% of patients. Nervous system manifestations are varied and include seizures, stroke, psychosis, migraines, and peripheral neuropathies, but are rarely the initial sign. Pericarditis is the most common cardiac manifestation of SLE, reported in 30% of patients.

9. **The most common finding in patients with Behçet syndrome is recurrent, painful genital aphthous ulcers. However the *hallmark* finding for this disease is:**

    a. Green sclera.
    b. Hypopyon uveitis.
    c. Bullous conjunctivitis.
    d. Optic neuritis and a "blueberry" spot on the retina.
    e. Recurrent, painful corneal ulcers.

    The answer is b. Recurrent, painful aphthous ulcers that involve the oral mucosa and genitals are clinically predominant, but the hallmark of Behçet's, a hypopyon uveitis, is seen rarely. Other eye involvement includes iritis, uveitis, and optic neuritis, all of which can lead to blindness. CNS vasculitis, resulting in meningoencephalitis, intracranial hypertension, or a multiple sclerosis-like syndrome, can also occur.

10. **You are evaluating a 35-year-old woman who complains of precordial chest pain. She has a long history of systemic lupus. You know that:**

    a. Libman-Sachs vegetations are infectious excrescences on the aortic valve, representing bacterial endocarditis.
    b. Lupus pericarditis requires high-dose steroid therapy.
    c. Pericardial effusions are found in more than half of lupus patients.
    d. Pericarditis is the most common cardiac manifestation of SLE.
    e. SLE patients have no increased risk of coronary artery disease.

    The answer is d. Pericarditis is the most common cardiac manifestation of SLE, reported in 30% of patients. Signs and symptoms include fever, tachycardia, chest pain, and transient rubs. Pericardial effusions, however, are found in only 20% of patients. Purulent pericarditis associated with *Staphylococcus aureus* and tuberculosis has occurred in patients taking steroids. Pericarditis in SLE is usually self-limited. Libman-Sachs vegetations on the mitral valve are noninfectious and related to autoimmune deposition. SLE patients are at a markedly increased risk of coronary artery disease, especially when they also have hypertension and hypercholesterolemia. Myocarditis is clinically apparent in only 10% of patients; however, it is present in 40% at autopsy.

11. **Acute HIV syndrome is characterized by nonspecific symptoms such as fatigue, weight loss, diarrhea, pharyngitis, and adenopathy, seen:**

    a. Within 24 hours of exposure.
    b. 1 week after exposure.
    c. 2–6 weeks after exposure.
    d. 12–24 weeks after exposure.
    e. 4–6 months after exposure.

    The answer is c. Acute HIV syndrome usually occurs 2–6 weeks after initial exposure and is characterized by multiple nonspecific symptoms such as fever, fatigue, adenopathy, diarrhea, pharyngitis, weight loss, and rash. These symptoms may last up to 3 weeks and usually resolve without the patient seeking medical advice.

12. **A 24-year-old man with AIDS complains of headache, fever, stiff neck, and confusion. You suspect cryptococcal meningitis, knowing that the most accurate diagnostic study will be:**

   a. CSF cryptococcus antigen.

   b. CSF fungal culture.

   c. CSF India ink stain.

   d. Serum cryptococcus antigen.

   e. Serum cryptococcus antibody.

   The answer is a. Of the diagnostic tests for cryptococcus, identifying cryptococcal antigen in the CSF is 100% sensitive and specific. India ink has a 60–80% sensitivity; fungal culture and serum cryptococcal antigen have a 95% sensitivity for identifying cryptococcus.

13. **In an AIDS patient with diarrhea, the pathogen most likely to lead to a bacteremia is:**

   a. *Campylobacter jejuni.*

   b. Enteroadherent *E. coli.*

   c. *Isospora* spp.

   d. *Salmonella* spp.

   e. *Shigella* spp.

   The answer is d. *Salmonella* is a particular problem in patients with HIV, often producing recurrent bacteremia and other significant clinical disease. Campylobacter infection usually causes a proctocolitis. *Isospora* and *Cryptosporidium* are protozoal infections that produce a chronic watery diarrhea. Cytomegalovirus is a viral opportunistic infection that is associated with diarrhea and other gastrointestinal disease (such as hepatobiliary) in patients with HIV.

14. **An otherwise healthy 45-year-old woman says she has suffered from hives daily for almost 3 months. She can recall nothing new in her environment that she can implicate as a cause. You know the most likely cause is:**

   a. Adult-onset food allergy.

   b. Idiopathic, with a possible underlying autoimmune process.

   c. Food preservative allergy.

   d. Hereditary angioedema (hereditary C1 esterase inhibitor deficiency).

   e. Food additive allergy.

   The answer is b. Eighty to ninety percent of cases of chronic urticaria can be classified as chronic idiopathic urticaria (CIU), with no identifiable cause. As many as 40–60% of cases of CIU are actually autoimmune in nature. These patients can have a factor in the serum that is capable of causing a wheal-and-flare response, and they may have specific autoantibodies to the high-affinity immunoglobulin E (IgE) receptor or IgE itself. Food allergy is rarely a cause of chronic urticaria and is usually suspected or known by the patient. Allergy to food additives or preservatives can be an occult cause of chronic urticaria, but this is quite rare, occurring in no more than 3–4% of patients. Hereditary angioedema is extremely rare and is characterized by angioedema without urticaria.

15.   The best treatment for the patient in the previous question is probably:

a. Long-term prednisone therapy.

b. Cyclosporine.

c. A second-generation H1 blocker such as cetirizine, desloratadine, fexofenadine, or loratadine.

d. An H2 blocker such as cimetidine, ranitidine, or famotidine.

e. Aspirin.

The answer is c. The first-line treatment for chronic urticaria is an H1 antihistamine. The second-generation H1 blockers have a much better safety profile than do the first-generation H1 blockers. Cetirizine causes sedation in 10% of patients. Desloratadine, fexofenadine, and loratadine cause sedation at a rate similar to placebo (approximately <5%). Long-term therapy with corticosteroids, such as prednisone, should be avoided unless absolutely necessary because of adverse systemic effects. Cyclosporine is a potentially toxic drug that should be reserved for use when all conventional therapies have failed, and it should be used only by a specialist skilled in its use. H2 blockers, such as ranitidine, can be helpful as adjuncts to H1 antihistamines but are not effective when used alone. Aspirin is not known to be of benefit in urticaria, and it can exacerbate the condition in some patients. The H1 blockers clearly have the best cost–benefit ratio in this patient group.

16.   When evaluating a patient with a bee sting, which of the following could represent an anaphylactic reaction?

a. Metallic taste.

b. Dizziness.

c. Uterine contractions.

d. Bronchospasm.

e. All of the above.

The answer is e. All of the listed symptoms can be a result of an anaphylactic reaction to a bee sting. Reactions to bee stings can be limited to local reactions from the venom—redness, swelling, tenderness, and pain. These reactions are usually self-limited, resolving in a few hours. Anaphylactic reactions usually are the result of secondary infections and are IgE mediated. Epinephrine should be used if the reaction is beyond skin manifestations.

17.   Choose the correct statement about urticaria of pregnancy (pruritus gravidarum):

a. The rash is limited to the palms of the hands and soles of the feet.

b. It is almost exclusively a third-trimester condition.

c. In most cases, there is no visible rash.

d. Antihistamines are not useful.

e. Mucous membrane involvement mandates high-dose steroid therapy.

The answer is c. Pruritus gravidarum is a poorly defined condition associated with itching but without an obvious dermatosis. It classically occurs in the first trimester.

18.   You are seeing an AIDS patient with vision change and determine that she probably has a cytomegalovirus infection. You should treat her with:

a. Intravenous amphotericin B.

b. Intraocular amantadine.

c. A fourth-generation fluoroquinolone.

d. Intravenous ganciclovir.

e. Famciclovir eyedrops.

The answer is d. Ganciclovir is an antiviral medication used to treat or prevent cytomegalovirus (CMV) infections and is marketed under the trade names Cytovene and Cymevene. Ganciclovir for ocular use is marketed under the trade name Vitrasert. Ganciclovir is indicated for sight-threatening CMV retinitis in severely immunocompromised people. It is considered a potential human carcinogen, teratogen, and mutagen, and its use is limited to sight-threatening infections.

19. **Concerning the treatment of gout:**

    a. Allopurinol increases uric acid elimination and is useful during an acute attack.
    b. Colchicine should not be used prophylactically.
    c. If NSAIDs are contraindicated, intramuscular injections of ACTH are useful.
    d. Probenecid lowers uric acid by diminishing production.
    e. Response to colchicine is diagnostic for the disease.

    The answer is c. Colchicine is effective for gout, pseudogout, and other crystal arthritides, so it cannot be used to make the specific diagnosis of gout. Long-term therapy of gout is designed to decrease serum uric acid levels either by decreasing production (allopurinol) or increasing excretion (probenecid). ACTH is also recommended for those patients with contraindications to NSAIDs. The dose of ACTH is 40–80 IU given IM. Uric acid lowering agents should not be started during an acute attack. Colchicine may be given prophylactically for 6–12 months to suppress flare-ups.

20. **Pseudogout differs from gout in that:**

    a. Indomethacin is contraindicated.
    b. The attack is more severe.
    c. The crystals cannot be identified using microscopy.
    d. The knee is the most commonly involved joint.
    e. The typical patient is younger.

    The answer is d. In a patient with pseudogout, the knee is the joint most commonly involved, followed by the wrist, ankle, and elbow. The average attack is not as severe as acute gout. In general, these patients are between the sixth and eighth decades that have a previous history of arthritic attacks. Joint fluid examination shows the weakly positive birefringent crystals of calcium pyrophosphate dihydrate. The crystals appear rhomboidal on regular light microscopy. Treatment for an acute attack is similar to the therapy for acute gout: NSAIDs or oral colchicine, although the latter is not as effective as with gout.

21. **The treatment of Kawasaki Syndrome is intended to prevent:**

    a. Coronary artery aneurysms.
    b. Fistula formation from the draining lymph nodes.
    c. Fulminant liver failure.
    d. Meningoencephalitis.
    e. Paraplegia or quadriplegia.

    The answer is a. The treatment of Kawasaki syndrome is directed toward the amelioration of symptoms and the prevention of coronary aneurysms. Gamma-globulin 2 g/kg intravenously should be administered over 12 hours, followed by high-dose aspirin therapy (100 mg/kg/24 h PO given in divided doses every 6 hours for 14 days). Low-dose aspirin therapy (3–5 mg/kg/24 h PO) should continue until acute phase reactants return to normal over 3–5 months. A pediatric cardiologist should follow children to monitor cardiac status.

CHAPTER 10

Systemic Infectious Emergencies

Mark Saks, MD, MPH

1. **Which of the following is true regarding malaria?**

    a. Cerebral malaria is a common, life-threatening complication of *Plasmodium ovale* infection.

    b. There is little reported resistance to chloroquine phosphate and it remains the drug of choice in the initial treatment of malaria worldwide.

    c. Although blood cultures may be normal, a peripheral smear is diagnostic.

    d. A characteristic finding is leukocytosis and thrombocytosis.

    e. All patients with malaria require hospitalization.

    The answer is c. There are four species of *Plasmodium* that cause malaria in humans: *P. vivax, P. malariae, P. falciparum*, and *P. ovale*. All are transmitted by the bite of an infected female anopheles mosquito. *P. falciparum* is most likely to cause severe disease in humans including cerebral malaria, profound anemia, waxing/waning fevers, and, possibly, death. Clinical manifestations include paroxysms representing the erythrocytic stage of rigors: severe febrile episode, defervescence, and diaphoresis. The white blood cell count may be normal or slightly decreased. Blood cultures are not helpful. The diagnosis is established by visualization of the parasite on a thin or thick peripheral smear. However, smears may be negative secondary to RBC sequestration and treatment should be initiated if malaria is clinically suspected. Malaria may be managed as an outpatient with oral chloroquine if infection is not due to *P. falciparum*. Patients with *P. falciparum* infection or greater than 3% parasitemia should be hospitalized and treated with oral quinine and doxycycline or intravenous quinidine (intravenous quinine is not available in the United States).

2. **You are evaluating a 74-year-old man whose wife says he has increasing lethargy and somnolence over the past 12 hours. Prior to this, he had complained of chills, headache, neck pain and stiffness, and the light bothering his eyes. His rectal temperature is 102.6°F and you find nuchal rigidity when you examine him. Which statement is correct concerning this patient?**

   a. If he has a severe penicillin allergy, you should give him chloramphenicol to cover for *Listeria monocytogenes*.

   b. Because of his age, empiric treatment of *Neisseria meningitidis* is not indicated.

   c. You should delay antibiotics until you can perform lumbar puncture and obtain cerebrospinal fluid for culture and other important studies.

   d. You should avoid therapy with corticosteroids due to associated hyperglycemia and immune system dysfunction.

   e. You should prescribe an antibiotic to cover *Streptococcus pneumoniae*, which is the most common pathogen in adult patients.

   The answer is e. The most common cause of meningitis in neonates is group B *Streptococcus* (GBS) along with *E. coli* and *L. monocytogenes*. Therefore, antibiotic therapy with ampicillin and gentamicin should be initiated in this age group. During preschool years (>3 months but <7 years) *H. influenzae, S. pneumoniae*, and *N. meningitidis* predominate, and treatment with cefotaxime or ceftriaxone should be initiated in this age group. In patients older than 7 years, treatment includes cefotaxime or ceftriaxone plus ampicillin if *L. monocytogenes* is suspected (typically in patients older than 55 years). Because of the increasing prevalence of drug resistant *S. pneumoniae*, the addition of vancomycin to the above is recommended. *S. pneumoniae* is the most common bacterial organism in patients older than 12 years. Alternative treatment with chloramphenicol and vancomycin is indicated if there is a history of severe penicillin allergy. The antimicrobial therapy should be modified once the antimicrobial susceptibilities are available.

3. **Which of the following statements regarding spinal epidural abscess is correct?**

   a. CSF analysis (Gram stain and culture) is sensitive but not specific.

   b. In the majority of cases the source of infection is not identified.

   c. A nerve-root pain syndrome implicates disk disease and therefore effectively excludes the diagnosis.

   d. The classic triad of back pain, fever, and a neurologic deficit is present in a small minority of patients.

   e. They are more commonly found in the cervical spine than in the thoracolumbar spine.

   The answer is d. Spinal epidural abscess is classically described as the triad of back pain, fever, and a neurologic deficit. However, these are present in a minority of patients and a high index of suspicion must be maintained to make the diagnosis. Although still rare, the incidence of spinal epidural abscess has been increasing in recent years due to increased rates of IV drug abuse, spinal surgery, immunosuppression (diabetes, HIV, etc.) and the overall aging of the population. Although in some cases the original source of infection is not identified, most cases of spinal epidural abscess have been attributed to either direct extension from nearby tissues or hematogenous spread from distant sites. The diagnosis of spinal epidural abscess remains problematic. Laboratory tests may reveal nonspecific indicators of infection or inflammation. Lumbar puncture is not routinely recommended as CSF analysis is usually negative and culture results are rarely positive. Additionally, there is the risk of placing the spinal needle into and through the abscess area. Plain films and radionuclide scanning lack sensitivity. Thus diagnosis is typically made with either a CT scan or MRI with and without contrast. MRI has the advantage of being able to provide both transverse and longitudinal images and is therefore the recommended study, if available.

4. **You are evaluating a 30-year-old previously healthy man for fever and confusion. His roommate tells you that he has complained of headache, nausea, vomiting, and photophobia. You suspect bacterial meningitis. Choose the correct statement regarding his diagnosis:**

    a. Kernig and Brudzinski signs are present in 95% of patients with bacterial meningitis.

    b. The culture of his cerebrospinal fluid (CSF) that is obtained promptly and prior to the administration of antimicrobials may yield the causative agent, as it does in at least 50% of cases.

    c. A CSF with numerous Gram-positive diplococci but a neutrophil count of only 18 cells/mL is a good prognostic sign.

    d. His appearance and level of mental function upon presentation indicate that this is most likely viral meningitis.

    e. If the Gram stain of his CSF reveals Gram-negative diplococci, suspect an underlying basilar skull fracture.

    The answer is b. In a young, previously healthy adult, a diminished level of consciousness, the presence of seizures, and a low CSF cell count in the presence of a high bacterial load all are poor prognostic signs. It is critical to remember that empiric antibiotic treatment should be initiated as soon as possible during any workup for meningitis. The diagnostic results will not be affected by such treatment but morbidity and mortality will clearly be improved. Basilar skull fractures are associated with meningitis caused by *Streptococcus pneumoniae* and less commonly by *Haemophilus influenzae*.

5. **A 9-year-old boy has had fever, muscle aches, nausea, vomiting, and diffuse abdominal pain for the past 5 days. Two days ago, his mother noted a rash consisting of multiple 2 to 3 mm blanching, erythematous macules around his wrists and ankles that spread to his chest, back, arms, and thighs today. Choose the true statement regarding this patient:**

    a. This rash rarely involves the palms or soles.

    b. The classic triad of fever, rash, and tick bite occurs in more than 75% of cases.

    c. A history of tick bite can be elicited in 95% of cases.

    d. Patients younger than 20 years account for 20% of cases.

    e. The causative organism is an obligate intracellular bacterium.

    The answer is e. This patient has Rocky Mountain spotted fever, an acute febrile tick-borne illness caused by *Rickettsia Rickettsii*. RMSF is most common in the states of the mid-eastern seaboard but has been reported in nearly every state. The female dog tick, *Dermacentor variabilis*, is the vector in the east; the vector in the west is the wood tick, *D. andersoni*. The disease is seasonal, with most cases occurring from April to September. Sixty percent of cases occur in patients younger than 20 years. The onset is usually abrupt, with high fevers, shaking chills, myalgias, abdominal pain, and a severe headache. Variations from this pattern should not dissuade one from the diagnosis and the classic triad of fever, rash, and a tick bite is apparent in less than 5% of patients. Classically, a macular rash begins on the wrists, palms, ankles, and soles 2–6 days after the onset of fever and spreads centripetally. The rash evolves to dark, nonblanching, and petechial or ecchymotic lesions. Empiric treatment with doxycycline should be initiated prior to serologic tests or skin biopsy results. The mortality rate is 8– 20% for untreated patients.

6. **Which of the following statements regarding tularemia is true?**

    a. Deer flies, mosquitoes, ticks, and direct contact with infected animal tissue can transmit the disease.

    b. The most common manifestation is an atypical pneumonia and leukopenia.

    c. Person-to-person contact is common, and family members should be offered prophylaxis.

    d. Oral tetracycline for a minimum of 2 weeks is the treatment of choice.

    e. Many patients experience a Jarisch-Herxheimer reaction after appropriate treatment.

    The answer is a. Tularemia, a systemic disease caused by *Francisella tularensis,* is most often contracted during the summer as a result of tick bites. However, it has also been linked to the handling of infected rabbit carcasses and to contact with infected domesticated cats and dogs. The disease is not transmitted via person-to-person contact. There are six clinical presentations, depending on whether the symptoms are localized to the entry site, regionally invasive, or systemic. The most common is ulceroglandular fever in which an indurated ulceration at the site of inoculation develops with local lymphadenopathy. Glandular tularemia, the second most common type, is characterized by marked lymphadenopathy without the accompanying skin lesion. Oculoglandular tularemia is rare, but can result in conjunctivitis and corneal perforation. The most severe form is pneumonic tularemia, which has a case-fatality rate of up to 30%. Treatment for tularemia is with streptomycin IM bid for 7–14 days. Gentamicin may be used as an alternative. Infection generally results in life-long immunity. A vaccine is available that can be offered to high-risk patients to decrease the severity of infection, but it is not totally effective in preventing the illness.

7. **A 25-year-old medical student just returned from walking the Appalachian Trail. While in New Hampshire 18 days ago, he removed some deer ticks (*Ixodes dammini*) and took doxycycline100 mg twice daily for 2 weeks to prevent Lyme disease. Now he complains of malaise, high fevers, headache, and dark urine. You examine him and see no rash, but find hepatosplenomegaly. His laboratory results show pancytopenia with signs of hemolysis, elevated liver enzyme levels, and decreased haptoglobin. An intraerythrocytic parasite ("Maltese cross" formation) is noted on his peripheral blood smear. You should now:**

    a. Continue the doxycycline for another 21-day course as an outpatient.

    b. Switch the doxycycline to amoxicillin 500 mg orally 3 times daily for 21 days as an outpatient.

    c. Switch the doxycycline to penicillin G 20 million U/d intramuscularly for 28 days as an outpatient.

    d. Switch the doxycycline to chloramphenicol 1g intravenously every 6 hours for 21 days as an inpatient.

    e. Switch the doxycycline to clindamycin and quinine.

    The answer is e. This patient has babesiosis, an increasingly prevalent malaria-like illness that, in the United States, is caused by *Babesia microti* and *B. Gibson.* These protozoal organisms are similar in structure and have a similar life cycle to that of plasmodia. The major zoonotic reservoirs are domesticated mammals, rodents, and deer. *Ixodes* ticks, also the vector of Lyme disease, function as the principal vector. However, blood transfusions have also been implicated in the transmission of babesiosis. Patients with babesiosis develop fatigue, anorexia, malaise, myalgia, chills, high spiking fevers, sweats, headache, emotional liability, and dark urine. On examination, hepatosplenomegaly is common. Laboratory results will show anemia, thrombocytopenia, leukopenia, elevated liver enzymes, and signs of hemolysis with hyperbilirubinemia and decreased haptoglobin. Diagnosis is made by finding intraerythrocytic ring forms on a Giemsa-stained peripheral blood smear, though false-negative results can occur when the level of parasitism is low. The treatment of choice is with quinine and clindamycin. The other therapies listed are used in the treatment of Lyme disease. Approximately 20% of the patients with babesiosis have a concurrent infection with Lyme disease.

8. **Which of the following is correct regarding tetanus?**

    a. Tetanospasmin is an endotoxin that affects motor and sensory function.

    b. The disease is difficult to clinically differentiate from rabies because of the marked muscle spasm present in both.

    c. Tetanus immune globulin (TIG) neutralizes circulating tetanospasmin and should not be administered until the patient becomes symptomatic.

    d. Metronidazole is the antibiotic of choice to prevent additional toxin production.

    e. The case mortality for tetanus in the United States is 10%.

    The answer is d. *Clostridium tetani* is a Gram-positive, spore-forming anaerobic bacillus. It is ubiquitous in soil and dust and can survive for months to years. When introduced into an open wound, under anaerobic conditions, it matures and can produce the exotoxin tetanospasmin. This toxin invades unhealthy tissue and enters peripheral nerve endings and ascends to the spinal cord and brain (anterior horn cells) causing spastic paralysis. The toxin has no effect on sensorium. Trismus is the presenting symptom in 50% of cases. While it may take several weeks for the symptoms to germinate, in general a shorter incubation period means more severe disease. There is no known cure. Treatment consists of supportive care, airway management, benzodiazepines to control muscle spasms, surgical debridement of the affected tissue, tetanus immune globulin (TIG), tetanus toxoid, and metronidazole. Clinical disease does not provide immunity.

9. **A 27-year-old woman was bitten on the calf by a raccoon while she was camping 3 days ago. Which of the following would be a relative contraindication to giving her antirabies prophylaxis?**

    a. She is in the second trimester of pregnancy.

    b. She has a prior history of severe asthma.

    c. She has anaphylaxis when exposed to eggs.

    d. She is HIV positive.

    e. The raccoon that bit her was subsequently shot and autopsy results are pending.

    The answer is e. Worldwide, dogs are the most commonly infected animal and the principal reservoir of disease. In the United States, due to high levels of veterinary care, the principal reservoirs are wild raccoons, skunks, foxes, and bats. In the United States, most human cases of rabies are associated with bats. Following a bite, domesticated animals that are apparently healthy should be observed for 10 days; if the animal does not show signs of rabies, then no treatment is required. However, wild animals that are caught should undergo autopsy and antibody testing immediately. Victims should undergo prophylaxis, which can later be discontinued, unless results are immediately available. Postexposure rabies prophylaxis should consist of localized wound care, passive immunization with human rabies immunoglobulin (HRIG), and active immunization with human diploid cell vaccine (HDCV). HRIG 20 U/kg should be administered into the immediate wound, as much as possible, with the remainder given IM. HDCV should be given IM at a distal site (deltoid) on days 0, 3, 7, 14, and 28 (Gluteal injections are discouraged, as the drug may be inadvertently deposited in subcutaneous tissues). Patients with previous prophylaxis do not need HRIG and should get HDCV on days 0 and 3 only. Prophylaxis may be given during pregnancy and does not result in an increase in fetal wastage, congenital defects, or side effects and should not be withheld when indicated. Corticosteroids, antimalarials, and other immunosuppressives can interfere with the development of active immunity and should be withheld during the course of treatment, if possible. In immunosuppressed patients, it may be necessary to have antibody titers checked at 2 and 4 weeks to ensure a response. Egg allergy is a concern in influenza prophylaxis, where the vaccine is nurtured in eggs, but there is no concern when giving rabies postexposure prophylaxis.

10. **Regarding administration of the whole cell pertussis, diphtheria, and tetanus (DPT) vaccine, which of the following statements is true?**

  a. The acellular pertussis vaccine (DTaP) is less effective than the whole cell vaccine and adverse reactions are more common.

  b. Aseptic meningitis is a frequently reported complication.

  c. Local induration is common.

  d. Immunity to tetanus wanes, but immunity to pertussis and diphtheria is life-long.

  e. Previous local reactions preclude future use of tetanus toxoid vaccine.

  The answer is c. Local arthrus reactions may occur among patients with tetanus booster immunization. However, local symptoms do not justify withholding boosters. Urticaria, anaphylaxis, neuropathies, and aseptic meningitis are rare systemic reactions that are not necessarily dose-related. Contraindications to DPT include previous severe neurologic or hypersensitivity reactions. It has been shown that immunity wanes to all three components of the vaccine, therefore additional booster doses after childhood are advised. Safe in adults and adolescents, TdaP has largely replaced DPT, DT, and Td for these immunizations and boosters. Additionally, whole-cell pertussis vaccine is no longer recommended unless the acellular vaccine is not available. Patients older than 7 years should receive Td rather than DT because of severe reactions associated with the larger doses of diphtheria toxoid in the DT formulation (lower case "d," lower doses).

11. **A 6-year-old girl who recently emigrated from Sri Lanka with her parents complains of severe sore throat, headache, difficulty swallowing, and generalized weakness and malaise. Her previous medical history is not known. Her oral temperature is 103.2°F. You note prominent cervical lymph nodes and an adherent gray pseudomembrane in her posterior oropharynx. Treatment must include antitoxin therapy plus:**

  a. Active immunization.

  b. Passive immunization.

  c. Active immunization and antibiotics.

  d. Passive immunization and high-dose acyclovir.

  e. Active immunization and steroids.

  The answer is c. This patient has a classic case of diphtheria, a respiratory infection caused by *Corynebacterium diptheriae*. Management should focus on airway protection, limiting additional *C. diptheriae* growth and toxin production, and minimizing the effects of toxin that has already been produced. Equine serum diphtheria antitoxin should be administered promptly after the clinical diagnosis of respiratory diphtheria. Antitoxin can be obtained by contacting the CDC. The size and location of the membrane, the duration of illness, and the patient's overall degree of toxicity determine the dosage of antitoxin. The Committee on Infectious Diseases of the American Academy of Pediatrics (AAP) recommends 20,000–40,000 units for pharyngeal or laryngeal involvement of 48 hours' duration, 40,000–60,000 units for nasopharyngeal lesions, and 80,000–100,000 units for extensive disease of 3 or more days' duration or for diffuse swelling of the neck. In addition to antitoxin therapy, antibiotics should be administered for 14 days. Erythromycin, 40–50 mg/kg/d (up to 2 g) IV or orally in divided doses; intramuscular (IM) aqueous crystalline penicillin, 100,000–150,000 U/kg/d in four divided doses; or procaine penicillin, 25,000–50,000 U/kg/d in two divided doses for 14 days given IM every 12 hours is acceptable. Patients should be admitted to respiratory isolation.

12. A 76-year-old woman was found in her home with a decreased level of responsiveness. The patient's daughter last saw her yesterday morning, and the patient can provide no further information. Vital signs: rectal temperature 96.6°F, heart rate 120/min, respiratory rate 26/min, blood pressure 84/44 mm Hg, oxygen saturation 94% on room air. Your examination is significant for signs of dehydration and a diminished mental status. Laboratory values reveal WBC of 18.2 with 10% band forms, hemoglobin 9.6 g, hematocrit 28.8%, platelets 120,000, sodium 128 mEq/L, potassium 3.4 mEq/L, BUN 64 mg/dL, and creatinine of 2.8 mg/dL. Urinalysis is consistent with a urinary tract infection. Which of the following statements regarding this patient's condition is true?

    a. The patient may benefit from cortisol administration.

    b. Fluid resuscitation should be limited due to her decreased oxygen saturation and concerns for precipitating pulmonary edema.

    c. A serum lactate is of limited value.

    d. The patient should be transfused with packed red blood cells (PRBC) until her hematocrit is greater than 50%.

    e. A CVP less than 8 mm Hg is a good prognostic sign.

    The answer is a. Sepsis is defined as the presence of an infection and evidence of a systemic inflammatory response (SIRS) manifested by abnormalities in vital signs (temperature, pulse rate, and respiratory rate) or laboratory values (leukocytosis or bandemia). A complex series of pathophysiologic events are responsible for the transition from infection to SIRS to sepsis to septic shock. Increasing evidence seems to show that early goal-directed therapy (EGDT) aimed at reversing tissue hypoxia and decreasing tissue hypoperfusion combined with timely, broad-spectrum antibiotic administration leads to improved morbidity and mortality. Septic patients should undergo central venous (preferably internal jugular or subclavian placement) and arterial catheterization and should have central venous pressure (CVP), mean arterial pressure (MAP), and central venous oxygen sat (SvO_2) continually monitored and reassessed. Fluids should be given to keep CVP greater than 8 mm Hg. Vasopressors should be titrated to keep the MAP greater than 65 mm Hg. Transfusions of PRBC should be given to keep the hematocrit greater than 30%. Although the routine use of corticosteroids in sepsis has not yet been established, the use of supplemental corticosteroids in sepsis is common and may help correct underlying adrenal insufficiency. However, a hormone stimulation test or baseline cortisol level should be performed first.

13. **A patient with toxic shock syndrome (TSS) will likely exhibit:**

    a. Hypotension or orthostatic blood pressure changes and a fever higher than 102°F.

    b. Normal BUN, creatinine, and hepatic function tests.

    c. Thrombocytosis.

    d. A bleeding diathesis.

    e. Blood cultures positive for Group A *Streptococcus* (GAS).

    The answer is a. TSS was originally attributed to super-absorbent tampon use but can be associated with isolation of group A *Streptococcus* (GAS) from any sterile or nonsterile body site. Patients with TSS typically exhibit hypotension or orthostasis, a temperature >102°F, a diffuse macular erythroderma that involves the palms and soles and desquamates 1–2 weeks after the onset of illness, and evidence of multiple organ system dysfunction including (*at least three*): vomiting/diarrhea, myalgia, hepatitis, disorientation, mucosal inflammation, thrombocytopenia, and twofold increase in BUN/Cr. Clinically significant bleeding diatheses are uncommon in TSS, although thrombocytopenia, elevated PT, PTT, and FSP may be present. The case definition for TSS does not require a positive culture for GAS. However, patients should have serologic tests to exclude other diseases such as RMSF, leptospirosis, measles, HBV, VDRL, and infectious mononucleosis.

14. **Choose the true statement concerning toxic shock syndrome (TSS):**

   a. Early antimicrobial therapy has been shown to decrease the recurrence rate of TSS.
   b. The number of cases associated with persons other than menstruating women is decreasing.
   c. The case mortality is between 10% and 20%.
   d. Twenty percent of menstrual-related cases of TSS are caused by *S. aureus* strains that produce endotoxin.
   e. Diarrhea and vomiting are uncommonly associated with TSS

The answer is a. Antibiotic therapy does not affect the outcome of the acute syndrome, but it does decrease the recurrence rate of TSS (which can be as high as 60%). The source of infection (e.g., nasal pack, tampon) should be sought and removed. The most important principle is aggressive treatment of shock. Shock that is resistant to volume resuscitation may require pressor agents. Mild cases of TSS may go unrecognized. In severe cases, the onset is acute with fever, chills, profuse watery diarrhea, and vomiting. The characteristic diffuse erythematous rash is followed by desquamation of the palms, fingers, and feet. TSS can be associated with tampon use, childbirth, nasal packing, postoperative wound infections, and infection of superficial wounds. Menstrual-related TSS case mortality is less than 10%.

15. **Which of the following statements regarding sexually transmitted diseases (STDs) is correct?**

   a. *Treponema palladium* causes a painful genital ulcer and nontender bilateral inguinal lymphadenopathy.
   b. Treatment for *Haemophilus ducreyi* can be with either erythromycin 500 mg orally twice daily for 7 days, or a 1-time dose of azithromycin 1 g orally, or ceftriaxone 250 mg IM.
   c. *Chlamydia trachoma* causes painless perineal or anorectal ulcerations.
   d. Treatment for *Klebsiella granulomatis* (formerly *Calymmatobacterium granulomatis*) should be with intramuscular benzathine penicillin G.
   e. *Condylomata acuminata* (HPV) is rarely asymptomatic and is associated with massive lower GI bleeding.

The answer is b. *Treponema pallidum* is the agent causing syphilis. Early syphilis typically presents with a painless indurated genital ulcer with tender inguinal adenopathy. Benzathine penicillin G 2.4 million units IM is the primary treatment; however, doxycycline 100 mg orally twice daily for 2 weeks can be used as an alternative regimen. Diagnosis is based on dark field microscopy or serologic tests (RPR, VDRL, and FTA-ABS). *Haemphilus ducreyi* is the agent causing chancroid: painful nonindurated irregular genital ulcers and unilateral or bilateral inguinal adenopathy. Diagnosis can be made by culture or clinical features. *Chlamydia trachoma* causes LGV. It presents as small painful shallow anal or perianal ulcers with inguinal lymphadenopathy that evolves into painful inguinal buboes. Diagnosis is based on serologic tests and culture. Genital warts are often asymptomatic or may cause anal pruritus or scant bright red blood per rectum. Donovanosis, also known as granuloma inguinale, is characterized by painless genital ulcers, which can be mistaken for syphilis. The causative organism, *Klebsiella granulomatis*, was formerly called *Calymmatobacterium granulomatis*: prior to that it was called *Donovania granulomatis*. This reclassification under the genus *Klebsiella* was a drastic taxonomic change, because it also involved changing the organism's phylum. However, polymerase chain reaction (PCR) techniques using a colorimetric detection system showed a 99% similarity with other species in the *Klebsiella* genus.

16. **A 43-year-old woman who was recently treated for vaginal discharge now returns after she received a letter telling her that she had a positive VDRL. She recalls having had a painless ulcer 5 or 10 years ago that resolved without treatment. She has no complaints or physical findings on your examination. What is the treatment of choice for this patient?**

    a. Benzathine penicillin G, 2.4 million units IM weekly for 3 weeks.

    b. Benzathine penicillin G, 2.4 million units IM daily for 14 days.

    c. Aqueous crystalline penicillin G, 50,000 U/kg IV every 6 hours for 3 weeks.

    d. Procaine penicillin, 2.4 million units IM daily for 10–14 days and probenecid 500 mg orally 4 times daily for 17–21 days.

    e. Benzathine penicillin G, 2.4 million units IM, one dose only.

    The answer is a. Because she has likely had syphilis for longer than 1 year, this patient has late latent syphilis. During latent syphilis, there are no clinical symptoms and laboratory testing is the only means of identification. The positive VDRL should be confirmed with subsequent fluorescent treponemal antibody absorption (FTA-ABS) tests. Treatment with benzathine penicillin G 2.4 million units IM weekly for 3 weeks should be initiated. The patient should be advised to undergo HIV testing and her sexual partners should be evaluated for syphilis. Choice **d** is an acceptable treatment for neurosyphilis.

17. **A 24-year-old sexually active man, who admits to only variable use of condoms, complains of painful vesicles and ulcers on his penile shaft that have been present for 3 days. This is his first episode. Which of the following statements regarding the diagnosis and treatment of primary genital site herpes simplex virus (HSV) is correct?**

    a. The lesions are typically indurated and sharply demarcated and rarely coalesce.

    b. The prognosis is the same even if the isolate is found to be HSV type 1 (HSV-1).

    c. If he has subsequent relapses, the natural course of the episode almost always will be identical to the primary episode.

    d. Confirmatory testing and serology often is not helpful in this scenario.

    e. Early treatment with acyclovir or valacyclovir is curative.

    The answer is d. The diagnosis of genital herpes is usually made clinically based on the finding of painful grouped vesicles on erythematous bases that may coalesce to form shallow ulcerations. Genital herpes is incurable. Outbreaks are generally self-limited, although early antiviral therapy can decrease the severity and length of the outbreak and continued therapy may prevent recurrences. When relapse does occur, it is usually much milder than the first episode of disease. Treatment, however, does not affect the infectivity of the patient with active lesions. First-episode genital HSV is not infrequently type 1, which does not seem to be associated with relapsing disease. The first episode of HSV-2 disease can be milder if previous HSV-1 has occurred.

18. **A 32-year-old woman complains of weakness, lightheadedness, dry mouth, difficulty speaking, and double vision. Yesterday she was at a family gathering where she sampled some of her aunt's canned peaches. You suspect botulism. Physical findings that would confirm your suspicion include:**

    a. Distal muscles weakness with generalized sensory dysesthesias.

    b. Hypertension and decreased deep tendon reflexes.

    c. Ptosis, extraocular palsies, and pinpoint pupils.

    d. A normal gag reflex.

    e. Normal alertness with a descending, symmetrical flaccid paralysis.

    The answer is e. The patient with botulism is usually alert and afebrile with a descending, symmetrical flaccid paralysis. The muscles that are affected first are the cranial nerves and bulbar muscles. Therefore ocular signs are prominent and include ptosis, extraocular palsies, and markedly dilated and fixed pupils. The gag reflex is depressed or absent and patients often complain of dryness of the mouth, tongue, and pharynx and may have a red, dry appearance of their mucous membranes. Postural hypotension may be present. Upper extremity muscles are more affected than those of the lower extremity with proximal muscles weaker than distal muscle groups. A decrease in vital capacity to less than 30% of predicted is a standard criterion mandating mechanical ventilation. Deep tendon reflexes may be normal, symmetrically decreased, or absent. Sensory examination is normal. Treatment is focused on providing ventilator support and aggressive supportive care. Trivalent antitoxin should be given as early as possible, although it neutralizes only circulating toxin and has no effect on bound toxin. Saline enemas and cathartics have been recommended to cleanse the GI tract of residual toxin. Magnesium-containing cathartics should be avoided because magnesium can exacerbate muscle weakness. Antibiotics are not currently recommended for food-borne botulism, as they may increase cell lyses and promote toxin release.

19. **The antibiotic category considered safe for use at any time during pregnancy and lactation is:**

    a. Aminoglycosides.

    b. Fluoroquinolones.

    c. Penicillins.

    d. Sulfonamides.

    e. Tetracyclines.

    The answer is c. Penicillins as a group have been used extensively since the 1940s and are generally believed to be the safest antibiotics available for use during pregnancy. Macrolides are also widely considered to be safe in pregnancy. Sulfonamides (category B or C) may be used safely early in pregnancy but are contraindicated in near-term pregnancies because they have been associated with neonatal hyperbilirubinemia and kernicterus. Aminoglycosides (category C or D) such as gentamicin have been shown to cause nephrotoxicity in the fetus. Fluoroquinolones (category C) should be avoided during pregnancy as they may have detrimental effects on fetal cartilage and joint development. Tetracyclines (category D) have been associated with fetal liver, genitourinary, teeth, and bone abnormalities and should not be used during pregnancy unless no other alternatives are available.

20. **Patients with absent or nonfunctioning spleens can develop a fulminant pneumococcemia termed "overwhelming postsplenectomy infection" (OPSI). It is characterized by:**

    a. Meningitis, DIC, and hemorrhagic pancreatitis.

    b. Pituitary infarct, hemorrhagic thyroiditis, and asterixis.

    c. Septic shock, coronary artery occlusion, and fulminant hepatitis.

    d. Septic shock, adrenal hemorrhage, and DIC.

    e. Shock, rotatory nystagmus, and hemorrhagic hepatitis.

The answer is d. The spleen is one of the most important immunologic organs and is the site of IgM synthesis, the first immune response of the body. Patients with a surgical splenectomy or functional asplenia (as occurs in sickle cell disease) are at risk of developing severe infection with pneumococcus, other encapsulated organisms (*H. influenzae, N. meningitidis,* etc.), and Gram-negative bacteria (*E. coli, P. aeruginosa,* etc.). Overwhelming postsplenectomy infection (OPSI) is characterized by initial flu-like symptoms that rapidly progress to septic shock, multiorgan failure, adrenal hemorrhage, and DIC. Although no obvious source of infection is found in many cases, OPSI is believed to be a fulminant form of pneumococcemia. Asplenic children younger than 2 years are at the greatest risk of pneumococcal sepsis. All asplenic patients should be immunized against pneumococcus, *H. influenza* type B, influenza, and possibly *N. meningitidis.*

21. **A 32-year-old woman with a history of HIV (CD4 count of 43) presents to the ED with complains of 2 weeks of gradually worsening photophobia and blurry vision. She also complains of weight loss and diarrhea. She is not taking any antiretroviral medications. Her oral temperature is 102.3°F. The most likely cause of her symptoms is:**

a. Varicella-zoster virus.

b. Central retinal vein occlusion.

c. Cytomegalovirus (human herpesvirus-5).

d. Acute narrow angle glaucoma.

e. Toxoplasmosis.

The answer is c. Cytomegalovirus (CMV) infection in immunocompetent patient is generally sub-clinical and characterized by mild fever, lymphadenopathy, and pharynigitis. However, in neonates and immunocompromised patients, CMV infection can cause generalized disease with severe end-organ dysfunction such as hepatosplenomegaly, pneumonitis, colitis, and esophagitis. CMV retinitis occurs in 10–30% of HIV-infected patients and is the most common cause of blindness in patients with AIDS. With recent advances in highly activated antiretroviral therapy (HAART), reduced incidences of CMV retinitis have been observed, but discontinuation of HAART may result in intraocular inflammation. CMV retinitis typically produces severe necrotic vasculitis and retinitis. When present, it may be asymptomatic or cause diminished visual acuity, photophobia, scotoma, redness, or pain. It is diagnosed by its characteristic appearance on indirect ophthalmoscopy of fluffy white retinal lesions, often perivascular.

22. **The evaluation of sputum in a patient with suspected pneumocystis pneumonia (PCP) is:**

a. Highly specific.

b. The "gold standard" criteria for diagnosis.

c. Variably sensitive, depending on techniques and institution where it is performed.

d. Mandatory in all patients with negative bronchoscopy/bronchoalveolar lavage.

e. Discouraged because of potential exposure of health care workers.

The answer is c. Pneumocystis pneumonia (PCP) is caused by *Pneumocystis jiroveci,* a yeast-like fungus, and is one of the most common opportunistic infections seen in AIDS. Patients often have fevers, shortness of breath, and a nonproductive cough, and may be hypoxic. Chest x-ray may show a diffuse interstitial or perihilar "butterfly" pattern; the serum lactate dehydrogenase may be elevated. Establishment of a definitive diagnosis with sputum culture is difficult and not necessary to justify treatment. The sensitivity and specificity of induced sputum samples vary widely depending on the techniques at a particular institution. Prophylaxis against PCP with trimethoprim-sulfamethoxazole (TMP-SMX) is recommended for all patients with CD4 counts less than 200. For active PCP, treatment should be initiated as early as possible with TMP-SMX either orally or intravenously for 21 days. Alternative treatment consists of pentamidine, dapsone, atovaquone, or clindamycin plus primaquine. In addition, steroid therapy should be initiated in patients with decreased oxygen saturation or with an elevated alveolar-arterial gradient.

23.   **The most common cause of mortality from cryptococcal infection is:**

   a. Pneumonia.

   b. Meningoencephalitis.

   c. Acute respiratory distress syndrome (ARDS).

   d. Aplastic anemia.

   e. Splenic rupture.

   The answer is b. *Cryptococcus neoformans* is a fungal CNS infection that occurs in up to 10% of patients with HIV. Infection commonly causes a diffuse meningoencephalitis that presents with nonspecific symptoms such as fever, headache, dizziness, nausea, and vomiting. Focal cerebral, brainstem, and basal ganglia deficits can also be seen. Patients with focal findings are at risk of increased intracerebral pressure and herniation. Concurrent pulmonary involvement occurs in 33% of the patients; therefore, when an immunosuppressed patient presents with cryptococcal pneumonia, a lumbar puncture should be performed to rule out concomitant meningeal involvement. Classically the India ink stain was used to identify cryptococcus, but a serum antigen test is available. Oral fluconazole is an acceptable treatment for cryptococcal pneumonia in patients without meningeal involvement. Cryptococcal meningitis should be treated with IV amphotericin B with or without 5-flucytosine.

24.   **A 43-year-old man complains of severe lower abdominal pain and fevers (103.4°F) since yesterday. He rode his motorcycle to the ground a few days ago and skidded on his abdomen, but did not seek medical care because he thought he had "just a lot of scrapes." He then noted "blisters" on his lower abdomen and groin yesterday but that they are markedly larger and draining today. The patient is febrile and mildly hypotensive. You note a well-demarcated, erythematous, tender area on his lower abdomen with necrotic patches and bullae. Laboratory results are remarkable for a leukocytosis; abdominal CT scan shows subcutaneous gas. Choose the correct statement for this patient:**

   a. You must initiate antistaphylococcal antibiotics, taking care to cover community-associated MRSA.

   b. Perform local, bedside wound debridement as soon as possible.

   c. Place the patient on oral broad-spectrum antibiotics and have him return tomorrow for a wound check.

   d. Call your surgeon; this patient should go the operating room for wide debridement and excision.

   e. Wound cultures are likely to reveal a Gram-negative infection.

   The answer is d. This patient has necrotizing fasciitis. There are two general types: type 1 is polymicrobial and typically is found on the abdomen and perineum; type 2 is caused by group A beta-hemolytic streptococci and is typically found on the extremities. Treatment is focused on aggressive surgical debridement, fluid resuscitation, and broad-spectrum antibiotics. The cumulative mortality rate for this is approximately 34%. Diabetes mellitus, advanced age, two or more comorbidities, and a delay before surgery are all associated with greater mortality.

25. **A 30-year-old woman whose children have been sick with a viral syndrome complains of a fever (102.8°F), malaise, and loss of appetite for the past 2 weeks. She is on long-term phenytoin for a seizure disorder and had a breast biopsy 3 weeks ago. On skin examination, you note approximately 50 scattered pustular and/or necrotic skin lesions without mucosal involvement. You hear no heart murmur. Her right knee is swollen, painful, and hot. Examination of the joint fluid shows cloudy fluid without organisms or crystals. You send the fluid for culture, but results are pending. The following is the most likely diagnosis and appropriate therapeutic response is:**

    a. The patient has the dermatitis/arthritis syndrome of gonococcemia. Start ceftriaxone and admit her.

    b. The patient is experiencing a drug reaction to phenytoin (i.e., Stevens-Johnson syndrome). Start steroids and admit her to the intensive care unit.

    c. The patient has a shingles. Prescribe pain medications and send her home.

    d. The patient has staphylococcal bacteremia. Start antistaphylococcal treatment and admit her.

    e. The patient has a viral syndrome. No specific treatment is necessary; send her home.

    The answer is d. This patient has infective endocarditis (IE). Most people with bacterial endocarditis have a predisposing factor such as congenital heart disease, mitral valve prolapse, or a history of IV drug use or prior endocarditis. Lack of a heart murmur is common in the early stages of acute bacterial endocarditis. Symptoms associated with IE are nonspecific and include intermittent fever, malaise, confusion, cough, chest pain, headaches, and anorexia. A small percentage will have petechiae, splinter hemorrhages, Osler's nodes, and Janeway lesions, or Roth's spots. Pustular lesions are also consistent (as is almost any type of skin lesion) with IE and the resulting staphylococcal bacteremia. Major diagnostic criteria include positive blood cultures and echogardiographic evidence of endocardial vegetations, paravalvular abscess, or new valvular dysfunction. In early disseminated gonococcal infection (DGI), a tenosynovitis predominates without actual joint invasion such as occurs in the later variety of DGI. Stevens-Johnson syndrome is unlikely because of the lack of mucosal involvement. A viral syndrome usually produces polyarticular arthritis.

26. **A 55-year-old woman complains of chronic back pain and a temperature of 101°F. She has been ill for approximately 3 months, with low-grade fever and fatigue. She has been administered several courses of pain medications and antibiotics for low back pain, which was presumed to be secondary to a urinary tract infection. However, the back pain has worsened over the last 2 weeks. Now she is losing weight and reports intermittent soreness on urination. She appears chronically ill but you find no adenopathy. She has two small, painful nodular lesions at the base of her right big toe. She has a 2/6 systolic ejection murmur at the second left intercostal space. Her lower back is moderately tender to direct percussion. Her white blood cell count is mildly elevated. The sedimentation rate is 102 mm/h. Urinalysis shows 2 plus protein and 2–3 white blood cells with 30 red blood cells per high-power field (HPF). X-rays of the lumbosacral spine demonstrate mild degenerative joint disease. Her most likely diagnosis is:**

    a. Reactive arthritis.

    b. Chronic pyelonephritis.

    c. Musculoskeletal back pain.

    d. Infectious endocarditis.

    e. Acute pyelonephritis.

    The answer is d. Low back pain occurs with 15% of cases of subacute infectious endocarditis. The pain resolves with successful antibiotic treatment. The back pain does not seem to be due to direct infection of the sacroiliac joint. This case history is somewhat typical for this low-grade infectious process muted further by intermittent courses of antibiotics administered for a variety of reasons, which temporarily blunt the bacterial process.

27.   **A 6-year-old child has erythema, edema, and warmth in the area around his right eye. His mother states that an insect bit him in this area several days ago, but she noted no symptoms until yesterday after he woke up. Although his eye is swollen shut, his vision and ocular movement are unaffected if he holds his eyelid open. The most likely pathogen is:**

   a. *Staphylococcus epidermidis.*

   b. *Escherichia coli.*

   c. *Staphylococcus aureus.*

   d. *Bacteroides fragilis.*

   e. *Borrelia burgdorferi.*

   The answer is c. This patient has periorbital cellulitis. Differentiation of periorbital cellulitis from orbital cellulitis is the crucial clinical decision. Periorbital cellulitis is an infection lying anterior to the orbital septum and is associated with eyelid edema, discoloration, redness, and warmth. Vision, extraocular motion, and papillary findings are normal. In contrast, orbital cellulitis causes increased pain, tenderness, proptosis, and decreased ocular mobility. A CT scan may be helpful in distinguishing the two diagnoses. Early periorbital cellulitis may be treated with outpatient antibiotics with daily follow-up to make sure the infection is resolving. Treatment for orbital cellulitis involved admission for intravenous antibiotics and may require surgery if severe. The most likely organisms for both conditions are *S. aureus, Streptococcus pyogenes,* and *Haemophilus influenzae.*

28.   **A 22-year-old woman complains of cold symptoms for more than 2 weeks. She seemed to be getting better, but then developed a relapse, including headache, yellow nasal secretions, and bad breath. Although she had chills, and a probable fever, she did not take her temperature. You should:**

   a. Start amoxicillin 250 mg orally every 8 hours for 10 days.

   b. Order a Waters view to evaluate her maxillary sinuses.

   c. Refer the patient to an ear, nose, and throat specialist.

   d. Order a CT scan of the sinuses.

   e. Culture nasal secretions and prescribe delayed antibiotics depending on the results.

   The answer is a. It is important, but difficult, to distinguish between allergic and infectious sinusitis. Allergic sinusitis is related to allergen exposure and patients typically have had previous episodes. Their sinus pain and tenderness tends to be associated with sneezing, rhinorrhea, itchy, and watery eyes. Bacterial sinusitis is suggested by a biphasic course of illness, patients with a viral upper respiratory tract infection improve initially only to have worsening sinus congestion and discomfort. Nasal and nasopharyngeal cultures are frequently contaminated with normal flora and do not correlate with intrasinus cultures. Therefore, they are not recommended. The gold standard of sinus imaging is a coronal CT scan with or without IV contrast. Plain film radiography (Waters view) is much more sensitive in evaluating the maxillary sinus than the other sinuses. Patients who are not improving after 7 days or with strongly suspected bacterial sinusitis should be started on antibiotics with efficacy against *S. pneumoniae,* nontypable *H. influenzae,* and *M. catarrhalis.* Amoxicillin is still considered a first line agent but treatment failures due to beta-lactamase producing bacteria have been noted. Amoxicillin-clavulanate, clindamycin, trimethoprim-sulfamethoxazole, and a second- or third-generation cephalosporin are all acceptable as second-line agents for more complicated cases. CT scans of the sinuses and/or referral to an ENT specialist is appropriate if second-line treatment fails.

29.   **When using penicillin to treat a patient whom you have diagnosed with streptococcal pharyngitis, you may be preventing:**

   a. Spread of infection to others, but not pharyngeal space infections.

   b. Acute rheumatic fever, but not streptococcal pneumonia.

   c. Pharyngeal space infections, but not acute glomerulonephritis.

   d. Acute glomerulonephritis but not acute rheumatic fever.

   e. Streptococcal pneumonia but not spread of infection to others.

   The answer is c. No evidence suggests that treatment of streptococcal throat infection can prevent the development of acute glomerulonephritis. Appropriate antimicrobial therapy started within 9 days of the onset of streptococcal pharyngitis can prevent rheumatic fever. Antibiotic therapy decreases infectivity after 24 hours and reduces suppurative complications (i.e., pharyngeal space infections, pneumonia). Overall, however, antibiotic therapy does not seem to decrease the length of the patient's sore throat or any other symptoms.

30.   **Transmission of *Salmonella* to a susceptible host usually occurs by the:**

   a. Drinking from wilderness water sources.

   b. Inhalation of aerosol droplets.

   c. Occupational exposure to contaminated soil.

   d. Ingestion of contaminated food or drink.

   e. Travel to endemic areas in the United States.

   The answer is d. *Salmonella* is a flagellated Gram-negative bacterium. There are several species known to cause disease in humans: *S. enteritidis* and *S. typhimurium* cause 3–5 days of mild abdominal cramping, diarrhea, and fever known as salmonellosis, and *S. typhi* causes more severe symptoms known as typhoid fever. Treatment is largely supportive but ampicillin, ciprofloxacin, or trimethoprim-sulfamethoxazole may be started if symptoms do not resolve in 5–7 days. However, antibiotics may prolong the carrier state. Almost all *Salmonella* infections to a susceptible host occur through consumption of contaminated foods. Eggs and other poultry products are the single most common source of *Salmonella*; however, improperly prepared beef, fruits, vegetables, dairy products, and shellfish have also been associated with infection. *Salmonella* is also found in household pets such as dogs, cats, and reptiles. Prevention is of paramount importance: frequent hand washing, proper preparation of raw foods, and through cooking of eggs and poultry products limit the risk of transmission. All cases of confirmed or suspected *Salmonella* infection should be reported to local or state health departments.

31. **A 43-year-old woman with no significant past medical history complains of the acute onset of 10–12 episodes of loose, watery brown diarrhea over the past 36 hours. She also has nausea and mild diffuse abdominal cramping. She denies vomiting, fevers, or chills and has no known sick contacts or recent travel. Her vital signs are unremarkable and she does not appear dehydrated. The next step in the management of this patient is:**

    a. Reassure the patient, anticipatory guidance, and discharge to home.

    b. Begin an immunosuppression workup due to the severity of her symptoms.

    c. Perform rectal examination and, if heme positive, refer for inflammatory bowel disease workup.

    d. Perform rectal examination and, if heme negative, start her on antibiotics.

    e. Order stool studies for Gram stain, fecal leukocytes, toxins, ova, and parasites.

    The answer is a. In evaluating healthy patients with acute diarrhea, the clinical evaluation, combined with epidemiologic information, should be used to help guide laboratory evaluation and management. Healthy adults lacking specific epidemiologic risk factors (such as recent foreign travel, consumption of raw shellfish, prolonged antibiotic use, etc.) and who have fewer than 3 days of symptoms typically do not require laboratory testing unless they have signs and symptoms of dehydration. In patients with symptoms lasting for more than 5 days, fecal testing for inflammatory bowel disease should be considered. Patients with symptoms lasting for more than 1 week or with recurrent episodes should undergo fecal testing for ova and parasites and should also be tested for possible immunocompromise. The use of antidiarrheal agents remains controversial and is not generally recommended.

32. **A 47-year-old homeless woman complains of a cough for the past 2 months. She says that it was initially nonproductive, but she now is bringing up yellow sputum. The cough is associated with pleuritic chest pain and fevers/chills that are worse at night, but she denies shortness of breath or dyspnea. She also admits to a 15 lb weight loss during this period. She recently had tuberculin skin testing (PPD) at her shelter but states it was "negative." Vital signs are normal as her examination, CBC, and basic metabolic panel. Her x-ray shows a right upper lobe cavitary lesion. Which of the following statements is true concerning her diagnosis?**

    a. Place a repeat PPD in the ED to detect active clinical disease.

    b. Immediately begin treatment for tuberculosis (TB).

    c. Do not bother with sputum studies, as they have both low sensitivity and specificity.

    d. You must confirm the presumptive diagnosis of TB by culture.

    e. Remember that s normal chest x-ray excludes active TB.

    The answer is d. The PPD test remains the best test to identify latent TB infection but is of little utility in determining active disease. At least 20% of patients with active TB will have a falsely negative PPD. A normal chest x-ray has a high negative predictive value and is useful in screening for active pulmonary TB. However, depending on the clinical circumstances (such as HIV, immunosuppression, etc.) a normal chest x-ray does not always exclude active TB. Initial clinical or radiographic findings suggestive of active TB should be confirmed with acid-fast bacilli (AFB smear) on stained sputum examination. However, AFB smears have a low sensitivity because of a variable amount of sputum production and the fact that few bacilli may be present in the sputum. Therefore, the collection of early-morning samples on 3 consecutive days is recommended. A presumptive diagnosis of TB based on AFB smear should be confirmed by culture, which may take 1–8 weeks depending on culture method used. Routine laboratory studies are generally not specific, and of limited utility, but may show a normochromic, normocytic anemia, elevated erythrocyte sedimentation rate (ESR), hyponatremia, and hypercalcemia.

33. **For the patient described in the previous question, which of the following statements is true regarding her emergency department management?**

  a. If she is pregnant, pyridoxine (vitamin B$_6$) should be given in addition to her antibiotics.

  b. She should be started on single agent therapy with INH unless her cultures result in a drug-resistant strain.

  c. She needs respiratory isolation only because she is actively coughing and is therefore at higher risk of spreading TB.

  d. She should be placed on streptomycin and admitted to respiratory isolation.

  e. She is not at risk of hemoptysis because her x-ray does not show an effusion.

  The answer is a. ED management of tuberculosis is based on limiting contact with other patients or ED staff, managing emergent complications such as massive hemoptysis (defined as greater than 600 cc in the previous 24 hours), and initiating antituberculous medications. All patients suspected of having TB should immediately be placed in respiratory isolation, regardless of cough frequency or sputum production. Patients with hemoptysis should be evaluated for possible bronchoscopy, angiography, or surgical resection. Because of the high degree of noncompliance with antituberculous therapy, frequent comorbid immunosuppression, and the increased prevalence of multi-drug resistant strains, patients with suspected TB are typically admitted to respiratory isolation to begin medical therapy. The most commonly used first-line agents currently include isoniazid (INH), rifampin (RIF), pyrazinamide (PZA), and ethambutol (ETH). Streptomycin was once considered a first-line agent but drug resistance has limited its use and it is now considered a second-line agent. Because of its association with peripheral neuropathy and intractable seizures, INH is often given in conjunction with pyridoxine (vitamin B$_6$). Pyridoxine is especially recommended in pregnant, alcoholic, diabetic, and HIV-positive patients who are at higher risk of developing neuropathy. Although there are multiple regimens, all are designed to rapidly kill large numbers of bacilli, prevent the emergence of resistant strains, and prevent relapse. All last at least 6–9 months as shorter regimens are associated with unacceptably high failure rates.

34. **A 30-year-old previously healthy man presents with complaints of 2 days of myalgias and malaise. Yesterday evening he developed a cough, fever, and rapidly worsening dyspnea. He has a blood pressure of 90/ 40 mm Hg and is hypoxic on room air. The chest x-ray shows diffuse alveolar infiltration. He recently camped in rural areas of Arizona and spent a night in an abandoned barn. He most likely contracted his infection from:**

  a. The bite of an infected flea.

  b. The bite of an infected mosquito.

  c. The bite of an infected tick.

  d. Eating contaminated food.

  e. Inhaling aerosolized mouse droppings.

  The answer is e. This patient most likely has Hantavirus pulmonary syndrome. Hantavirus is carried by the deer mouse *Peromyscus maniculatus* and transmitted via aerosols of infected urine, hair, and droppings. In Asia and Europe, Hantavirus has long been known to cause a hemorrhagic fever with renal syndrome with more than 100,000 annual cases and a mortality rate of approximately 6%. In 1994 in the United States, a previously unknown Hantavirus was found to cause a pulmonary syndrome associated with profound hypoxia and respiratory distress. Since first identified, the majority of cases have occurred in the southwestern United States, however there have been sporadic cases throughout the country. Patients typically exhibit tachypnea, tachycardia, and hypoxia. Laboratory findings include hemoconcentration, thrombocytopenia, and leukocytosis with atypical lymphocytes. Chest x-ray shows bilateral fluffy interstitial infiltrates that are increased in dependant areas. This condition carries a significant morbidity and mortality and aggressive supportive care including early intubation and ventilatory support is warranted.

35.   **A 72-year-old male smoker complains of 5 days of fever to 103.2°F, malaise, lethargy, and a dry nonproductive cough. Three days ago, he noted diffuse cramping abdominal pain and multiple episodes of loose, watery stool. Laboratory testing is significant for: sodium 128 mEq/L, ALT of 52 IU/L, and an AST of 11 IU/L. There is no leukocytosis. Chest x-ray shows a nonspecific patchy infiltrate. The most likely etiologic agent is:**

   a. *Legionella pneumophila.*

   b. *Klebsiella pneumoniae.*

   c. *Mycoplasma pneumoniae.*

   d. *Chlamydia pneumoniae.*

   e. *Streptococcus pneumoniae.*

   The answer is a. After an incubation period of 2–10 days, Legionnaire's disease typically presents with nonspecific signs and symptoms including fever, chills, myalgias, malaise, headache, and a cough, which can be either dry or productive of sputum. Patients may also complain of diarrhea, although this finding is not as common as once believed. Immunocompromised patients may also exhibit extrapulmonary symptoms such as arthritis, meningitis, or encephalitis. Laboratory testing may reveal a lack of leukocytosis, abnormal liver function tests, or renal failure. Chest x-rays often show nonspecific patchy infiltrates. Urine antigen and sputum culture can be used to confirm the diagnosis. Treatment with azithromycin for 5–10 days or a fluoroquinolone for 10–14 days is recommended. All cases of confirmed or suspected *L. pneumophila* infection should be reported to local or state health departments.

36.   **A 20-year-old college student complains of 1 week of fevers, chills, and sweats and 5 days of a sore throat. She is not drooling, is able to speak easily, and tolerates oral fluids in the emergency department. Vital signs: temperature 102.4°F, heart rate 110 beats/min, respiratory rate 18/min, blood pressure 100/70 mm Hg. You see marked tonsillar edema and thick exudates. You also note bilateral tender posterior cervical lymphadenopathy. The most accurate laboratory test to confirm your suspicion of infectious mononucleosis (IM) is a:**

   a. Peripheral blood smear.

   b. Heterophile agglutination test for immunoglobulin M (IgM) antibodies.

   c. Hepatic function panel.

   d. Mononucleosis spot test.

   e. IgM antibody to viral capsid antigen.

   The answer is e. Positive results for IgM antibody to viral capsid antigen is useful to diagnose acute infection, particularly in cases that are heterophile negative as they develop in 100% of cases of IM. A mononucleosis spot test (Monospot) allows rapid ED screening for heterophile antibodies and is positive in up to 95% of adults and in most children older than 5 years. However, it is usually negative during the first week of illness and in children younger than 4 years. Heterophile agglutination test results are positive in 90% of affected adolescents and adults but may take several weeks after the onset of IM symptoms to become positive. A peripheral blood smear is nonspecific although it typically reveals relative and absolute lymphocytosis, with greater than 10% atypical lymphocytes. It may also show evidence of hemolytic anemia or thrombocytopenia. Liver function test results are abnormal in approximately 90% of cases of IM but are a nonspecific finding. It should be noted that Epstein-Barr virus (EBV) is primarily a pediatric infection in third world countries and causes a mild flu-like syndrome in these children. Delayed infection in industrialized countries results in the more severe IM syndrome seen in young adults.

37. **To prevent hookworm you should tell your patients to:**

    a. Avoid raw fish and shellfish.

    b. Reduce fecal contamination of water and food supplies.

    c. Cook meat thoroughly before eating.

    d. Filter drinking water and control crop irrigation.

    e. Wear shoes.

    The answer is e. Hookworm infection has been recognized as a major cause of iron deficiency anemia worldwide. The infective larvae are found in soil and can penetrate human skin, usually through the feet. Adult worms migrate to the intestines where they penetrate into the mucosa and feed, causing significant ongoing luminal blood loss. As with most helminthic infections, peripheral eosinophilia is common, however specific diagnosis requires identification of the characteristic ova in the stool.

38. **You have just diagnosed *Enterobius vermicularis* (pinworm) in a 35-year-old woman. Treatment involves:**

    a. Antihelminthics to the woman who tested positive, but family members do not require prophylaxis or treatment.

    b. Mebendazole to the patient and all members of her immediate family.

    c. One time treatment with praziquantel, which is more than 95% effective.

    d. Disposal of all bedclothes, burning all clothing worn within the past 7 days, and fumigation of the house.

    e. Metronidazole to the patient and all members of her immediate family.

    The answer is b. The primary symptom of this infection is severe perianal itching. Because pinworm infection is so highly contagious, it can be assumed that if one family member is infected, the entire family is infected. Therefore, simultaneous treatment of the whole family is necessary as well as cleaning the environment (e.g., bedding, carpets, etc.) to prevent reinfection. Mebendazole is the drug of choice for pinworm infection. It causes worm death by selectively and irreversibly blocking uptake of glucose and other nutrients in susceptible adult intestines where helminths dwell.

39. **A patient complains of a rapidly progressive hand and arm pain and ascending redness that she first noticed approximately 12 hours after her cat bit her in the back of her hand. The most likely causative organism is:**

    a. *Staphylococcus aureus.*

    b. *Pasteurella multocida.*

    c. *Pasteurella stomatis.*

    d. Alpha-hemolytic streptococci.

    e. Beta-hemolytic streptococci.

    The answer is b. Cat bites have a higher incidence of infection than dog bites, although the exact incidence is unknown due to reporting bias. *P. multocida* is found in the oral flora of 70–90% of healthy cats and causes a distinctive cellulitis. Although *S. aureus* and alpha- and beta-hemolytic streptococci are well known to cause cellulitis, this is usually not evident for 48–72 hours. *P. multocida,* on the other hand, causes a rapidly progressive cellulitis that may be apparent within 6 hours and is readily seen in 24 hours. It has also been associated with abscess formation, bacteremia, tenosynovitis, and synovial infection. Treatment with a penicillin, fluoroquinolone, or second- or third-generation cephalosporin should be initiated. Some resistance to vancomycin, clindamycin, and first-generation cephalosporins has been demonstrated. *P. stomatis* has been isolated from dog bites and tends to be less virulent.

40. A 73-year-old man complains of several days of severe burning and aching in his right mid-back. He also complaints of malaise but denies fevers and chills. This morning, his wife noted clusters of "clear blisters" on red bases in the same area of his pain. Which of the following is true regarding his diagnosis and management?

a. Clinical suspicion must be confirmed with tissue biopsy and culture.

b. Antiviral medications shorten the duration of viral shedding but do not reduce the severity of pain or speed healing.

c. Corticosteroids have been shown to reduce the development of postherpetic neuralgia but not acute pain.

d. Treatment with gabapentin may reduce the risk of postherpetic neuralgia.

e. Therapy with short-acting opioid pain relievers is appropriate, but the use of long-acting, controlled-release opioids is rarely required.

The answer is d. This patient has herpes zoster, a reactivation of the varicella-zoster virus. After initial infection, the virus remains dormant in dorsal-root ganglia for a variable period of time. Risk factors for reemergence include increasing age, immunosuppression, and neoplastic disease. This is followed by the eruption of a maculopapular rash that form clusters of clear vesicles on an erythematous base that resolve over 2–4 weeks after passing though stages of postulation, ulceration, and crusting. Characteristically, the rash has a dermatomal distribution and rarely crosses the midline. However, the presence of a few lesions outside of the primary dermatome is not unusual. Although during the prodromal phase, patients exhibit nonspecific, flu-like symptoms, the herpes zoster rash is sufficiently unique to make a clinical diagnosis. Complicating diagnosis, however, the pain, itching, or burning may precede the skin lesions by several days and postherpetic neuralgia may persist for extended periods following resolution of the lesions. Pain control with short- or long-acting opioids and sympathetic-nerve blockade is the mainstay of treatment. Antiviral medications (acyclovir, valacyclovir, famciclovir, etc.) have been shown to reduce the severity of pain, reduce the formation of new lesions, speed healing, and reduce viral shedding. Corticosteroids are not recommended for use without antiviral therapy but have been shown to reduce acute pain and increase healing. They have not, however, been shown to decrease postherpetic neuralgia. Treatment with centrally acting medications such as gabapentin, on the other hand, are not effective against acute pain but may be effective at reducing the risk of postherpetic neuralgia.

CHAPTER 11

Nontraumatic Musculoskeletal Emergencies

Joseph Lex, MD, FACEP, FAAEM

1. **Physical findings of an isolated L5 radiculopathy include:**

   a. Decreased patellar reflex.
   b. Paresthesias of the little toe.
   c. Weakness of the extensor hallucis longus tendon.
   d. Asymmetric Achilles tendon reflexes.
   e. Weakness of hip flexion.

   The answer is c. The motor innervation of the muscle group of the lower extremities is easily remembered since it progresses in a logical pattern. Individual testing and bilateral comparison of the muscle groups is strongly recommended. L3 is responsible for hip flexion. L4 innervates the quadriceps and a lesion at this level will cause a reduced patellar reflex and difficulty in squatting. L5 lesions cause weakness of foot dorsiflexion and great toe extension (difficulty in walking on the heels). S1 radiculopathy is manifested by the inability to flex the calf muscles (difficulty in walking on the toes) and an asymmetric Achilles tendon reflex. L4 compression causes radicular pain or paresthesias in the knee, anteromedial tibia and foot; L5 compression affects the great toe and midportion of the foot; and S1 compression affects the little toe and posterolateral calf.

2. **Which of the following techniques of joint aspiration is correctly described?**

   a. Knee: lateral to the distal edge of the patella, aim a 27-gauge needle in an inferior and cephalad direction, use 1% lidocaine with epinephrine.
   b. Wrist: dorsal wrist, superior to the ulnar styloid process, aim a 20-gauge needle just distal to the radial notch, use 1% lidocaine with epinephrine.
   c. First metatarsal–phalangeal joint: plantar surface of foot, aim a 20-gauge needle at the joint space just to the side of the extensor hallucis tendon, use 1% lidocaine with epinephrine.
   d. Shoulder: anterior shoulder, 2 cm medial to the acromial process, aim in cephalad direction with an 18-gauge needle, use 1% lidocaine with or without epinephrine.
   e. Elbow: lateral elbow, between the lateral epicondyle and the olecranon, aim toward the patient's thumb, use 1% lidocaine without epinephrine.

   The answer is e. The most devastating complication of joint aspiration is infection. Aspirations should not be made through areas of cellulitis or bursitis. Other complications are infrequent (e.g., transient arm numbness in shoulder aspirations from inadvertent anesthesia of the brachial plexus). Lidocaine with epinephrine should not be used for anesthesia when aspirating the joints of the fingers or the toes: the digits are supplied by end arteries and ischemic injury may result.

3.   **A 75-year-old woman with rheumatoid arthritis complains of fever and a swollen left knee. You aspirate her knee and find cloudy fluid; the Gram stain is positive for Gram-positive cocci. The drug of choice to treat her is:**

    a. Clindamycin.

    b. Trimethoprim-sulfamethoxazole.

    c. Ciprofloxacin.

    d. Vancomycin.

    e. Azithromycin.

The answer is d. Patients with inflammatory joint disease are at increased risk for developing septic arthritis due to *Staphylococcus aureus*. The Gram stain results are consistent with this diagnosis. Vancomycin should be used empirically because of the prevalence of methicillin-resistant strains of this bacterium.

4.   **Choose the correct radiographic descriptions of bone and joint diseases:**

    a. Advanced gout: "rat bite" subchondral erosions, relative preservation of the joint space, periarticular soft tissue swelling, involvement of the first metatarsal–phalangeal joint.

    b. Rheumatoid arthritis (RA): periarticular osteoporosis, joint swelling, marginal erosions, symmetric involvement of the knees and hips.

    c. Charcot joint: preservation of the normal anatomy and joint spaces.

    d. Osteoarthritis: loss of joint space, hypertrophic bone spurs, decreased bone density, involvement of proximal interphalangeal (PIP) joints of hands.

    e. Acute septic arthritis: fragmentation of cartilage, joint effusion.

The answer is a. The most consistent radiographic finding in acute septic arthritis is effusion and soft tissue swelling. Cartilage is radiolucent and not seen on conventional x-rays, but loss of cartilage is indirectly seen as a narrowing of joint space. Acute gout may show minimal x-ray findings. Chronic tophaceous gout is characterized by periarticular densities (tophi) that cause subchondral erosions with preservation of the joint space. The first manifestations of RA are bilateral, symmetrical periarticular swelling and osteopenia. The inflamed synovium causes erosions beginning at the edge of the cartilage (marginal erosions). The PIP joints are most commonly involved. Osteoarthritis (OA) is characterized by a narrowing of the joint spaces secondary to mechanical cartilage loss and a reactive bone sclerosis and a bone spur formation. OA may be idiopathic, hereditary, posttraumatic or secondary to certain metabolic diseases. Diabetes is the most common cause of a Charcot (neuropathic) joint: typically the midfoot joints are involved. With neuropathic injury, the joint resembles a pulverized "bag of bones." Syphilis and syringomyelia are other causes of neuropathic joints.

5.   **A 45-year-old right-hand dominant carpenter complains of a recurrent right palm numbness and loss of grip strength. The physical finding most consistent with carpal tunnel syndrome is:**

    a. A positive Phalen test.

    b. A positive Finkelstein test.

    c. A positive Thompson test.

    d. Thenar hypertrophy.

    e. Carpal bone atrophy on wrist radiograph.

The answer is a. Repetitive trauma, pregnancy, diabetes, hypothyroidism, and rheumatoid arthritis are causes of carpal tunnel syndrome. Physical examination is conducted to exclude vascular insufficiency and to detect thenar atrophy or weakness (inability to abduct and oppose the thumb). Percussion over the carpal tunnel (Tinel test) or flexion of the wrist for 1 minute (Phalen test) may reproduce symptoms such as tingling radiating to the hand or shoulder. X-rays are usually negative. Initial treatment consists of a wrist splint and NSAIDs. Surgical decompression may be necessary. Finkelstein test may be positive in de Quervain tenosynovitis.

6. **Choose the correct statement about acute arthritis:**

   a. The most likely cause of an acutely red, swollen, and tender joint in an elderly woman with no previous medical history is infection.
   b. In adults, rheumatic fever presents with monoarticular joint disease and is often associated with fever.
   c. A synovial cell count of 1000–10,000 WBCs/mm^3 with a lymphocytosis in a patient with polyarticular joint pain and swelling suggests gout.
   d. A synovial cell count of 100,000 WBCs/mm^3 with a predominance of PMNs usually indicates a bacterial infection.
   e. Gram stain of synovial fluid in cases of acute bacterial arthritis is positive in 75% of cases.

   The answer is d. Pseudogout, or calcium pyrophosphate deposition disease (CPPD), is characterized by the acute onset of monoarticular joint pain and swelling, usually affecting the large joints. X-rays reveal chondrocalcinosis. Confirmatory data include the positive birefringent, rhomboid-shaped crystals. NSAIDs are effective therapy. Rheumatic fever presents with more striking joint findings in adults than children. A heart murmur should be excluded in adults with polyarthritis, particularly those younger than 30 years. High PMN cell counts may occur in any acute inflammatory condition, such as gout or rheumatoid arthritis. However, very high cell counts, monoarthropathy, and upper extremity involvement should raise suspicions of infection, particularly in the absence of crystals of pseudogout or gout. The Gram stain is positive in a minority of patients with septic arthritis. The serum ANA, ESR, or ASO titer may be useful in evaluating arthropathies.

7. **The key sign of spinal stenosis is:**

   a. Genital numbness and stool incontinence.
   b. Hyperreflexia and poor anal "wink."
   c. Hyporeflexia and a negative cremasteric reflex.
   d. Lower extremity pain exacerbated with walking and relieved with sitting.
   e. Urinary incontinence and stocking anesthesia.

   The answer is d. Spinal stenosis complaints usually come from older patients. Pain is diffuse, usually involves the back, and often radiates down one or both legs, associated with paresthesias. Rest usually resolves it, although it takes longer to resolve than true vascular claudication. Patients also note pain relief with back flexion. A typical story involves the patient who is able to walk uphill without pain but develops pain walking downhill when the back is extended. Impotence and incontinence can also be present with severe spinal stenosis.

8.   **A 52-year-old man complains of severe right knee pain. He recalls no trauma, but attended a wine tasting party last weekend. He denies past medical history and is afebrile with normal vital signs. Physical examination reveals a swollen, red, painful right knee. Radiograph shows an effusion, but no bony erosions. You perform arthrocentesis and obtain 27 mL of cloudy straw-colored fluid, which you send to the laboratory for studies. The cell count is 50,000 WBCs/mm^3 with 85% PMNs, glucose 120 mg/dL (serum 130), protein 3.5 g/dL. The Gram stain shows numerous WBCs, but is negative for organisms. Evaluation for crystals shows numerous needle-shaped crystals with negative birefringence. A good treatment plan would be:**

   a. Oral colchicine 0.5 mg every hour until relief is obtained or to a maximum of 6 mg or when diarrhea occurs.

   b. Subcutaneous colchicine 1 mg plus oral probenecid 250 mg bid for 1 week.

   c. Sublingual colchicine 2 mg followed by oral steroids tapered over 5 days.

   d. Intra-articular triamcinolone injection.

   e. Oral allopurinol 500 mg tid for 1 week.

   The answer is a. Gout may be precipitated by liberal intake of alcohol or food. Generally, attacks have an acute onset, occur during the night, and involve a single joint of a lower extremity. Aspiration of joint fluid reveals an inflammatory effusion, with more than 10,000 WBCs (greater than 80% PMNs), a normal glucose, and numerous needle-shaped crystals. Coexistent infection is rare in acute gout and pseudogout, but cultures are prudent. Treatment is with oral or intravenous colchicine, which is most effective if administered shortly after the onset of symptoms. Extravasation of colchicine results in skin necrosis and tissue loss. Many consider NSAIDs such as indomethacin or naproxen the treatment of choice, although recent literature makes a strong case for the initial use of oral corticosteroids. Allopurinol and uricosuric drugs such as probenecid are not indicated in the acute treatment phase of gout. Patients should be instructed to refrain from alcohol use and to have adequate oral fluid intake.

9.   **Choose the correct pairing for the two most common sites and organisms responsible for septic arthritis in children:**

   a. Knee, wrist → *S. aureus, S. pyogenes.*

   b. Hip, knee → *S. pyogenes, Salmonella* sp.

   c. Knee, hip → *S. aureus, H. influenzae.*

   d. Knee, elbow → *H. influenzae, S. aureus.*

   e. Wrist, knee → *S. pneumoniae, H. influenzae.*

   The answer is c. Traumatic injury is the most common cause of acute joint pain and swelling in children. The most frequently involved joints in trauma are the knees, wrists, and elbows. Bilateral joint involvement suggests inflammatory arthritides, such as viral or juvenile rheumatoid arthritis. The knee and hip are the most commonly involved joints in pediatric septic arthritis. Fever or chills are usually present. The earliest x-ray finding in a septic hip is asymmetric joint-space widening from effusion. The most common organisms are *S. aureus* and *H. influenzae.* In sickle cell patients, *Salmonella* is an important consideration in all bone and joint infections. Early aspiration and intravenous antibiotics are essential to preserve joint function.

10.   **A 70-year-old woman complains of low back pain radiating to the anterior and posterior thighs. Prolonged standing or sitting exacerbates the pain and it is worse at night. She notes morning stiffness. Bilateral sacral tenderness is elicited with palpation and with compression of the iliac wings. Which of the following statements about this disorder is true?**

   a. The disorder is characterized by pain radiating to the distal lower extremities.

   b. A pelvis radiograph is diagnostic in symptomatic patients.

   c. An associated finding may be instability of the pubic symphysis.

   d. Morning stiffness is not characteristic of this disorder.

   e. Initial treatment of this condition is surgical.

The answer is c. Characteristic findings of sacroiliitis usually allow it to be distinguished from lumbar pain. Low back pain radiating to the anterior or posterior thighs is common, but unlike lumbar pain, it rarely radiates below the knees. Pain increases at night, or with prolonged sitting or standing, and is associated with morning stiffness. Pain is elicited by direct palpation or by stressing the joints. Pelvic x-rays may be negative in early stages. Later stages may reveal sclerosis or loss of the sacroiliac joint. Films of alternate leg weight bearing may show subluxation of the pubic bone. Initial treatment consists of bed rest, anti-inflammatory drugs, and heat. Septic arthritis of the SI joint should be considered in a patient with unilateral low back or sacral pain and fever.

11. **Patients with flexor tenosynovitis:**

    a. Almost never recall a precipitating event.
    b. Have a negative Kanavel sign.
    c. Have exquisite pain with finger flexion.
    d. Have no pain when the proximal tendon sheath is palpated.
    e. Present with diffuse fusiform swelling.

    The answer is e. Flexor tenosynovitis is a surgical emergency that must be diagnosed promptly by the examining physician and managed aggressively by both the emergency physician and the hand surgeon. Recognizing the classic clinical findings described by Kanavel makes the diagnosis. The four cardinal signs are tenderness over the flexor tendon sheath, symmetric swelling of the finger, pain with passive extension, and a flexed posture of the involved digit at rest.

12. **A 65-year-old man lifts a cardboard box of old magazines at a local yard sale and develops acute lower back pain radiating to his left leg. You suspect a herniated disk at the L4-5 level, knowing that:**

    a. Findings on lumbar spine x-rays can confirm the diagnosis.
    b. Demonstrating sciatic pain down the left leg with straight-leg-raising (SLR) maneuver is pathognomonic for disk herniation.
    c. Demonstrating a left SLR and a cross-straight-leg-raising (CSLR) sign is specific for disk herniation in this age group.
    d. A negative "strum" sign (the sciatic nerve plucked behind the knee) in association with an SLR and CSLR, would probably be very significant.
    e. Flexion of the head or dorsiflexion of the foot will increase pain if irritation of the sciatic nerve root is present.

    The answer is e. Plain x-rays are often normal in acute herniations. Abnormal radiographs may not correlate with physical findings such as depressed reflexes or muscle group weakness. The SLR and the CSLR tests are most indicative of disk herniation and nerve root impingement in a young patient when a very positive SLR, or a positive SLR and CSLR are present. The tests are less specific in the elderly. Positive tests suggest a radicular component (i.e., from osteophyte impingement or other degenerative change). Actions that stretch the nerve roots and reproduce or increase symptoms provide additional evidence of radicular disease and nerve impingement. Elective CT scans, MRI, or myelography will provide additional information.

13.   **A 27-year-old man complains of a nontraumatic, red, painful, and swollen knee. He denies illicit drug use. He says he was treated for VD last week and is on his last day of doxycycline. He is afebrile and has a right knee effusion. The remainder of his examination is unremarkable. Synovial fluid analysis shows 3500 WBCs/mm³ with 50% PMNs, protein 3.2 g/dL, no crystals, negative Gram stain, and glucose 100 (serum glucose 105). The laboratory informs you that the culture specimen has been discarded and they need another sample. You should now:**

a. Prescribe crutches, aspirin, or an NSAID for presumptive treatment of reactive arthritis and discharge the patient for outpatient follow-up.

b. Explain to the patient the need for a culture; reaccess the joint injecting and aspirating nonbacteriostatic saline for the sample if necessary, then discharge the patient home on crutches and indomethacin, emphasizing the need for follow-up.

c. Admit the patient for high-dose aspirin therapy.

d. Reaspirate the joint, obtain urethral and pharyngeal cultures, and admit for intravenous antibiotic treatment.

e. Reaspirate the joint and admit for intravenous antibiotic treatment with a penicillinase-resistant penicillin active against *S. aureus.*

The answer is d. Reactive arthritis is diagnosed by the findings of urethritis, conjunctivitis, psoriatic-like skin lesions (palms and soles), and mono- or oligoarthritis (usually of the knees, ankles, or feet). The treatment is rest and NSAIDs. Partially treated infections may alter the synovial fluid analysis. Gonococcus may be recovered from urethral, rectal, and pharyngeal cultures.

14.   **There is an association between degenerative cervical spine disk disease and:**

a. Odynophagia.

b. Ptosis, miosis, and anhydrosis.

c. Urinary incontinence.

d. Contralateral shoulder pain.

e. Ipsilateral diaphragmatic paralysis.

The answer is b. Anterior cervical osteophytes that impinge on the esophagus may cause dysphagia. Posterior disk herniation may produce cord compression and cause urinary retention. The most common site of degenerative disk disease is of C5-C6 (C6 nerve root). This root is responsible for innervating the proximal shoulder muscles (deltoid, biceps) and the skin of the upper shoulder. Because the cervical sensory and motor nerves may exit separately through the neural foramina, painless motor weakness or radicular pain without motor findings may occur. Osteophytes at other sites can cause Horner's syndrome or vertebrobasilar insufficiency symptoms. The phrenic nerve arises from C3-C5; unilateral paralysis would be a distinctly unusual complication of degenerative disk disease.

15.   **A 34-year-old man says he twisted his neck in a wrestling match. His left arm is draped over his head. The pain radiates to his left forearm and middle finger. If he leaves his arm by his side the pain increases. You expect to find that:**

a. Vertical pressure (axial loading) on top of his skull will decrease his symptoms.

b. Cervical spine films including oblique views will reveal the pathognomonic abnormalities.

c. If his triceps strength is normal, his sensory complaints cannot be due to a cervical nerve radiculopathy.

d. Gentle neck traction is not recommended.

e. Objective sensory abnormalities may be difficult to elicit.

The answer is e. Acute cervical disk herniation may result in compression and cord myelopathy. A posterior herniation results in lower extremity hyperreflexia, a positive Babinski sign, and occasionally loss of sphincter control. More commonly, acute disk herniations occur in a posterolateral direction, particularly at the right C5-C6 (C6 root) level, or as in this patient the left C6-C7 (C7 root) level. Plain x-ray films may be normal in acute herniation. The dorsal sensory and ventral motor roots may remain separated in the posterior intervertebral foramina in the cervical spine in 50% of patients (this does not occur in the rest of the spine). Therefore, isolated motor or sensory abnormalities may occur in patients with cervical osteophytes or disk disease. Triceps (C7 motor) strength may be intact while paresthesias occur in the distribution of the C7 dermatome (the middle finger is innervated by C7). The tricep reflex will be reduced. Various maneuvers may increase or decrease root irritation and symptoms.

16. **A felon:**

    a. Can be treated by the emergency physician using incision and drainage followed by antibiotics.

    b. Is most commonly caused by group A *Streptococcus*.

    c. Is the same as a paronychia.

    d. Requires hospital admission.

    e. Requires nail bed removal.

    The answer is a. A felon is a subcutaneous pyogenic infection of the pulp space of the distal finger or thumb. The patient presents with marked throbbing pain and a red, tense distal pulp space. *Staphylococcus aureus* is the most common organism, but *Streptococcus* species, anaerobes, and Gram-negative organisms are also encountered. Most felons can be drained adequately with a limited incision and drainage procedure. Most felons have significant associated cellulitis that should be treated with oral antibiotics. A first-generation cephalosporin or antistaphylococcal penicillin should be prescribed for 7–10 days or until the infection has abated.

17. **The most sensitive laboratory study for detecting rhabdomyolysis is:**

    a. Serum BUN and creatinine.

    b. Serum myoglobin.

    c. Urine myoglobin.

    d. Serum CPK.

    e. Urine hemoglobin.

    The answer is d. CPK is the most sensitive test for diagnosing rhabdomyolysis, with 5 times the upper limit of normal considered the threshold for making the diagnosis. CPK levels rise almost immediately after injury (2–12 hours), are easily measured, and remain elevated, as this enzyme is not cleared rapidly. The higher the CPK level, the greater the mortality. Although myoglobin typically rises more quickly than CPK, its half-life is only 1–3 hours, and it can completely disappear from the plasma within 6 hours of injury. Urine tests using guaiac or orthotolidine can detect both hemoglobin and myoglobin in the urine, but cannot differentiate the two. False-negative tests for myoglobinuria can occur because of rapid clearance of myoglobin from the urine, with as many as 25% of patients with proven rhabdomyolysis having a urine dipstick negative for hemoglobin or myoglobin.

18.   **You suspect that a patient has suffered an injury to the motor branch of his ulnar nerve since he is unable to:**

a. Abduct his fingers.

b. Extend his fingers.

c. Extend his wrist.

d. Flex his fingers.

e. Flex his wrist.

The answer is a. The dorsal interosseous muscles abduct the fingers away from the midline. The ulnar nerve innervates them. Wrist and finger extension is under control of the radial nerve, while the median nerve controls flexion.

19.   **A 14-year-old boy complains of pain in his groin, which sometimes goes to his thigh and knee. The pain is dull, vague, intermittent, or continuous, and is exacerbated by physical activity. He walks with his leg in external rotation, and has an antalgic gait. You strongly suspect the child has:**

a. Legg-Calvé-Perthes disease.

b. Osgood-Schlatter disease.

c. Septic arthritis.

d. Slipped capital femoral epiphysis.

e. Transient toxic synovitis.

The answer is d. Children with a stable slipped capital femoral epiphysis have symptoms of intermittent limp and pain of several weeks to months duration. Stable slips make up approximately 90% of all cases. The pain of SCFE may be localized to the hip but more commonly is poorly localized to the thigh, groin, or knee. With continued slippage, internal rotation, flexion, and abduction are lost; and parents and children may note progressive external rotation and shortening of the involved lower extremity with subsequent difficulty in daily activities such as tying shoes. On examination, children initially experience a slight loss of internal rotation and experience pain only at the extremes of motion. The gait is antalgic and muscle atrophy is minimal. As the slip becomes more severe, the gait becomes more antalgic, internal rotation is lost, abduction and flexion of the hip increase, thigh and gluteal muscle atrophy is more pronounced, and leg length discrepancy develops.

20.   **An 83-year-old woman complains of severe bilateral shoulder pain worsening over the past several months. She denies trauma. You are suspicious she has a:**

a. C4 radiculopathy.

b. C5 radiculopathy.

c. C5 myelopathy.

d. C6 radiculopathy.

e. C6 myelopathy.

The answer is d. C6 lesions are frequent and may cause pain along the upper neck, down the biceps, along the lateral forearm, and into the dorsal radial aspect of the hand. Motor weakness usually involves the biceps or wrist extensors, making elbow flexion and wrist extension difficult.

21. **A 25-year-old man complains of sudden onset of right leg pain. On examination, he appears moderately ill. He has a fever of 102.3°F and is normotensive. His entire right lower leg is swollen, red, and exquisitely tender. You see no break in the skin and he denies any trauma. He felt well prior to falling asleep last night. He and his girlfriend spent yesterday in a bay swimming and harvesting oysters. Which of the following is accurate?**

    a. This probably is not cellulitis. A different etiology is the most likely cause of the symptoms.

    b. This is compatible with cellulitis. Because of the severe symptomatology, this patient needs evaluation for underlying immunocompromise.

    c. This is unlikely to be cellulitis because the skin is intact by inspection.

    d. This may be cellulitis even though the skin is intact by inspection. The patient needs parenteral nafcillin because of the severe symptomatology. Nafcillin treats streptococcal and staphylococcal infections.

    e. This may be cellulitis even though the skin is intact by inspection. The patient needs parenteral antibiotic (piperacillin/tazobactam) and doxycycline because of the severe symptomatology. This covers infection with *Streptococcus, Staphylococcus,* and *Vibrio* species.

    The answer is e. Patients with cellulitis often do not provide a history of skin trauma. Inspection of the skin may or may not detect an injury; microscopic tears can provide a portal of entry for bacteria. Consider immunocompromise in a patient if an unusual organism is cultured or the patient has repeated episodes of cellulitis. The patient's symptomatology is consistent with cellulitis. However, the rapid progression of infection is usually not observed in streptococcal or staphylococcal infections. As the patient was in brackish water and could have injured his foot on oyster shells, *Vibrio vulnificus* may be the infecting organism. The rapid progression of symptoms is compatible with vibrio infections. A fulminant course is not uncommon and can be limb and/or life threatening if not quickly treated. Doxycycline and piperacillin/tazobactam are appropriate antibiotics. Both treat streptococcal and staphylococcal infections. Vibrio infections should be treated with more than one antimicrobial.

22. **Carpal tunnel syndrome is characterized by:**

    a. Improvement with repetitive motion.

    b. Negative Tinel sign.

    c. Positive Finkelstein test.

    d. Positive Phalen test.

    e. Radial nerve palsies.

    The answer is d. The most sensitive provocative test to diagnose carpal tunnel syndrome is the wrist flexion test, or Phalen test (sensitivity 76%, specificity 80%). The patient fully flexes the wrists for 60 seconds while the forearms are held in a vertical position. The test is positive if paresthesias or numbness develops in the median nerve distribution. Another test, Tinel sign, is positive if light tapping or percussion over the median nerve at the wrist produces pain or paresthesias in the median nerve distribution. Finkelstein test is positive in de Quervain tendonitis.

23.   **A 64-year-old woman complains of diffuse muscle pain, especially in her thighs and upper arms, along with low-grade fevers, and generalized fatigue. Laboratory studies show a mild anemia and elevated ESR. You strongly suspect she has:**

a. Systemic lupus.

b. Influenza.

c. Dermatomyositis.

d. ACE inhibitor-induced rhabdomyolysis.

e. Polymyalgia rheumatica.

The answer is e. Polymyalgia rheumatica (PMR) is an inflammatory condition of the muscles, usually of the neck, shoulders, and hips. The average age at diagnosis is 70 years, and women are affected more frequently than men. Its cause is unknown, and no test in pathognomonic for its diagnosis. While erythrocyte sedimentation and C-reactive protein tests are usually elevated, they are certainly not diagnostic for PMR.

24.   **Your treatment for the patient in the above question should be:**

a. Stat plasmapheresis.

b. High-dose oral steroid therapy and arrange for temporal artery biopsy.

c. Saline cathartics to rapidly clear the toxin.

d. Discontinue all medications and admit for observation.

e. Rapid infusion of concentrated hydroxocobalamin.

The answer is b. Approximately 50% of patients diagnosed with PMR also have giant cell arteritis (temporal arteritis). Once the diagnosis is made, patients should be started on oral prednisone therapy and referred for temporal artery biopsy.

CHAPTER 12 Neurologic Emergencies

Joseph Lex, MD, FACEP, FAAEM

1. **Which of the following statements is true?**

    a. Herpes zoster is often associated with motor dysfunction with or without a rash.

    b. Acute rabies infection typically begins as a Ramsay-Hunt syndrome before progressing to severe throat spasm and to cardiac and renal failure.

    c. Weakness or diplopia when fatigued may be the only complaint with multiple sclerosis.

    d. Treatment for polymyositis is early administration of systemic steroids.

    e. Serum calcium should be measured in patients with recurrent generalized weakness that follows periods of heavy exertion or that is present upon awakening.

    The answer is c. Ramsay-Hunt syndrome refers to herpes zoster involving the tympanic membrane, ear canal, and other areas in the distribution of the sensory branches of the facial nerve. Herpetic zoster may result in motor abnormalities in up to 25% of cases. Weakness or diplopia only on exertion is a common complaint in early cases of multiple sclerosis. Another early presenting sign is retrobulbar neuritis; in fact, 50–75% of cases occur in patients who develop multiple sclerosis. Steroids may transiently exacerbate weakness in patients with polymyositis and should not be started on patients who will be discharged from the ED. Acute periodic paralysis appears to involve abnormalities in cellular function, possibly related to potassium transport. The disease is most common in young men. No specific physical findings may be found and it is often misdiagnosed as hysterical in origin.

2. **A 34-year-old woman with known myasthenia gravis presents in respiratory distress. She is unable to move without assistance. Her vital signs are: temperature 36°C (96.8°F), heart rate 50/min, blood pressure 100/60 mm Hg, respiratory rate 35/min and shallow. She is drooling and has upper airway rhonchi and bilateral wheezing. Her respiratory rate appears to be decreasing. You immediately:**

    a. Administer 2–4 mg of intravenous edrophonium.
    b. Perform endotracheal intubation.
    c. Administer 1 mg of atropine; if there is an improvement in her wheezing, administer pralidoxime.
    d. Start an intravenous atropine drip.
    e. Arrange emergent hyperbaric therapy.

    The answer is b. You should be able to differentiate a myasthenic crisis from a cholinergic crisis. Both can present with progressive muscle weakness and respiratory depression, dysphagia, and other physical signs. Bradycardia, wheezing, and salivation suggest cholinergic crisis. A common error is to mistake a cholinergic as a myasthenic crisis and administer additional acetylcholinesterase inhibitor. The immediate treatment for either type is ABCs and intubation at the first clinical signs of respiratory failure. In a cholinergic crisis, atropine can be used for the muscarinic symptoms, but it is not a substitute for airway management and ventilatory assistance.

3. **The initial diagnostic test to perform in a patient who presents with severe headache is:**

    a. Magnetic resonance angiography.
    b. Magnetic resonance imaging.
    c. Computerized tomography with contrast.
    d. Computerized tomography without contrast.
    e. Digital subtraction angiography.

    The answer is d. The CT scan without contrast remains the imaging procedure of choice for the ED initial examination of the patient with suspected intracranial disease. It is more sensitive than MRI for detecting acute intracranial bleeding and it is useful for detecting masses, hematomas, and hydrocephalus. MRI has greater sensitivity for tumors, acute infarctions, chronic subdural hematomas, and imaging the posterior fossa and the pituitary region. MRI is generally less available than CT scan, and for critically ill patients, MRI offers less access to the patient.

4. **Choose the true statement concerning migraine headache:**

    a. Auras in patients with migraine may include hemiplegia, ataxia, or visual field defects.
    b. The pain is typically unilateral and rarely becomes bilateral.
    c. The site of recurrent migraine headaches typically varies somewhat with each episode of pain.
    d. Migraines are often unpredictable and typically cause severe, sharp bitemporal pain.
    e. The prodrome occurs before the aura and is usually manifested by symptoms of depression, elation, or hunger.

    The answer is e. Migraine often occurs in a predictable time pattern for each patient. The prodrome precedes the actual attack by hours to days and is manifested by emotional feelings such as depression, elation, or hunger. The aura immediately precedes the headache. One model is that arterial vasoconstriction within a particular cerebral region dictates the nature of the aura, whether it be visual scintillating scotoma (occipital ischemia), hemiplegia (middle cerebral territory), or ataxia (posterior circulation). Arterial vasodilation then follows resulting in throbbing headache usually starting on one side but often becoming bilateral. Nausea and vomiting are typical symptoms.

5. **A previously healthy 32-year-old man is brought to the ED "confused" and complaining of a severe headache for at least 12 hours despite over-the-counter pain medication. Because of his presentation, you suspect a subarachnoid hemorrhage, knowing that:**

    a. A plain CT scan will diagnose 97% of subarachnoid hemorrhages.

    b. If the patient has no papilledema, you can safely perform lumbar puncture prior to CT scanning.

    c. If the patient has a subarachnoid hemorrhage, the spinal fluid will be xanthochromic.

    d. MRI offers no significant advantage over CT scan in this setting.

    e. Blood pressure should be reduced if the diastolic pressure is greater than 100 mm Hg.

    The answer is d. The most common site of a ruptured cerebral aneurysm is the anterior circle of Willis. A ruptured aneurysm causes an acute frontal headache that is aggravated by movement and recumbency. Intraparenchymal hemorrhage is frequently present. CT scan may be negative in up to 5% of cases of "fresh" subarachnoid hemorrhage; and, the percentage of false-negative studies is higher as the time from bleeding to CT scan increases. A lumbar puncture (LP) may be required to detect blood. Xanthochromia may develop within 4–6 hours. Papilledema may be a late (12–18 hours) finding and may not develop in some individuals. Other findings may include projectile vomiting, anisocoria, fluctuating mental status, hemiplegia, and diplopia. Acute treatment focuses on preserving cerebral perfusion. Blood pressure should not be acutely reduced unless diastolic pressures remain greater than 120 mm Hg. Vasodilator therapy (calcium channel blockers) has met with mixed success.

6. **Choose the correct statement about the treatment of status epilepticus in adults:**

    a. Phenytoin is the initial drug of choice in status epilepticus.

    b. The therapeutic agent for refractory seizures is pancuronium bromide.

    c. Magnesium must be administered in conjunction with intravenous phenytoin in patients who have second- and third-degree heart block.

    d. The mortality of status epilepticus is related to seizure-induced hypercarbia and electrolyte alterations.

    e. Intravenous pyridoxine may stop seizures due to isoniazid overdose.

    The answer is e. The mortality of status epilepticus is high and depends upon the etiology. Initial pharmacologic therapy for status epilepticus is IV lorazepam or diazepam. Additional pharmacologic intervention includes IV phenytoin, phenobarbital, or general anesthesia. Phenytoin may impair cardiac conduction and should not be administered in patients with second- or third-degree heart blocks. Seizures secondary to INH are treated with IV pyridoxine.

7.   **Choose the true statement about trigeminal neuralgia:**

   a. The pain is brief and radiates along the distribution of the first or second divisions of the trigeminal nerve.

   b. The pain is stabbing and, while initially unilateral, often becomes bilateral.

   c. Active suicidal ideation secondary to trigeminal neuralgia may resolve with a trial of a benzodiazepine.

   d. Pain may be precipitated by stimulation of a trigger zone (e.g., tapping the mandible, cheeks, maxillary sinus, or infraorbital rim).

   e. The differential diagnosis includes multiple sclerosis, migraine headache, giant cell arteritis, temporomandibular joint syndrome, and odontogenic disorders.

   The answer is d. The pain of trigeminal neuralgia is typically brief and radiates along the distribution of the second or third divisions of the trigeminal nerve. The typical patient with trigeminal neuralgia is a woman of approximately 50 years of age. Paroxysms of pain may be induced by gentle stimulation of a trigger zone (e.g., by chewing). Unlike migraine, there is no associated nausea, vomiting, or parasympathetic manifestation. Pain involving all three divisions of the trigeminal nerve makes the diagnosis unlikely. Untreated, the pain of trigeminal neuralgia may cause severe depression. Medical therapy consists of opioids for acute pain in addition to carbamazepine (side effects include bone marrow depression). If refractory to pharmacologic therapy, surgical radiotherapy with destruction of the trigeminal ganglion may be effective.

8.   **Choose the true statement concerning epilepsy:**

   a. Generalized seizures typically begin with rigid extension of both upper and lower extremities and progress to adduction and internal rotation of the shoulders associated with loss of consciousness.

   b. Temporal lobe seizures are easily diagnosed.

   c. Hypokalemia can cause seizure activity.

   d. Patients with isolated frontal lobe seizures may experience auditory hallucinations.

   e. All parts of the brain are equally susceptible to epileptogenic activity.

   The answer is d. The temporal lobe is the area of the brain most sensitive to hypoxia, hypoglycemia, and abnormal epileptic discharges. Primary seizure activity results from an idiopathic epileptogenic focus. Secondary causes of seizures include endocrine, toxic, metabolic, traumatic, infectious, and neoplastic disorders. The different areas of the brain vary in the sensitivity to seizures as well as in the manifestations. Temporal lobe (hallucination, memory, and emotional lability) seizures are perhaps the most easily misdiagnosed. The occipital lobe is least susceptible to seizure activity.

9.   **A 13-year-old girl presents with a 3-day history of malaise, low-grade fever, and double vision with unilateral ptosis. The potential diagnosis of botulism is best supported by finding:**

   a. Acute renal failure.

   b. Cardiac failure.

   c. Bilateral numbness of hands and feet.

   d. Acute urinary retention.

   e. Pseudomembranous pharyngitis.

   The answer is d. Both botulism and diphtheria may present with acute bulbar nerve palsies, weakness of any or all extremities, and cholinergic manifestations, such as urinary retention and colicky pain. In both diseases, the most common early neurologic findings are ptosis, double vision, and difficulty in accommodation. Diphtheria is an acute febrile illness. A primary symptom is a severe pseudomembranous pharyngitis presenting with severe throat pain and excessive saliva production. In diphtheria, cardiotoxic and renal abnormalities are direct results of the elaborated bacterial toxin.

10. **A 34-year-old woman with myasthenia gravis presents with flank pain and fever of 103.4°F. She is allergic to penicillin, and despite boluses of intravenous fluid and antibiotic therapy, she becomes hypotensive. A medicine that you can safely use in her management is:**

    a. Gentamicin.

    b. Vecuronium.

    c. Lidocaine.

    d. Procainamide.

    e. Succinylcholine.

    The answer is c. Aminoglycoside and polymyxin antibiotics have some curare-type effects on the motor endplate; if they are used in the myasthenic patient, the physician should be prepared to treat paralysis and respiratory arrest. Obviously, these patients are more susceptible to muscle-paralyzing agents as well. Phenytoin, quinidine, procainamide, and lithium can also adversely affect patients with myasthenia gravis.

11. **You can isolate the function of the seventh cranial nerve by:**

    a. Having the patient raise his eyebrows.

    b. Having the patient whistle or purse his lips.

    c. Having the patient open his mouth and say "ah."

    d. Testing the corneal reflex.

    e. Looking for asymmetry of tongue extension.

    The answer is b. The seventh cranial nerve controls all facial muscles except those of mastication. Peripheral lesions of the seventh nerve cause ipsilateral facial muscle weakness, but upper motor neuron lesions (brainstem and above) cause only ipsilateral lower facial weakness. Asymmetry of the nasolabial folds is a sign of dysfunction of the seventh nerve. The corneal reflex is mediated by a sensory (fifth nerve) arc in addition to the motor arc of the seventh nerve. Thus, unilateral suppression of the corneal reflex does not necessarily indicate a lesion of the seventh nerve.

12. **Choose the correct statement about headache:**

    a. Pain fibers arising from periventricular white matter as well as from intracranial arteries and veins may contribute to headache.

    b. A tumor below the tentorium will generally cause referred pain to the base of the skull.

    c. Unlike more superficial tumors, headache is an early symptom of brain lesions that lie deep within the cortex.

    d. Acute CSF outflow obstruction is generally painless.

    e. Headache of intracranial origin, unlike pain from extracranial structures, will generally remain unchanged with any maneuver such as direct pressure to the temporal area or head shaking.

    The answer is b. Pain from intracranial structures above the tentorium is mediated through the fifth nerve and will generally be felt in its distribution (i.e., in the area anterior to a frontal plane extending through the external auditory canals). Infratentorial pain is mediated by fibers of the ninth, tenth, and eleventh cranial nerves and may be perceived as infraoccipital or neck pain. The brain itself is devoid of nociceptors; therefore, a headache is caused by displacement, obstruction, or pressure on innervated areas. Lesions arising in certain areas of the brain (e.g., tumors of the frontal lobe) may alter the appreciation of pain.

13. Neuropathy is differentiated from myopathy in that:

   a. Neuropathies progress proximally.

   b. Myopathies affect distal and proximal muscle groups equally.

   c. Myopathies and neuropathies both have prominent sensory findings.

   d. Myopathies often have striking weakness of the small muscles of the hands.

   e. Myopathies have relatively preserved deep tendon reflexes.

   The answer is a. Neuropathies tend to have the following characteristics: proximal progression of symptoms, sensory deficits often in a stocking glove distribution, and early loss of DTRs. Myopathies characteristically present with proximal motor weakness, myalgias, and delayed loss of DTRs; CPK enzymes may be elevated. There are exceptions to these generalizations.

14. A 32-year-old man complains of a chronic, dull orbital headache. The pain is constant and made worse by head movements. Sleeping helps, but the pain may be present in the morning. Neurologic examination reveals only a right plantar extensor response. The most likely cause of this headache is:

   a. Sinus infection.

   b. Supratentorial tumor.

   c. Infratentorial tumor.

   d. Muscle tension.

   e. Metabolic.

   The answer is b. Characteristics of a headache from a space-occupying intracranial lesion include a dull, constant, boring quality, often increased by coughing or straining. The pain may be noted on awakening. Depending on the site of the lesion, focal localizing signs may be absent or transient. In muscle tension or other extracranial headaches, pressure over the area inhibits nociceptor impulses in the spinal cord and provides relief (e.g., massaging the forehead and neck in muscle tension headaches). CT scan is indicated in patients with a history of a prolonged or unexplained headache.

15. The best way to differentiate pseudoseizure or hysterical seizures from epileptic seizures is:

   a. The presence of urinary incontinence.

   b. The presence of plantar extensor responses in the postictal period.

   c. The presence of epileptogenic focus on EEG.

   d. The depth and duration of the postictal state.

   e. The presence of tongue biting or self-injury.

   The answer is c. The term epileptic seizure describes the abnormal behavior from paroxysmal abnormal cortical activity. In epileptic seizures, plantar responses are often upgoing, self-injury is common, and corneal reflexes are absent. In nonepileptic seizures, the seizure pattern often has an atypical appearance and incontinence is rare. The EEG is the best tool for differentiating the two conditions.

16. The average duration of a tonic–clonic seizure is:

   a. 15 seconds.

   b. 28 seconds.

   c. 60 seconds.

   d. 120 seconds.

   e. 148 seconds.

The answer is c. In a typical tonic–clonic seizure, electroencephalogram changes last an average of 59.9 seconds, and behavioral changes last only a few second longer. Thus, a seizure lasting 5 minutes is more than 17 standard deviations beyond the "typical" seizure.

17. **Choose the correct interpretation of reflexes:**

    a. Patient with root and grasp reflexes → brainstem lesion.
    b. Delayed deep tendon reflexes (DTRs) in all extremities → hypothyroidism.
    c. Brisk DTRs in upper and lower extremities → diffuse cortical lesion.
    d. Weak DTRs in upper and lower extremities → high spinal cord lesion.
    e. Right upper and right lower extremity DTRs 3+; left upper and lower extremity DTRs 1+ → Brown-Séquard lesion.

    The answer is b. Deep tendon reflexes are most helpful when they are asymmetric between extremities. Symmetrical DTRs and a normal neurologic examination are considered a normal variant. In hypothyroidism, the deep tendon reflexes are delayed, which is a different quality than decreased. Asymmetrical DTRs suggest a cortical lesion; asymmetrical DTRs of the upper and lower extremities would be suggestive of a cord lesion. Pure Brown-Séquard syndrome is associated with (1) interruption of the lateral corticospinal tracts—ipsilateral spastic paralysis below the level of the lesion, Babinski sign ipsilateral to lesion, abnormal reflexes and Babinski sign may not be present in acute injury; (2) interruption of posterior white column—ipsilateral loss of tactile discrimination, vibratory, and position sensation below the level of the lesion; and (3) interruption of lateral spinothalamic tracts with contralateral loss of pain and temperature sensation.

18. **A 40-year-old man complains of a unilateral periorbital headache accompanied by rhinorrhea and lacrimation. The most effective abortive therapy to treat this headache seems to be:**

    a. Transnasal sumatriptan.
    b. High-flow oxygen using a nonrebreather mask.
    c. Intravenous ketorolac.
    d. Valsalva maneuver while squatting.
    e. Papaya juice.

    The answer is b. Cluster headaches share with migraine headaches of a vascular origin and recurrent nature. Men are afflicted far more often than women. The age of onset, unlike that of migraine, is usually the mid-thirties to mid-forties. There is no aura, nausea, or vomiting. A cluster headache has recurrent characteristics of time, location, and duration. The pain has a boring quality and localizes to the frontal region. Unlike a migraine headache, it does not become bilateral or extend posteriorly to the scalp. A nocturnal onset is a characteristic but not invariable finding. Accompanying autonomic signs include ipsilateral lacrimation, rhinorrhea, and flushing. Intranasal drugs are usually not well absorbed because of the mucosal swelling. High-flow oxygen therapy using a nonrebreather mask can abort the attack in less than 1 minute.

19. **A 32-year-old patient is brought by his fiancée after she saw him have a tonic–clonic seizure. The patient has retrograde amnesia and complains of a headache and fatigue. He has no prior history of neurologic illness. Physical examination, laboratory studies, and a head CT scan are normal. You should now:**

    a. Administer a loading dose of phenobarbital and phenytoin and discharge with a prescription for both and follow-up.

    b. Give a loading dose of carbamazepine and discharge for follow-up.

    c. Admit the patient for observation despite his full recovery.

    d. Discharge the patient with instructions for prompt medical follow-up and instruct not to drive until further notice.

    e. Obtain an EEG in the ED.

The answer is d. The management of the patient with a first seizure is controversial. The goal is to reduce the risk of recurrent seizures. The etiology of the seizure and EEG results (not usually available in the ED) are the most important predictors of reoccurrence. Patients with no history of neurologic disease and who have a normal neurologic examination require individual risk–benefit analysis (pending EEG results, side effects, costs, alternatives) prior to initiating anticonvulsant therapy (good choices are carbamazepine or phenytoin). The patient should be referred to his primary care physician for additional treatment and diagnostic studies. Patients with a prior history of neurologic disease or who exhibit an abnormal neurologic examination should generally receive an anticonvulsant. This subgroup has a high risk of recurrence. Treatment can reduce the risk of recurrent seizures by half.

20. **There may be an indication for surgery in a patient with cerebellar hemorrhage and:**

    a. Hematoma more than 4.5 cm maximum in diameter.

    b. Glasgow Coma Scale score of 12 or greater on admission.

    c. Abnormal brainstem reflexes.

    d. Abnormal primitive reflexes.

    e. Hypotension.

The answer is c. Indications for surgery in patients with cerebellar hemorrhage are controversial. Ventriculostomy is indicated in patients with hemorrhage and hydrocephalus. Suboccipital craniotomy with clot evacuation is indicated in patients with altered level of consciousness and a large clot (>30 mm but not greater than 40 mm). Patients with a large central clot and absent brainstem reflexes have a poor prognosis. In these cases, some advocate supportive therapy only.

21. **Which of the following conditions is paired correctly?**

    a. History of camping → flaccid ascending paralysis.

    b. Proximal muscle pain and weakness → myasthenia gravis.

    c. Febrile upper respiratory infection → bilateral lower extremity weakness and hyperreflexia.

    d. Guillain-Barré syndrome → flaccid descending paralysis and muscle tenderness.

    e. Botulism → hyperreflexia, lower extremity weakness.

The answer is a. Clinically, the onset of tick paralysis is similar to Guillain-Barré syndrome, and both conditions should be considered in patients with ascending paralysis (which sometimes includes the bulbar muscles). In Guillain-Barré syndrome, weakness usually starts distally and ascends, paresthesias may be present, and the cerebrospinal protein is elevated. Tick paralysis is associated with an ascending paralysis and lacks bulbar involvement. Both wood and dog ticks can cause the disease, and their removal is curative. Guillain-Barré syndrome may occur after infections and in patients with collagen vascular disease. Polymyositis is a generic term and it has many underlying etiologies. Collagen vascular disease, toxoplasmosis, endocrinopathies, and occult cancer are part of the differential diagnosis. Although most neuropathies are chronic, a few have a rapid onset. Temporal arteritis is frequently associated with polymyalgia rheumatica. Botulism must be differentiated from other illnesses that cause paralysis. In myasthenia gravis, eye signs are also prominent, but pupillary response is preserved, no autonomic symptoms are present, and weakness responds to the administration of edrophonium. Diphtheria can be distinguished by the prolonged interval between pharyngitis and neurologic symptoms. Eaton-Lambert syndrome does not usually involve bulbar muscles.

22. **A 25-year-old patient is unresponsive. Serum glucose is normal and head examination shows no trauma. There is no response to intravenous naloxone. You perform cold caloric diagnostic maneuvers, knowing that:**

    a. Tonic deviation of both eyes toward the tested ear → intact cortex with brainstem dysfunction.

    b. Bilateral nystagmus → consider psychiatric diagnosis.

    c. No eye movement → intact brainstem.

    d. Fast phase of nystagmus away from the tested ear → cortical dysfunction.

    e. Tonic deviation of only the ipsilateral eye → hypothermia.

    The answer is b. In the comatose patient, oculovestibular testing or cold calorics may differentiate cortical and brainstem lesions. If the brainstem and cortex are both intact (patient is physiologically intact and awake), nystagmus will develop with the fast component away from the tested ear. If the cortex is not intact but the brainstem is functioning, the eyes will tonically deviate toward the tested ear. If both the cortex and brainstem are impaired, the eyes will not move in response to testing. If only the ipsilateral eye moves in response to testing, an internuclear ophthalmoplegia is present indicating structural damage to tracts in the brainstem.

23. **A 70-year-old man is brought by ambulance from home. He has an acute left hemiplegia affecting the leg more than the arm and face. He has grasp and suck reflexes and he perseverates. The most likely vascular territory of his stroke is in the distribution of the:**

    a. Middle cerebral artery (MCA).

    b. Posterior cerebral artery (PCA).

    c. Anterior cerebral artery (ACA).

    d. Vertebrobasilar artery.

    e. Cerebellar infarction.

    The answer is c. ACA strokes usually affect the leg more than the arm or face. MCA infarctions predominantly affect the face and upper extremity. PCA infarctions cause visual field deficits. Vertebrobasilar syndrome can present in numerous ways but there are usually crossed signs. There may be an ipsilateral cranial nerve deficit associated with contralateral hemiplegia. Cerebellar infarcts usually present as ataxia associated with nausea and vomiting. Cranial nerve findings may also be evident.

24. A 30-year-old diabetic woman with a history of severe gastroparesis presents obtunded and diaphoretic. Her vital signs are: rectal temperature, 103.4°F; heart rate, 140/min; respiratory rate, 36/min; blood pressure, 105/60 mm Hg. She has leukocytosis (WBC 18,000/mm³) and when the nurse inserts an indwelling catheter, the urine is the color of strong tea and dips strongly positive for hemoglobin. Serum total creatine kinase is 45,000 IU. The most specific treatment would include:

a. Dantrolene.

b. Edrophonium.

c. Systemic antibiotics.

d. Fluids and stress-dose steroids.

e. Physostigmine.

The answer is a. Neuroleptic malignant syndrome (NMS) is characterized by fever, altered mental status, and muscle rigidity. Patients can have marked elevation of their CPKs and develop myoglobinuric renal failure. Patients require the ABCs, cooling, and volume replacement. Treatment includes intravenous dantrolene every 6 hours for muscle relaxation. Bromocriptine, a direct dopamine agonist, may help treat hyperthermia.

25. While the pathophysiology of transient global amnesia (TGA) is unknown, it commonly occurs after physical exertion, emotional stress, pain, cold-water exposure, sexual intercourse, and Valsalva maneuver. The suspected common physiologic feature is:

a. Increased venous return to the superior vena cava.

b. Transient hypoxia.

c. Cholinergic surge.

d. GABA receptor hyperstimulation.

e. Internal jugular vein valvular incompetence.

The answer is a. The exact mechanism that produces TGA is unclear. Some evidence favors a migraine variant, as patients who suffer from a TGA event have a slightly higher incidence of a previous migraine, but patients with TGA rarely report an associated headache, nausea, photophobia, or phonophobia. Partial complex seizure (e.g., temporal lobe) is also unlikely, as TGA events are not associated with alteration of consciousness or stereotypical movements and EEG does not demonstrate epileptiform activity. Transient ischemic attacks (TIA) is also unlikely, as studies have demonstrated that patients with TGA have fewer cerebrovascular risk factors than those with known cerebrovascular or coronary artery disease; in addition, the prognosis for TGA is often better than for TIAs. While no sex predilection has been observed, triggers differ between men and women. For men, TGA occurs more often after a physical precipitating event, such as sexual intercourse. In women, episodes may be more associated with emotional precipitating events, a history of anxiety, or pathological personality. TGA event triggers have the common physiologic feature of increased venous return to the superior vena cava. The significance of this feature is still unclear.

26. A 55-year-old man with a recent upper respiratory illness presents with dizziness. His diagnosis is most likely peripheral rather than central vertigo because he has:

a. Tinnitus and pain on percussion of his ethmoid sinus.

b. Lateral, vertical, and rotary nystagmus.

c. Vertigo with nystagmus and diplopia on Hallpike maneuver.

d. Nystagmus that does not inhibit with ocular fixation.

e. Ataxia on finger-to-nose and heel-to-shin tests.

The answer is a. Classically, peripheral vertigo is characterized by prominent nausea and vomiting, unidirectional nystagmus that is aggravated by head position (Hallpike maneuver), a latency period, and inhibition by ocular fixation. It is often preceded by an upper respiratory illness or sinus condition. In contrast, central vertigo is characterized by minimal nausea; nystagmus that is not related to head position; no latency period; multidirectional, and is not inhibited by ocular fixation. Central vertigo may be associated with other brainstem signs such as diplopia, dysarthria, facial numbness, or limb weakness.

27. **A 65-year-old man with diabetes complains of painful right-sided ptosis and pupil-sparing, partial third cranial nerve palsy. He probably has:**

    a. Right posterior communicating aneurysm.

    b. Left anterior communicating aneurysm.

    c. Right carotid-cavernous fistula.

    d. Increased intracranial pressure.

    e. Diabetic right third-nerve palsy.

    The answer is e. Painful ophthalmoplegia due to isolated oculomotor or abducens palsy is fairly common in patients with diabetes. As a rule, cerebral aneurysms cause internal ophthalmoplegia before or along with involvement of the extraocular muscles. This is because the parasympathetic fibers that carry the pupillomotor information (to constrict the pupil) travel close to the surface of the oculomotor nerve and are spared by diabetes. Compressive lesions, such as aneurysms, thus first affect these fibers.

28. **A 38-year-old woman had an 8-mm saccular (berry) aneurysm of the left anterior communicating artery clipped surgically 6 days ago. She had no postoperative neurologic deficits and went home yesterday. She now returns by ambulance agitated, combative, and with right-sided hemiparesis (arm > leg). The most likely cause is:**

    a. Early hydrocephalus.

    b. Late hydrocephalus.

    c. Vasogenic edema.

    d. Vasospasm.

    e. Rebleeding.

    The answer is d. Vasospasm is the most feared and most devastating complication of SAH. It is responsible for 14–32% of deaths and permanent disability in SAH. A large amount of blood in the basal cisterns is a predictive factor for developing vasospasm. Once present, the mainstay of therapy is intravascular expansion (triple H therapy) to maintain perfusion in the narrowed vessel segments. Highly specialized centers offer intravascular interventions (e.g., local papaverine injection, angioplasty) for the treatment of vasospasm. Hydrocephalus presents with headache, decline in mental status, and other signs of increased intracranial pressure. Focal neurologic deficits are usually not a part of the presentation. Rebleeding is another major complication with a risk of 1% per day for the first 3 weeks after the initial bleed.

29. **The features of the neurologic examination which are most reliable in differentiating spinal cord infarction from the other apoplectic and acute causes of paraparesis such as cord compression by tumor or hematoma, demyelinating transverse myelitis, or epidural infection are:**

   a. Areflexia due to spinal shock.

   b. Urinary retention.

   c. Preservation of position and vibratory sensation.

   d. Bilateral Babinski reflex responses.

   e. Sparing of sacral sensation.

   The answer is c. A pattern of sensory dissociation characterized by loss of perception of pain and temperature below the level of the lesion and retention of position and vibratory sensation and even of light touch is characteristic of the ischemic lesion of spinal cord, also termed spinal artery thrombosis and myelomalacia. This is because, in transverse or axial orientation, ischemic lesions of the cord usually affect the vascular territory of the anterior spinal artery or its clinical equivalent, the central watershed territory, and spare the posterior columns, which carry proprioceptive and vibratory sense. Keep in mind that to affect bowel/bladder function bilateral involvement of the nervous system is required (brain, brainstem, spinal cord, nerve roots). Unilateral lesions will not cause problems in the bowel/bladder systems.

30. **The most common clinically recognized "lacunar syndrome" is:**

   a. Nonanatomic sensory paresis.

   b. Pure motor hemiparesis.

   c. Thalamic pain syndrome of Dejerine-Roussy.

   d. Hemiballismus.

   e. Proprioceptive symptoms only.

   The answer is b. Pure motor hemiparesis was the first clinically recognized lacunar syndrome and is also the most common of the lacunar syndromes, accounting for approximately one-half to two-thirds of the cases in several series. In the original definition, pure motor hemiparesis was described as "a paralysis of face, arm and leg on one side, unaccompanied by sensory signs, visual field defect, dysphasia or apractagnosia." Subsequently, this definition has been expanded to include patients without involvement of the face and with transient numbness or subjective heaviness of the affected limbs at the onset of the motor deficit. Pure sensory strokes, on the other hand, are limited to "a persistent or transient numbness and mild sensory loss over one side of the body, including face, arm, and leg," without associated hemiparesis, visual field defect, brainstem dysfunction, memory loss, dyslexia, or other deficits. Pure sensory strokes are less common than pure motor hemiparesis, occurring in approximately 6–7% of patients in an examined series of lacunar infarctions.

31. **Match the correct brain region with findings expected in a patient experiencing an intracerebral hemorrhage (ICH) in that region of the brain:**

   a. Brainstem → contralateral hemiparesis, contralateral sensory loss, contralateral conjugate gaze paresis, homonymous hemianopia, aphasia, neglect, or apraxia.

   b. Thalamus → contralateral sensory loss, contralateral hemiparesis, gaze paresis, homonymous hemianopia, miosis, aphasia, or confusion.

   c. Cerebellum → contralateral hemiparesis or sensory loss, contralateral conjugate gaze paresis, homonymous hemianopia, abulia, aphasia, neglect, or apraxia.

   d. Putamen → quadriparesis, facial weakness, decreased level of consciousness, gaze paresis, ocular bobbing, miosis, or autonomic instability.

   e. Lobar → ataxia, usually beginning in the trunk, ipsilateral facial weakness, ipsilateral sensory loss, gaze paresis, skew deviation, miosis, or decreased level of consciousness.

The answer is b. Clinical manifestations of ICH are determined by the size and location of hemorrhage, but may include hypertension, fever, cardiac arrhythmias, neck rigidity, subhyaloid retinal hemorrhages, altered level of consciousness, anisocoria, or focal neurologic deficits. These deficits vary depending on the region of brain affected:

- Putamen—contralateral hemiparesis, contralateral sensory loss, contralateral conjugate gaze paresis, homonymous hemianopia, aphasia, neglect, or apraxia.
- Thalamus—contralateral sensory loss, contralateral hemiparesis, gaze paresis, homonymous hemianopia, miosis, aphasia, or confusion.
- Lobar—contralateral hemiparesis or sensory loss, contralateral conjugate gaze paresis, homonymous hemianopia, abulia, aphasia, neglect, or apraxia.
- Caudate nucleus—contralateral hemiparesis, contralateral conjugate gaze paresis, or confusion.
- Brainstem—quadriparesis, facial weakness, decreased level of consciousness, gaze paresis, ocular bobbing, miosis, or autonomic instability.
- Cerebellum—ataxia, usually beginning in the trunk, ipsilateral facial weakness, ipsilateral sensory loss, gaze paresis, skew deviation, miosis, or decreased level of consciousness.

32. **The National Institutes of Health Stroke Scale (NIHSS):**
    a. Offers no prognostic information.
    b. Measures motor and sensory defects only.
    c. Does not include a measurement of level of consciousness.
    d. Includes vision changes, but not language.
    e. Can help identify patients who are likely to respond to fibrinolytic therapy.

    The answer is e. The NIHSS can be used easily, is reliable and valid, provides insight to the location of vascular lesions, and can be correlated with outcome in patients with ischemic stroke. It focuses on six major areas of the neurologic examination: (1) level of consciousness, (2) visual function, (3) motor function, (4) sensation and neglect, (5) cerebellar function, and (6) language. The NIHSS is used most by stroke teams. It enables the consultant to rapidly determine the severity and possible location of the stroke. A patient's score on the NIHSS is strongly associated with outcome, and it can help identify those patients who are likely to respond to thrombolytic therapy and those who are at higher risk to develop hemorrhagic complications of thrombolytic use.

33. **A 24-year-old college student with a known seizure disorder failed to take any phenytoin for the last week because of final examinations. He had three seizures today and was brought by his roommate for treatment. The patient weighs approximately 220 lb, and his serum phenytoin level is 0. You need to give him a loading dose of approximately:**
    a. 800 mg.
    b. 1000 mg.
    c. 1200 mg.
    d. 1500 mg.
    e. 1800 mg.

    The answer is e. Phenytoin is the primary drug used in the management of status epilepticus after initial benzodiazepine therapy. It may also be used as primary therapy for patients whose seizures are less frequent. The recommended loading dose is 18–20 mg/kg IV, and so for this 100-kg patient, a dose of 1800–2000 mg is appropriate. Infusion should be limited to 50 mg/min due to the cardiotoxicity of the diluent. Patient should be on a cardiac monitor.

34.   **Yesterday you saw a 27-year-old man who had "the worst headache of his life." After a normal brain CT scan, you performed lumbar puncture. You instructed the patient to remain flat for 2 hours. The results of the spinal tap are negative, and you sent the patient home with appropriate analgesia. Twenty-seven hours later he returns, saying he has an even worse headache than before. You suspect postdural puncture headache (PDPH):**

a. An autologous blood patch will relieve the headache in a majority of patients with this condition.

b. The headache is from a hyperstimulatory overproduction of cerebrospinal fluid and can be relieved by a second tap with removal of more fluid.

c. This is an uncommon complication, occurring in less than 10% of patients.

d. You had correctly used a large needle to minimize the amount of time needed to remove fluid, and this should have prevented the headache.

e. You realize you should have had him stay flat for at least 2 more hours to avoid this complication.

The answer is a. Headache is the most common complication of lumbar puncture, occurring in up to 40% of patients. The amount of time a patient remains recumbent after lumbar puncture does not appear to affect the incidence of headache. Certain factors have been implicated as causes of PDPH, including the size or diameter of the spinal needle, the orientation of the bevel during the procedure, and the amount of fluid withdrawn. Smaller-diameter needles will cause less leakage, and it is postulated that inserting the needle with the bevel up (i.e., bevel pointing up when the patient is in the lateral position) will minimize damage to the dural fibers. Using atraumatic needles or pencil-point needles (e.g., Whitaker or Sprotte) has also been shown to significantly reduce the incidence of PDPH. Most PDPH headaches resolve spontaneously within a few days with bed rest and mild analgesics. For persistent headaches, oral caffeine 300 mg every 4–6 hours or caffeine sodium benzoate (500 mg in 1 L of fluid) may be effective. For severe headaches lasting more than 24 hours, an epidural blood patch (autologous blood clot) will relieve the headache in the majority of patients.

Obstetric and Gynecologic Emergencies

CHAPTER 13

Thomas B. Barry, MD

1. **When attempting to make the diagnosis of pregnancy:**

   a. If the urine has a specific gravity of 1.020 or greater, the sensitivity of a urine immunologic test for pregnancy is equal to IRA of serum beta-hCG.

   b. An intrauterine gestational sac, if present, can be reliably detected by ultrasound when the quantitative serum beta-hCG reaches 1200 mIU.

   c. A complex adnexal mass or free fluid in the cul-de-sac seen with ultrasound and a positive pregnancy test is pathognomonic for ectopic pregnancy.

   d. Transvaginal ultrasound will show a viable intrauterine pregnancy not earlier than 7 weeks of gestation.

   e. An intrauterine pregnancy is reliably distinguished from the decidual reaction in the normal menstrual cycle by the presence of a double white line around the gestational sac.

   The answer is e. The reliability of urine pregnancy tests is affected by the concentration of the urine. When a test sensitive to 25 IU/L is used, a negative test 1 week after the "missed period" virtually guarantees that the woman is not pregnant. The gestational sac can be detected by transvaginal ultrasound by approximately 5 weeks, and transabdominal at 6 weeks. The fetal heartbeat appears shortly after the sixth week. The absence of a heartbeat may indicate a missed abortion if a fetus is seen, or a blighted ovum if only a sac is present. If the serum beta-hCG is greater than 1600–1800 mIU and no intrauterine gestational sac is seen on transvaginal ultrasound, ectopic pregnancy is likely. The definitive diagnosis of ectopic pregnancy by ultrasound requires visualizing a fetus or fetal heartbeat outside the uterus.

2.   **During normal vaginal delivery, the accepted method for delivering the baby's shoulder is:**

   a. Gentle traction upward on baby's head to deliver the posterior shoulder, then traction downward to deliver the anterior shoulder.

   b. Gentle traction upward to deliver the posterior shoulder, deliver the posterior arm, then traction downward to deliver the anterior shoulder.

   c. Hook an index finger in baby's anterior axilla to deliver the anterior shoulder and arm, then gentle traction to deliver the posterior shoulder.

   d. Gentle traction on baby's neck downward to deliver the anterior shoulder, then traction upward to deliver the posterior shoulder.

   e. Gentle traction on baby's head downward to deliver the anterior shoulder, then traction upward to deliver the posterior shoulder.

   The answer is e. With one hand on the baby's head and while instructing the mother not to push, the covered second hand lifts the chin up posterior to the maternal anus (modified Ritgen maneuver). After delivering the head, palpating the neck for the umbilical cord, and suctioning the airway, both hands are applied to the baby's head and downward traction is applied to deliver the anterior shoulder from beneath the pubic symphysis. Flexing the hips or applying suprapubic pressure may aid in disimpacting the anterior shoulder at this point. After the anterior shoulder appears, gentle upward traction is used to deliver the posterior shoulder (remember: head up-down-up.) Brachial plexus palsies or rectal lacerations may occur if too much force is used.

3.   **Normal cardiovascular changes in pregnancy include:**

   a. Decreased heart rate.

   b. Increased cardiac output in the supine position during the third trimester.

   c. Increased systolic and diastolic blood pressures during the second trimester.

   d. Increased supraventricular ectopy.

   e. Decreased plasma volume.

   The answer is d. Physiologic changes occur in pregnancy that may be confused with abnormal medical conditions or, in the case of trauma, hypovolemia, and internal hemorrhage. The heart rate normally increases during pregnancy, reaching 15–20 beats above the nonpregnant rate in the late third trimester. Blood pressure falls by 10–15 mm Hg by the second trimester; blood plasma volume increases by 33% (450 mL) and blood volume by 45%. A physiologic anemia is the result, and this increased plasma volume should be considered when managing fluids in the pregnant trauma patient. Because the uterus will compress the inferior vena cava in the supine position later in pregnancy, cardiac output will fall and may result in hypotension.

4.   **Following spontaneous vaginal delivery, excessive bleeding can be managed by:**

   a. Performing uterine massage.

   b. Administering fresh frozen plasma.

   c. Giving intramuscular oxytocin.

   d. Administering recombinant factor VIIa.

   e. Transfusing packed red cells.

The answer is a. Transfusion alone does not address the cause of the hemorrhage, and appropriate management of postpartum bleeding will most often prevent it from being needed. The placenta should be allowed to separate spontaneously in most cases, since traction risks cord rupture or uterine inversion. Uterine atony is responsible for many cases of postpartum bleeding and can often be controlled with uterine massage, intramuscular methylergonovine, or intravenous oxytocin. Adequate venous access should be assured and the patient typed and cross-matched. If the bleeding continues, emergent obstetrical consultation should be obtained because uterine curettage may be needed. Direct bimanual uterine compression or uterine packing is rarely needed. Recombinant factor VIIa has not been studied in postpartum bleeding.

5. A 21-year-old woman, G2P0Ab1, whose last menstrual period (LMP) was 6 weeks ago, complains of vaginal spotting for 1 week and a 3-day history of right lower quadrant pain. Choose the true statement concerning appropriate diagnostic steps:

    a. Urine pregnancy tests are rarely positive before 5 weeks of amenorrhea.
    b. In a normal pregnancy, pelvic sonography can demonstrate an intrauterine sac with a fetal pole by 4 weeks gestation.
    c. Tubal pregnancies are uncommonly visualized with pelvic ultrasound.
    d. Abdominal examination is rarely normal in a patient with ectopic pregnancy.
    e. An adnexal mass rules out an intrauterine gestation.

    The answer is c. In any patient presenting with complaints of vaginal bleeding and abdominal pain, ectopic pregnancy must be ruled out. The diagnosis of pregnancy can be made with the new urine pregnancy tests at the time of the first day of missed menses provided the urine is concentrated. Ultrasound can demonstrate a gestational sac in the uterus by 5 weeks gestation and a fetal pole by 6 weeks. The definitive diagnosis of tubal pregnancy (gestational sac with a fetal pole and cardiac motion in the adnexa) by ultrasound is uncommon. In patients with a serum hCG level of 1500 mIU/mL and fluid in the pouch of Douglas or an adnexal mass (and no IUP), ectopic pregnancy is virtually certain. Early ectopic pregnancies may exhibit minimal physical findings. An adnexal mass may represent the normal corpus luteum of an intrauterine pregnancy.

6. A 36-year-old woman, G8P7, whose LMP was 12 weeks ago, complains of bleeding and cramping. Her urine pregnancy test is positive. She denies passage of tissue. On examination, her cervix is closed and the uterus is 18 weeks in size. On ultrasound, heterogeneous tissue in a "snowstorm" pattern is seen to fill the uterus, and large bilateral cystic ovaries are seen. Her diagnosis is:

    a. Leiomyomata of the uterus.
    b. Molar pregnancy.
    c. Missed abortion.
    d. Endometrial cancer.
    e. Hematometrium.

    The answer is b. The scenario is a classic presentation of complete hydatidiform mole. A high quantitative serum beta-hCG level is expected. The large cystic ovaries (theca lutein cysts stimulated by the high beta-hCG levels) are common in molar pregnancy, along with a uterine size larger than would be expected by dates. Following successful D&C, the cysts regress and the beta-hCG levels fall. Neoplastic disease develops in approximately 15% of molar pregnancies with molar tissue persisting after evacuation. Metastatic disease may develop.

7. **A drug inappropriate to use during pregnancy is:**

    a. Erythromycin base.
    b. Heparin.
    c. Warfarin.
    d. Prednisone.
    e. Prochlorperazine.

    The answer is c. Warfarin crosses the placenta and is associated with a high rate of fetal malformation with first-trimester exposures. Use in the third-trimester results in fetal hemorrhagic complications. Heparin is the anticoagulant of choice in pregnancy because it does not cross the placenta. There have been associations noted with the use of unfractionated heparin and fetal osteoporosis, thrombocytopenia, miscarriage, and prematurity, but untreated maternal venous thrombosis is felt to be a greater risk. Low molecular weight heparin appears to show less risk of fetal osteoporosis and thrombocytopenia. Erythromycin estolate is associated with cholestatic hepatitis in the pregnant mother, but no adverse effects have been noted with therapeutic use of erythromycin base, prednisone, or prochlorperazine.

8. **The laboratory finding which reflects the normal physiologic changes in pregnancy is:**

    a. Leukopenia.
    b. Elevated transaminases.
    c. Increased BUN and creatinine.
    d. Increased PT and aPTT, leading to coagulopathy.
    e. Decreased P_{CO_2}.

    The answer is e. As a result of an increased glomerular filtration rate (GFR), the BUN and creatinine normally decrease during pregnancy. The alkaline phosphatase may double or triple as a result of placental production. A leukocytosis, with WBCs reaching 18,000 in the second and third trimester, is common, along with a mild anemia, which is the result of an expanded plasma volume. Fibrinogen and factors VII, VIII, IX, and X all increase during pregnancy and thus increase both the sedimentation rate and the risk of deep venous thrombosis. The PT and PTT are both shortened. There is an increased awareness of a need to breathe from early pregnancy onward. During pregnancy, tidal volume increases with the diaphragm ascending 4 cm and a 2-cm increase in the transverse diameter of the thorax. The increased tidal volume reduces P_{CO_2}.

9. **In the absence of continuous fetal heart rate monitoring, the most acceptable method of evaluating fetal heart rate during labor is:**

    a. Checking fetal heart rate for 1 minute every hour in early labor, then once every 15 minutes during pushing.
    b. Checking fetal heart rate every 15 minutes during the first stage of labor, every 5 minutes during the second stage of labor.
    c. Checking fetal heart rate every 15 minutes during the first and second stages of labor, then every 5 minutes during the third stage.
    d. Checking fetal heart rate during every contraction during the first and second stages of labor.
    e. Checking fetal heart rate every hour during early labor, then every 5 minutes during pushing.

    The answer is b. Intermittent auscultation with a Doppler fetoscope or fetal stethoscope is necessary if electronic fetal monitoring is not available. The accepted standard of care is to check every 15 minutes during stage I (prior to complete cervical dilatation), then every 5 minutes during the second stage (complete dilatation to delivery). If fetal bradycardia occurs (rate <120/min), the mother should be turned on her left side, given oxygen, and an intravenous fluid bolus. The possibility of prolapse of the umbilical cord should be checked for during vaginal examination.

10. **Choose the correct statement concerning the use of ultrasound in third-trimester bleeding:**
    a. Ultrasound frequently can make the definitive diagnosis of abruptio placentae.
    b. In a patient with third-trimester bleeding, an ultrasound examination should be performed prior to vaginal examination.
    c. If found during the second trimester, placenta previa requires the patient to have a therapeutic abortion.
    d. An extremely full bladder is needed to make the correct diagnosis of placenta previa.
    e. The number of ultrasounds performed during the third trimester should be limited, as they have been implicated in the occurrence of excessive bleeding after delivery.

    The answer is b. Ultrasound should be performed prior to vaginal examination in the patient with third-trimester bleeding to exclude the diagnosis of placenta previa. If previa is absent, the next most common cause of third-trimester bleeding is abruptio placentae. This diagnosis is not accurately made by ultrasound. Most important is stabilizing the patient and obtaining emergent consultation. Early in pregnancy, placenta previa is seen frequently but disappears due to growth of the lower uterine segment and is of no clinical significance. An extremely full bladder can deform the lower uterine segment and result in a false-positive diagnosis of placenta previa. The scan should show the internal cervical os or cervical canal, or be done in the plane of the vagina to ensure a midline scan is performed.

11. **When evaluating the results of hCG testing it is important to remember that:**
    a. Urine pregnancy test can detect pregnancy only as early as a week after the first missed menses.
    b. Serum beta-hCG approximately doubles every 3–4 days in a normal pregnancy.
    c. Beta-hCG should be undetectable within 2 weeks of a therapeutic abortion.
    d. Beta-hCG may be detected in the serum up to 35 days after a spontaneous abortion.
    e. Transvaginal ultrasound usually cannot detect a gestational sac until the serum beta-hCG is 1800 IU.

    The answer is d. Standard urine pregnancy tests can detect beta-hCG at levels of 25–50 IU. This means that a pregnancy can be diagnosed around the first missed menses. The serum beta-hCG doubles every 2 days and peaks at 60 days postimplantation. It can be detected up to 21 days after delivery and persist for 2 months after an abortion. In experienced hands, transvaginal ultrasound can visualize a gestational sac when the serum beta-hCG is above 800 mIU/mL and vaginal ultrasound should still be considered when the serum hCG level is below 1000 mIU/mL.

12. **A 38-year-old woman complains of 4 days of heavy vaginal bleeding, at the rate of 6–10 pads per day. Her periods are usually light and regular. Pregnancy test is negative and there are no signs or symptoms of anemia. You should:**
    a. Prescribe oral conjugated estrogen with no further treatment if bleeding stops.
    b. Order coagulation studies and a liver function panel even in the absence of petechiae, ecchymosis, or previous bleeding problems.
    c. Reassure the patient and refer for follow-up testing by gynecology.
    d. Check CBC and repeat in 24 hours.
    e. Reassure the patient that the bleeding will likely stop in a day or two.

    Answer is c. Nonovulatory cycles may be quite heavy. Menorragia from anovulation is seen in 10–15% of women. If bleeding persists for more than 9 days or recurs in less than 21 days further testing is required. Heavy bleeding may be due to malignancy, adenomyosis, polyps, fibroids, and endometrial hyperplasia. Idiopathic heavy bleeding without pathology responds to medical treatment in less than 50% of cases. In nonpregnant women older than 35 years, follow-up usually includes endometrial biopsy.

13.   **A 27-year-old female, G1P0, at 24 weeks gestation complains of difficulty breathing and severe wheezing. She has a history of asthma, but stopped her medicines when she found she was pregnant, for fear of harming her baby. Your treatment of this patient should:**

a. Avoid oxygen, as it can cause placental shunting.

b. Not include steroids unless her life is in danger.

c. Include all standard therapies she would receive if not pregnant.

d. Include subcutaneous epinephrine only if her life is in danger.

e. Include prophylactic magnesium sulfate to prevent premature labor.

The answer is c. Asthma management in the pregnant patient differs little from the nonpregnant patient. Beta$_2$-agonists are first-line therapy. Epinephrine may decrease uteroplacental blood flow. Steroids remain a core treatment in the pregnant patient. Oxygen should be administered to all symptomatic pregnant asthmatics. The fetus is even more sensitive to hypoxia than the mother. Magnesium is often used in treatment of refractory asthma and eclampsia. During labor, it should be used with caution as it relaxes smooth muscle in the uterus.

14.   **Regarding the treatment of urinary tract infections during pregnancy:**

a. Asymptomatic bacteriuria is a normal variant and does not require therapy.

b. Any urine with bacteria or leukocytes should be cultured during pregnancy.

c. Nitrofurantoin is contraindicated during the first trimester.

d. If treated appropriately, there is a low rate of recurrence during the same pregnancy.

e. Pyelonephritis, but not cystitis, increases the risk of preterm labor and delivery.

The answer is b. Asymptomatic bacterial cystitis and pyelonephritis need to be aggressively diagnosed and treated in the pregnant patient because they increase the risk of miscarriage and premature delivery. Thirty percent of women with asymptomatic bacteriuria may develop pyelonephritis if left untreated. Pregnant patients with pyelonephritis have increased morbidity and require admission. Because urinary infections have a high rate of recurrence, patients require close follow-up.

15.   **Bacterial vaginosis often includes the presence of:**

a. Diffuse vaginal erythema.

b. Thick pink-yellow discharge.

c. Vaginal pH less than 4.5.

d. Negative amine test.

e. Clue cells.

The answer is e. The Amsel criteria require that three of four of the following be present for the diagnosis to be made: a thin homogeneous discharge; pH of discharge greater than 4.5; positive amine odor (whiff) test; presence of clue cells. A diffusely erythematous vaginal mucosa is more commonly associated with trichomonas vaginitis.

16. **A 23-year-old woman, G1P0, at 27 weeks gestation complains of right upper quadrant pain. Vital signs: blood pressure, 140/90 mm Hg; heart rate, 95/min; respiratory rate, 22/min; temperature, 37.5°C. The CBC shows: WBC, 12,000/mm³; hemoglobin, 10.5; platelets, 90,000; schistocytes are seen on the peripheral smear. Bilirubin is 1.4 mg/dL and SGOT is 120. Her probable diagnosis is:**

  a. Cholecystitis with a common duct stone.

  b. HELLP syndrome.

  c. Hepatitis.

  d. Gastritis.

  e. Fitz-Hugh-Curtis syndrome.

  The answer is b. The HELLP syndrome is an acronym for hemolysis, elevated liver enzymes, and low platelets (less than 100,000). It is an uncommon presentation of preeclampsia, which includes hypertension, edema, and proteinuria. It develops in 5–10% of women with preeclampsia. These patients frequently have right upper quadrant or epigastric pain. Treatment is the same as preeclampsia: magnesium sulfate (6 mg bolus followed by a 2 g/h drip) and hydralazine (5–10 mg IV) for diastolic blood pressure above 105 mm HG.

17. **When assessing the urine dipstick test in a young woman with suspected UTI one should remember:**

  a. Urine nitrite test is more than 90% specific but 50% sensitive.

  b. Urine leukocyte esterase test is 50% specific but 90% sensitive.

  c. A negative test for both leukocyte esterase and nitrites excludes the possibility of UTI.

  d. Bacteria counts in urine are stable at room temperature.

  e. Consider a catheterized specimen as there is no risk of causing UTI and increases accuracy.

  Answer is a. Urine nitrite specificity is greater than 90% making it a good confirmatory test. Its 50% sensitivity makes it a poor screening tool. Leukocyte esterase sensitivity is 48% with usual levels of pyuria but is 80–90% specific. Negative dip does not exclude the possibility if UTI. One to two percent of patients will develop a UTI after a single catheter insertion. Bacteria in urine double each hour at room temperature.

18. **You have diagnosed a patient with preeclampsia and started appropriate therapy with intravenous magnesium sulfate. You now monitor her for signs of toxicity, which include:**

  a. Fever.

  b. Respiratory depression.

  c. Hyperreflexia.

  d. Hypotension.

  e. Tachycardia.

  The answer is b. Magnesium administration should always be accompanied by clinical observation for loss of reflexes (which occurs at approximately 10 mg/dL) or respiratory depression (which occurs at levels over 12 mg/dL.) The infusion should be stopped if signs of hypermagnesemia are seen, as it may result in respiratory depression requiring ventilatory support. Calcium gluconate, 1 g IV given slowly will reverse the adverse effects of hypermagnesemia.

19. **Perimortem cesarean section is recommended only when:**

    a. An obstetrician is available to perform the procedure.

    b. Fetal heart sounds are present.

    c. Resuscitation of the mother has stopped or been determined to be futile.

    d. The fetus is at 26 weeks of gestation or greater.

    e. Ultrasound confirms fetal gestation time and viability.

    The answer is b. Perimortem cesarean section in the ED should be performed if uterine size exceeds the umbilicus and fetal heart tones are present. Bedside ultrasound may also be used to quickly assess the presence of a fetal heart rate. No physician has been found liable for performing a perimortem cesarean. Time since maternal circulation ceased is the critical factor in fetal outcome. It is a difficult decision for the clinician to make but hesitation decreases chances for fetal survival. Reports show that 70% of children who survive perimortem cesarean sections are delivered in less than 5 minutes of ED arrival. Rapid extraction avoiding further injury to the mother or fetus is the goal. Maternal CPR is continued. A vertical incision is made from umbilicus to pubis. The bladder is retracted and a 5 cm vertical incision is made in the lower uterus and extended superiorly to the fundus with scissors, using one's fingers to protect the fetus.

20. **A 30-year-old African American woman complains of abdominal pain during menses. Her pregnancy test is negative. She was once told that she might have fibroids and is worried because she does not know how dangerous that might be. You tell her:**

    a. Fibroids are uncommon in African Americans.

    b. Fibroids may cause pain and bleeding but are not malignant.

    c. Fibroid degeneration is likely and you will test for it.

    d. Fibroids often cause pain with menses and this is what she is experiencing.

    e. Surgical removal of fibroids provides a permanent cure.

    The answer is b: Fibroids are benign muscle cell tumors. They occur in 25% of white women and 50% of African American women. Up to 30% of patients with leiomyomas (fibroids) have pain and abnormal bleeding. Degeneration from rapid growth and loss of blood supply occurs almost only during early pregnancy. There is a 25–30% recurrence rate after surgical removal.

21. **Anti-D immunoglobulin is definitely indicated in first trimester Rh-negative women with:**

    a. Threatened abortion and scant vaginal bleeding.

    b. Complete abortion.

    c. Lower abdominal pain.

    d. Vomiting lasting beyond 48 hours.

    e. Urinary tract infection untreated for 5 days.

    The answer is b. The American College of Obstetrics and Gynecology (ACOG) regards Rh immunization as the result of first trimester threatened abortion as "exceedingly rare." Many British authorities regard it as unnecessary with a viable fetus before 12 weeks gestation. The need for prophylaxis after a complete spontaneous abortion is not as controversial and is a level A recommendation by the ACOG. (Level B by The American College of Emergency Physicians [ACEP].) ACOG treats the management of ectopic pregnancy the same as any first trimester termination.

22. **The correct dose of Rh immune globulin (RhoGAM) for maternal bleeding during a particular time during pregnancy is:**

   a. First trimester: Rh negative—50 μg.

   b. First trimester: Rh positive—50 μg.

   c. Second trimester: Rh negative—50 μg.

   d. Second trimester: Rh positive—300 μg.

   e. Third trimester: Rh positive— 300 μg.

   The answer is a. Administration of at least one prophylactic dose of RhoGAM may be indicated with Rh-negative pregnant patients who have vaginal bleeding. Each 10 μg of RhoGAM protects against 1 mL of fetal blood. Since a first trimester fetus contains no more than a teaspoon (5 mL) of blood, 50 μg is sufficient. Bleeding during second trimester or later requires the higher dose of 300 μg, which protects against 30 mL of fetal blood.

23. **You have just diagnosed ectopic pregnancy in a 25-year-old woman. She is hemodynamically stable. She asks about methotrexate therapy, but you inform her she is not a candidate because she has:**

   a. A fever.

   b. An ovarian, rather than tubal, pregnancy.

   c. An allergy to eggs.

   d. Free fluid in the cul-de-sac.

   e. Fetal cardiac activity.

   The answer is e. Methotrexate is a potent folate antagonist that inhibits the enzyme dihydrofolate reductase, blocking DNA synthesis prior to cell division. Certain prognostic factors have been identified that are associated with a higher failure rate of methotrexate treatment including higher hCG concentrations (greater than 10,000 mIU/mL) and presence of fetal cardiac activity.

24. **A 23-year-old woman G2P1 complains of vaginal spotting and is fearful that she may be miscarrying. You perform bedside ultrasound and confirm an intrauterine pregnancy and show the patient the presence of fetal heartbeats. You now know the risk for her to miscarry is:**

   a. More than 20%.

   b. More than 15%.

   c. Approximately 5–15%

   d. Less than 1%.

   e. Unknown.

   The answer is c: Once fetal heart tones are identified, the risk of miscarriage is approximately 5% in all women and up to 15% in patients with vaginal bleeding.

25.   A patient with a molar pregnancy:

a. Requires laparoscopic biopsy for definitive diagnosis.

b. Usually presents because of hyperemesis gravidarum.

c. Almost always aborts before 12 weeks.

d. Is usually clinically apparent by 8 weeks.

e. Has a uterine size larger than expected by dates approximately 40% of the time.

The answer is e. Early molar pregnancy is usually not clinically apparent. Bleeding or intermittent bloody discharge or failure to hear fetal heart tones during the second trimester is usually the first indication. If spontaneous abortion occurs with molar pregnancy, it is usually during the second trimester (before 20 weeks), and the patient may note passage of grapelike vesicles. Uterine size is larger than expected by dates in approximately 40% of patients. Theca lutein cysts may be present on the ovaries as a result of excessive hormonal stimulation and torsion of the ovary may occur. The diagnosis of hydatidiform mole is based on the characteristic sonographic appearance of hydropic vesicles within the uterus ("snowstorm" appearance).

26.   When evaluating a patient for premature rupture of membranes (PROM) and trying to differentiate amniotic fluid from vaginal discharge it is helpful to remember that amniotic fluid:

a. Has a pH of 7–7.5.

b. Has a pH of 4.5–5.

c. Leaves nitrazine paper yellow.

d. Does not show ferning when dried on a slide.

e. Is always more watery than vaginal secretions.

The answer is a. Amniotic fluid has a pH of 7–7.5 and turns the nitrazine paper from yellow to green or blue. Vaginal secretions have a pH of 4.5–5. False-negative tests may be caused by small amounts of amniotic fluid being diluted by vaginal secretions. False-positives may occur with vaginal secretions mixed with blood or semen or affected by bacterial vaginosis.

27.   When assessing for urinary tract infections in young women:

a. Suprapubic discomfort during urination is more likely to indicate UTI than perineal burning during urination.

b. Cloudy urine is likely due to WBCs.

c. Dysuria and frequency without vaginal discharge is only 70% predictive.

d. The relation of intercourse to UTI is an oldwife's tale—there is no correlation.

e. Cultures must always be done prior to treatment.

The answer is a. Burning suprapubic pain is more associated with UTI than external dysuria. Urine cloudiness is usually not due to WBC but to amorphous phosphate crystals or proteins. Dysuria with frequency is 90% predictive in the young, sexually active woman without vaginal discharge. Bacterial concentration in the bladder may increase tenfold during intercourse because of milking action on the urethra. Treatment of suspected UTI on the basis of symptoms alone is proving both cost-efficient and cost-effective in patients without complicating factors.

28. **Vaginal bleeding during the third trimester:**
    a. Indicates labor will soon occur.
    b. May be considered a normal variant.
    c. Necessitates a digital examination to determine cause.
    d. Should always be considered an emergency.
    e. Indicates fetal demise.

    The answer is d. Hemorrhagic exsanguinations can occur in minutes. Placenta previa and placenta abruptia are typical causes though bleeding from vaginal, rectal, or cervical lesions is possible. Placenta previa occurs in 1/180–390 deliveries and is characterized by vaginal bleeding with little or no pain. Abruptio placenta occurs in 1/200 pregnancies and has a mortality rate of 25%! It is typically accompanied by varied amounts of abdominal pain and may be associated with DIC. Digital examination is contraindicated until placenta previa can be excluded.

29. **When evaluating a vaginal discharge:**
    a. Gonorrhea or chlamydia are the usual causes.
    b. Symptoms allow confident differentiation of causality.
    c. Candidiasis is usually associated with a pH of greater than 5.
    d. Wet mount is seldom useful in making the diagnosis.
    e. Gardnerella is always pathologic.

    The answer is c. Symptoms alone do not allow confident diagnosis of the cause of vaginosis, although lack of itch makes candida less likely and lack of odor makes bacterial vaginosis unlikely. Gardnerella may be part of the normal vaginal flora. Thirty percent of women with vaginal complaints go without clear diagnosis even after examination with techniques more comprehensive than usually available in the emergency department. An association between Chlamydia and discharge has not been confirmed. Wet mount remains the best way to make a diagnosis.

30. **The most common cause of maternal death during the first trimester of pregnancy is:**
    a. DVT with PE.
    b. Ectopic pregnancy.
    c. Eclampsia.
    d. Hyperemesis gravidum.
    e. Abruptio placenta.

    The answer is b. Ectopic pregnancy remains the most common cause of maternal death and serious morbidity during the first trimester.

31.   **The most important risk factor for ectopic pregnancy is:**

   a. Previous ectopic pregnancy.

   b. History of salpingitis.

   c. Medically stimulated ovulation.

   d. In vitro fertilization.

   e. History of abortion.

   The answer is d. In vitro fertilization remains the most important risk factor. Previous ectopic, salpingitis, and tubal surgery are also risks factors. No relationship has been found between stimulated ovulation or number of implanted embryos and ectopic pregnancy, but heterotopic pregnancy does increase with ovarian stimulation and is related to the number of implanted embryos.

32.   **A 17-year-old woman complains of 4 days of heavy vaginal bleeding with cramping. A friend gave her some ibuprofen for her cramps. You plan your workup with pregnancy test and pelvic examination and inform the patient that ibuprofen:**

   a. Interferes with platelet function and should never be used during heavy bleeding.

   b. May help the cramping but will make the bleeding worse.

   c. Is fine for regular periods but should be avoided with heavy flow.

   d. May help the cramping and bleeding of anovulatory bleeding.

   e. Will likely cause stomach ulcers.

   The answer is d. NSAIDs may be useful with dysmenorrhea and ovulatory as well as anovulatory bleeding. Their prostaglandin inhibitory effect can increase vasoconstriction, and they can increase levels of thromboxane A_2 increasing vasoconstriction and platelet aggregation. They can reduce blood loss by 20–50%.

CHAPTER 14

Psychobehavioral Emergencies

Manish Garg, MD, FAAEM

1. The police bring you a disheveled 32-year-old woman who is wearing a soiled "Jesus for President" sweatshirt. They tell you she was standing outside a restaurant yelling at the customers about a CIA plot to poison their food. She is wearing an elaborate headpiece made of aluminum foil, which she refuses to remove because "then they'll know what I'm thinking." Her vital signs are normal. You are almost certain that her problem is psychiatric rather than organic because she:

   a. Is not ataxic.
   b. Is emotionally labile.
   c. Is not lethargic.
   d. Is oriented to day and date.
   e. Has visual hallucinations.

   The answer is d. Patients often present with an apparent acute psychosis that is secondary to an organic (medical) rather than a functional (psychiatric) etiology. Distinguishing the two can be difficult. Factors that suggest an organic etiology include disorientation, age of onset older than 35 years, visual hallucinations, lethargy, altered level of consciousness, and abnormal vital signs. Other factors that indicate a psychosis due to an organic etiology include tremor, ataxia, aphasia, occasional periods of perception or lucidity, sudden onset of symptoms, emotional lability, social immodesty, and an abnormal physical examination. Psychiatric patients, on the other hand, tend to be awake and alert, with appropriate orientation to time, place, and person. They will typically have normal vital signs. They demonstrate social modesty, intelligible speech, flat affect, auditory hallucinations, and a gradual onset of their symptoms.

2. **A 32-year-old man is standing in the hallway of the emergency department cursing loudly and screaming that no one is paying attention to him. One of the nurses recognizes him from another hospital as someone who frequently is admitted for psychiatric illness. Your initial action is to:**

    a. Introduce yourself and ask him how you can help him today.

    b. Call hospital security and place him in four point restraints.

    c. Ignore him.

    d. Order the nurse to give him ziprasidone 10 mg IM.

    e. Order the nurse to give him lorazepam 2 mg PO.

    The answer is a. If a patient is potentially dangerous, but not in need of immediate restraint, a psychiatric interview should take place in an open area with nearby security personnel. The physician should begin with an introduction and express the desire to help the patient. If sedation is necessary, haloperidol is the most widely used drug rapid tranquilization, although the recently approved atypical antipsychotics ziprasidone can be an alternative. Many physicians also use droperidol, but the FDA has now issued a warning against the use of this drug based on reports of adverse cardiovascular events including cardiac arrest and torsade de pointes. Lorazepam and other benzodiazepines may be used as adjuncts to neuroleptics for rapid tranquilization. For violent patients, temporary use of physical restraints may be necessary while rapid tranquilization is initiated.

3. **A 37-year-old woman with a history of chronic schizophrenia, hypertension, hyperlipidemia, and seasonal allergies complains of neck pain and stiffness. She is unable to turn her head to the left. She takes several medications, but the one most likely to be causing her present symptoms is:**

    a. Haloperidol.

    b. Lovastatin

    c. Amlodipine.

    d. Doxazosin.

    e. Benztropine.

    The answer is a. Acute dystonia, the most common adverse effect seen with neuroleptic agents, occurs in 1–5% of patients. It involves the sudden onset of involuntary contraction of the muscles of the face, neck, or back. The patient may have protrusion of the tongue (buccolingual crisis), deviation of the head to one side (acute torticollis), sustained upward deviation of the eyes (oculogyric crisis), extreme arching of the back (opisthotonos), or rarely laryngospasm. Dystonic reactions should be treated with IM or IV benztropine (Cogentin), 1–2 mg, or diphenhydramine (Benadryl), 25–50 mg. IV administration usually results in an almost immediate reversal of symptoms. Patients should receive oral therapy with the same medication for 48–72 hours to prevent recurrent symptoms.

4. **A 47-year-old man is brought by his caregivers from a boarding home. They tell you that he's had fevers up to 104°F for the past 24 hours. The patient has difficulty following your commands and is unable to provide a clear history. He is tachycardic, pale, and diaphoretic. He can move at will, but his muscles are rigid. When you review his list of medications, you find that he takes haloperidol. Your treatment for his current condition should include:**

    a. Benztropine (Cogentin).

    b. Carbamazepine (Tegretol).

    c. Dantrolene (Dantrium).

    d. Diphenhydramine (Benadryl).

    e. Phenytoin (Dilantin).

The answer is c. Treatment of neuroleptic malignant syndrome consists of fever reduction, intravenous rehydration, and supportive measures. Dantrolene, a direct-acting muscle relaxant, should be used in severe cases.

5. **A 23-year-old woman recently started taking haloperidol for newly diagnosed schizophrenia. Two days ago, the clinic physician increased her dose from 2 mg twice a day to 4 mg twice a day. She is now extremely restless and pacing the examination room, but is not agitated or psychotic. She tells you, "I can't help myself, doc. I've just gotta keep moving." You need to:**

   a. Change her haloperidol to chlorpromazine (Thorazine) and arrange outpatient follow-up.
   b. Give her dantrolene (Dantrium) and a bolus of intravenous normal saline.
   c. Increase her haloperidol dose until the symptoms are controlled.
   d. Lower her dose of haloperidol and start her on propranolol or benztropine.
   e. Physically restrain her if necessary and consult psychiatry for definitive evaluation.

   The answer is d. Akathisia is a state of motor restlessness characterized by a physical need to move constantly. It occurs most often in middle-age patients during the first few months after the initiation of therapy. Patients are usually observed pacing the room and expressing a sense of inner tension that is not relieved by activity. This reaction can easily be mistaken for a decompensating psychosis, leading to a vicious cycle in which more medication is given to treat a side effect caused by the same drug. Avoid this misdiagnosis with careful evaluation for the exacerbation of positive psychotic symptoms. These are not increased by akathisia. Akathisia is treated with beta-blockers (e.g., propranolol, 30–60 mg/d) or anticholinergic drugs (e.g., benztropine, 1 mg twice to 4 times daily).

6. **A 78-year-old man complains of appetite loss and weakness. While you are interviewing him, he starts to cry and tells you that his wife of 57 years died last month. On closer questioning, he admits that he has a pistol in the closet table and has thought about putting it in his mouth and pulling the trigger. You offer the patient psychiatric hospitalization, but he refuses. Your next step should be to:**

   a. Ask why he does not wish to be hospitalized.
   b. Involuntarily commit him using restraint as necessary.
   c. Physically or chemically restrain him until a psychiatrist can evaluate him.
   d. Start an antidepressant and discharge him.
   e. Start antipsychotic medications and discharge him.

   The answer is a. As an elderly man with a recent personal loss, this gentleman is at high risk for suicide. He may ultimately require involuntary commitment because he represents a significant danger to himself. Many depressed patients, though, may be reticent to accept hospitalization on account of anger or fear. When a patient is reluctant to accept hospitalization, the physician should attempt to identify and address the specific reasons. Family or friends may help convince the patient to accept psychiatric care.

7.   **A 35-year-old woman complains of dysmenorrhea, a lump in her throat, vomiting, shortness of breath, alternating diarrhea and constipation, poor sleep, and a burning sensation in her vagina intermittently for 3 years. She most likely has:**

   a. AIDS.

   b. Bipolar disease.

   c. Conversion disorder.

   d. Hyperthyroidism.

   e. Somatization disorder.

   The answer is e. The typical patient with somatization disorder is a woman in her forties with a 25- to 30-year history of multiple vague complaints. The symptoms that may best discriminate between patients with and without somatization disorder are (1) dysmenorrhea, (2) the sensation of a "lump" in the throat, (3) vomiting, (4) shortness of breath, (5) burning in the sex organs, (6) painful extremities, and (7) amnesia lasting hours to days. Tested prospectively among patients displaying at least two of these seven symptoms, the diagnosis of somatization disorder is correctly predicted with a sensitivity of 93% and a specificity of 59%. When four or more of these seven symptoms are present, the specificity rises to 100%.

8.   **The mother of a 2-year-old boy says that he won't stop vomiting. The child looks happy and normal, his vital signs are normal, and his physical examination reveals no pathology. The mother insists that the child is very ill and needs to be hospitalized "again." You ask for old records and find five prior admissions with similar complaints, but no organic diagnosis has ever been uncovered. In addition, no one other than the mother has ever seen the child vomit. You expect the mother:**

   a. To depart immediately when the child is admitted.

   b. To demonstrate frank psychosis.

   c. To have a background in health care.

   d. To have antisocial personality disorder.

   e. To ignore the child.

   The answer is c. The caretaker in Münchausen syndrome by proxy is the biologic mother in 98% of cases. Many have a background in health professions or social work. Depression, anxiety, and somatization are common, but frank psychotic behavior is atypical. The perpetrators of Münchausen syndrome by proxy are typically pleasant, cooperative, and appreciative. They often will stay in the hospital with their child and cultivate close relationships with hospital staff.

9.   **The mother of a 4-month-old boy tells you that he was in a bath seat in the sink when she turned away to get some soap and he turned on the hot water. The child has second-degree burns on both feet and ankles to just above the malleoli. Your management is to:**

   a. Admit the child and consult child protective services.

   b. Attempt to corroborate the history by contacting another caretaker.

   c. Call the state welfare agency to arrange a home visit.

   d. Teach the mother about burn prevention and water safety.

   e. Treat the burns and arrange outpatient follow-up.

The answer is a. A 4-month-old child does not possess the motor skills to turn on a water faucet. Scald burns are most commonly a result of partial immersion in hot water, and this is the typical distribution. All 50 states and the District of Columbia have mandatory reporting laws for suspected child abuse. A report must be filed with state or county child protective services. The family should be told that abuse is suspected and that a report has been filed. This conversation should demonstrate an attitude of seeking to help the child and family and so avoid vindictiveness.

10. **You are seeing an 84-year-old demented woman who is brought from a local nursing home for a feeding tube change. She has multiple deep bedsores and appears malnourished. You notice several bruises on her face and back. You suspect this may be elder abuse, so legally you are required to:**

    a. Ask the patient if she is abused and call the police if she answers affirmatively.

    b. Call the police to arrest the nursing home manager.

    c. Consult social services or case management.

    d. Do nothing, especially if the patient denies abuse.

    e. Admit the patient and file a report with the state department of health and human services.

    The answer is e. Laws have been enacted that pertain to the reporting and investigation of elder abuse in all 50 states and the District of Columbia. In 46 of the states, physicians are mandated to file a report if they know or reasonably suspect that elder abuse has occurred. Many states grant immunity to reporting physicians. Most state laws include a penalty for failure to report.

11. **Your state recognizes "living wills." A confused patient is accompanied by a friend who states that the patient's wife died last month. The patient has been depressed and took an overdose of sleeping pills. In the patient's possession is a properly executed living will dated 1 week ago. He refuses treatment. Your most appropriate action is to:**

    a. Follow the provisions of the living will.

    b. Question the friend concerning the patient's competency.

    c. Contact the patient's closest living relative to obtain consent.

    d. Obtain an emergency psychiatric consultation to determine the patient's competency.

    e. Treat the patient.

    The answer is e. The emergency physician has an obligation to treat suicidal mentally incompetent patients. Choice **a** is incorrect because the intent of the living will does not encompass suicide attempts. Choices **b**, **c**, or **d** might be appropriate in other situations in helping to arrive at a decision on treatment. In this case, any refusal of treatment by the patient would not be a competent refusal and no further evidence is necessary, nor consent needed, to treat him. Living wills become operative only if the patient is terminally or severely ill and treatment would merely postpone death.

12. **Choose the correct statement concerning major depression:**

    a. It is more common in men than in women.

    b. It is more common in patients with a family history of suicide.

    c. It is diagnosed when a patient exhibits direct or indirect signs of depression for more than 1 week.

    d. It is associated with a 5% lifetime risk of suicide.

    e. It is easily diagnosed.

    The answer is b. A 2-week history of sadness or apathy toward most normal activities is classed as major depression. Depression from medications (e.g., from reserpine) is more properly termed organic affective disorder. Major depression is more common in women and in persons with a family history of suicide or history of other psychiatric or medical disorders. The lifetime risk of suicide in people with a primary depressive episode is 15%. The disorder responds well to antidepressant therapy, but recurrences are common. The disorder masquerades as anxiety, insomnia, chronic fatigue, and other somatic complaints commonly heard in the ED. A useful mnemonic for eliciting signs of depression is IN SAD CAGES (Interest, Sleep, Appetite, Depressed, Concentration, Activity, Guilt, Energy, Suicide).

13. **Documenting a chain of evidence means:**

    a. Ascertaining that all entries in a medical record that pertain to a legal case are properly signed and dated, and all erroneous entries lined out, initialed, and dated.

    b. Establishing in a malpractice case which physicians and other personnel were directly responsible for a patient's care at each stage of the evaluation and treatment.

    c. Properly recording all treatment and medication changes in the medical record.

    d. Properly labeling a blood sample you have drawn for a blood alcohol determination in a suspected drunk driving case for the police, personally handing it to the arresting officer, getting a receipt.

    e. Documenting in a rape case that samples of vaginal fluid were taken for examination, labeling and initialing the sample, and sending it to the laboratory for analysis.

    The answer is d. The phrase "chain of evidence" has a very specific legal meaning. In cases in which the physician will be asked to provide the police with actual samples of blood, urine, or vaginal fluids for analysis, or when such samples will be sent to the laboratory with test results to be used later in court, the sample must be clearly identified as coming from the patient and each person handling the sample must be identified so as to prevent allegations of possible tampering in subsequent legal proceedings. In such cases, clearly label and date each sample, deliver it personally to the next person in the chain of custody, document the disposition of the sample, and obtain a receipt.

14. **You are evaluating a 26-year-old man who has been brought to the emergency department by his family for "acting bizarre." The patient told his family that he was rescued from a sinking ship where he was "king of the world." The family has always thought the patient was "eccentric" and on examination you also find the patient to have grossly disorganized behavior and speech. You diagnose the patient as having schizophrenia because:**

    a. Through further questioning he also meets criteria for a mood disorder.

    b. He has a stable level of functioning at work and with self-care.

    c. He has had the presence of delusions and disorganized behavior and speech for 1 week without treatment.

    d. He recently started abusing amphetamines after he was started on antianxiety medicine that was abruptly discontinued.

    e. He has also had continuous signs of "negative symptom" disturbance for at least 6 months.

The answer is e. The DSM-IV (*Diagnostic and Statistical Manual of Mental Disorders IV*) criteria for schizophrenia include the following: (1) Mood disorder or schizoaffective disorder with psychotic features has been ruled out. (2) A sharp deterioration from prior baseline level of functioning such as in work, grooming, or interpersonal relationships. (3) The presence of two or more positive symptoms: hallucinations, delusions, grossly disorganized speech, or behavior (or catatonic behavior); and negative symptoms such as flattened affect, poverty of speech, or inability to perform goal-directed activities. (4) Symptoms not caused by substance abuse, medications, or a general medical condition. (5) Symptoms of continuous signs (including prodromal/negative symptoms) for at least 6 months.

15. **A new 20-year-old mother comes to the emergency department after watching an afternoon talk show concerned that she may have "the hot topic that's sweeping the nation" of postpartum depression. The patient has been "feeling down" for a couple of days since she was discharged 3 days ago from the hospital with her baby. You reassure her that she has the "baby blues" and a decreased risk of developing postpartum depression since she:**

    a. Has a very stable, controlled history of bipolar disease.

    b. Is experiencing this with her first child.

    c. Has a stable job at a local fast-food restaurant.

    d. Is functioning independently as she has no family.

    e. Has symptoms different from that of a majority of mothers.

    The answer is c. Postpartum depression has a higher prevalence in patients with a history of mood disorders and/or suicidal thoughts, unemployment, and patients with no support for infant care. In previous studies, more than half of mothers reported some depressed mood after childbirth. Although less than 2% of mothers report thoughts of suicide, a careful screening should be done in new mothers and any ideation should be taken seriously and followed with a mental health care specialist.

16. **You are examining a 24-year-old man who has just jumped off the roof of a one-story house. You determine he has no major injuries, but are worried because he is wearing a Superman t-shirt and he tells you he is "going to fly and save the world." You also learn that he recently has maximized his credit card limit with shopping sprees. His roommate says he's been "talking all fast," and that he has been having "one night stands" with multiple partners. You feel confident in his diagnosis because you also learn:**

    a. He sleeps all the time.

    b. He is writing an epic novel.

    c. He is using methamphetamines.

    d. He has been having the symptoms for 1 week.

    e. He would still be able to work at his job.

    The answer is b. This patient is having a manic episode. The overall prevalence of the disease is 1.6% in both men and women. The DSM-IV criteria for manic episode includes the following: (1) Three or more of the following seven general categories of symptoms that have persisted: inflated self-esteem or grandiosity; insomnia; increase in goal-directed activity (writing a novel) or psychomotor agitation; pressured speech; flight of ideas; excessive hedonistic/pleasurable activities (money and sex); and easy distraction to trivial stimuli. (2) At least 2 weeks of persistently elevated, expansive, or irritable mood. (3) Symptoms not caused by substance abuse, medications, or a general medical condition. (4) Disease process is severe enough to cause impairment in social and occupational settings or hospitalization. (5) Symptoms do not meet criteria for a "mixed episode" (e.g., bipolar disorder).

17. **You are evaluating a 27-year-old woman with a past history of bipolar disease; her history makes you believe she is suffering from acute mania, but she has no psychotic behavior. You complete your primary and secondary surveys, which are negative, and offer the patient psychiatric evaluation. She declines, but is willing for you to start her on a medication and "I'll follow up when I calm down." You write a prescription for:**

a. Valproic acid.

b. Haloperidol.

c. Gabapentin.

d. An SSRI.

e. Electroconvulsive therapy.

The answer is a. Bipolar disorder can be treated primarily with mood stabilizing medications such as valproic acid, lithium, or carbamazepine. Valproic acid is a highly effective mood stabilizing medication and can be given rapidly for patients with acutely manic bipolar disorder. Haloperidol can be used adjunctively to control psychotic behavior. Gabapentin has a limited role in the treatment of mania and should not be used as a single agent. SSRIs or other antidepressants can be used for depressive episodes in bipolar patients, not manic episodes. ECT can be used adjunctively in bipolar disorder after at least partial response to initial mood stabilizing medications after 3 weeks of time.

18. **You are evaluating a 26-year-old woman who complains of palpitations, dry mouth, and prickling sensations of her fingertips and around her mouth after she saw a neighbor's new dog running around her yard. She has been "deathly afraid" of dogs after she read a book in school about a "big red dog" that was too big for the house. You diagnose a specific phobia and plan to send her for psychiatric follow-up for cognitive behavior therapy. You should acutely manage her symptoms with:**

a. Selective serotonin reuptake inhibitors (SSRIs).

b. Tricyclic antidepressants (TCAs).

c. Monoamine oxidase inhibitors (MAOIs).

d. Buspirone.

e. Benzodiazepines.

The answer is e. Most anxiety disorders are best treated long term with cognitive behavioral therapy. Benzodiazepines offer an efficacious short-term therapy in a patient who is cooperative, otherwise socially adjusted at work and at home, and is aware of her problems. Benzodiazepines seem to have the best pharmacotherapy in the treatment of specific phobia. Benzodiazepines, SSRIs, and MAOIs seem to have good efficacy in the treatment of panic disorder, generalized anxiety disorder, social phobia, PTSD, and OCD. TCAs have efficacy in panic disorder, generalized anxiety disorder, and PTSD (clomipramine can be used in OCD). Buspirone generally has efficacy in generalized anxiety disorder and OCD (in adjunct with an SSRI). Remember that TCAs and MAOIs have important restrictions and side effects.

19. **A 30-year-old insulin-dependent diabetic man was brought to the ED against his will after he had a hypoglycemic episode. The patient told the prehospital ambulance crew that he didn't want to go to the hospital because it makes him very anxious. You evaluate the patient and manage his glucose appropriately and there are no further diabetes-related issues. The patient tells you he feels intensely anxious because he feels like he will "never get out of the hospital." The patient tells you he "avoids the hospital at all costs" because he will "never escape." You suspect he also has:**

    a. Panic disorder.

    b. Social phobia.

    c. Anxiety disorder caused by a general medical condition.

    d. Agoraphobia.

    e. Generalized anxiety disorder.

    The answer is d. Agoraphobia is anxiety about or avoidance of situations or places from where escape might be difficult. Panic attack is a sudden and intense fear or terror often associated with feelings of impending doom. Social phobia is anxiety brought on by social or performance situations leading to avoidance behavior. Anxiety disorder caused by a general condition is associated with anxiety as a direct physiologic consequence of a general medical condition. In this patient, the diabetes has no relevance to his anxiety. Generalized anxiety disorder is associated with at least 6 months of persistent and excessive anxiety.

20. **A 22-year-old woman complains of intractable pain and vomiting from gastroparesis. She confides that she has a hard time feeling good about herself with feelings of emptiness and has in the past been reckless with spending money and sexual relations. One month ago you admitted her for mutilating herself. After you finish the history and physical examination, the patient will not let you leave the room because she needs you to know her entire history with the disease. After you communicate your intent to treat her symptoms, she showers you with praise and affection as her favorite physician. After your treatment plan is complete and her symptoms improve, the patient demands to see you and throws a temper tantrum for abandoning her as you now plan on discharging her from the hospital. The patient is exhibiting signs of:**

    a. Antisocial personality disorder.

    b. Borderline personality disorder.

    c. Bipolar mania, type II.

    d. Histrionic personality disorder.

    e. Schizoaffective personality disorder.

    The answer is b. Borderline personality disorder is characterized by poor self-image and emptiness, impulsiveness, instability of personal relationships alternating between idealization and devaluation, inability to control intense anger, efforts to avoid abandonment, and mood instability. Antisocial personality disorder is characterized by a pattern of reckless disregard and deceitfulness, violation and lack of remorse toward others since the age of 15. Dependent personality disorder is characterized by a pervasive and excessive need to be taken care of that leads to submissive behavior and fear of separation. Histrionic personality disorder is characterized by excessive emotionality and attention-seeking behavior using inappropriate seduction and overdramatization. Narcissistic personality disorder is characterized by a selfish and inflated self-importance or grandiosity and the need for admiration or entitlement at the expense of others.

21. **A 25-year-old woman has a history of seizures. Just after you introduce yourself, she casually states that she is about to "catch a seizure" and shows you a tremor in her right hand that gets more intense until her whole body is involved. You note that the patient's head moves side to side, she has uncoordinated movements of the extremities which you can halt, and she has wild pelvic thrusting which requires more people to assist in her care. The patient's episode is complete and she has no postictal phase and she seems unconcerned about whole experience. You make a diagnosis of pseudoseizure, which falls under the category of:**

 a. Somatization disorder.

 b. Factitious disorder.

 c. Malingering.

 d. Conversion disorder.

 e. Münchausen syndrome.

The answer is d. A conversion disorder is characterized by a sudden onset of a dramatic single symptom that typically is painless and neurologic in origin. The symptoms are not under voluntary control of the patient and there is no pathophysiologic explanation for the disease. The disorder has a gender predilection toward women and half the patients will show a lack of concern (*la belle indifference*) regarding the body dysfunction. Somatization disorder involves pain at different sites, gastrointestinal, genitourinary, and neurologic symptoms that are not intentionally produced or explained by a medical condition. Factitious disorder involves signs and symptoms that are intentionally produced in the absence of external incentives. Malingering involves signs and symptoms of that are intentionally produced motivated by external incentives. Münchausen syndrome is a rare type of factitious disorder where patients try to gain admission to the hospital during times in the week with limited consultant involvement and primary physician accessibility with presentations that often require lengthy and advanced workups and finally refusing discharge.

22. **You evaluate a 77-year-old man who is sent from Communist Martyrs Nursing Home for "change in mental status." The patient has a history of Alzheimer dementia and the nursing note only states that he is "not acting like himself" for a few days. You know that he is suffering from delirium rather than a progression of his dementia because:**

 a. He is not able to learn new information or to recall previously learned information.

 b. He fails to carry out motor activities despite having intact motor function.

 c. He fails to recognize or identify objects.

 d. He has a language disturbance and cannot plan, organize, or sequence.

 e. He is unable to focus his attention and has perceptual disturbances (i.e., hallucinations or delusions).

The answer is e. Delirium is defined as an acute or subacute condition of cognitive dysfunction due to an underlying condition and involves disturbances in consciousness (focusing attention), cognition (disorientation and memory deficits), and perception (hallucinations or delusions). Dementia is defined as a gradually progressive deterioration of cognitive function involving memory impairment (choice **a**), apraxia (choice **b**), agnosia (choice **c**), aphasia or disturbances in executive functioning (choice **d**). The cognitive deficits cannot be caused as a result of delirium and should cause significant impairment in social or occupational functioning.

23. **One of your security guards grabs you as you come through the door to start a shift and says, "You've got to give this guy something to calm him down." You see a disheveled middle-age man being held down by two officers. You learn that the patient has been in substance abuse rehabilitation but you don't know what drugs he abused. The rehab center did send a note stating that he had a seizure moments before they called the police and that he has had no access to acutely ingesting anything. The patient is tachycardic, hypertensive, tremulous, diaphoretic, and hallucinating, yelling "the demons are on me, get rid of the demons." For rapid tranquilization you choose to administer:**

 a. Lorazepam.
 b. Haloperidol.
 c. Olanzapine.
 d. Risperidone.
 e. Phenytoin.

 The answer is a. Lorazepam, a benzodiazepine, would be the first-line treatment for psychotic agitation in this patient who likely is suffering from alcohol withdrawal. Haloperidol is the most widely used medication for rapid tranquilization in the United States and is effective against tension, anxiety, and hyperactivity; however, it should not be used a sole agent in alcohol withdrawal. Olanzapine and risperidone are atypical antipsychotic agents with a broad spectrum of response with fewer side effects than haloperidol, but require a dissolvable oral formulation, which would be technically difficult in the above patient. Additionally, they would not help the withdrawal seizures. Phenytoin, an anticonvulsant would not be the first-line medication in alcohol withdrawal seizures and would not be effective in this patient's agitation and sympathetic overdrive.

24. **The family of a 74-year-old woman pulls you aside and says, "Mother is depressed." The patient has a history of dementia, but the family thinks the problem is more related to her "depression." You explain to them that if she did in fact have pseudodementia, you would expect to see:**

 a. No previous psychiatric history.
 b. Symptoms beginning gradually over a long time.
 c. A variable performance on similar tasks/tests.
 d. An unconcerned demeanor with loss of social skills.
 e. A chronic, progressive course with no response to medical therapy.

 The answer is c. Pseudodementia is the most common and treatable of the dementias. It is not uncommon for a person who is mildly demented to be a little depressed, but there are distinguishing features between dementia and depression. Pseudodementia is characterized by patients with previous psychiatric history and a more precise and rapid onset of symptoms. You expect to see variable performance on similar tasks/tests and a distressed person who emphasizes deficits and has intact social skills. Finally, pseudodementia does respond to medical therapy.

25.   **A 30-year-old medical student bypasses triage and comes directly to you saying, "I have a carotid artery dissection." He has chronic headaches and has determined from the shape of his head and neck that he has a dissection, which will cripple his chances of being a great physician. He has seen other physicians for this and has had "normal diagnostics" and received "shots of medicine in my neck" but his symptoms only come back. You palpate his neck and feel increased spasms of the muscles which the makes the patient state, "See, I'm right. It's a dissection." You realize he has:**

a. Somatization disorder.

b. Body dysmorphic disorder.

c. Pain disorder.

d. Hypochondriasis.

e. A vertebral artery dissection.

The answer is d. Hypochondriasis has four features: (1) The patient's symptoms are typically disproportionate to physical examination findings of organic disease. (2) A preoccupation with one's own body. (3) A compulsive insistence on being labeled as "sick" and subsequently crippled. (4) Continuous and unsatisfactory pursuit of medical care and opinion with a history of intervention yet eventual return of symptoms.

CHAPTER 15

Renal and Urogenital Emergencies

Mark Saks, MD, MPH

1. **A 37-year-old woman has a 2-week history of intermittent headache and general malaise. Over the last 24 hours, she has developed back pain, hematuria, vomiting, fever, and confusion. She denies recent travel or insect bites. There is no history of dysuria, urgency, frequency, or kidney stones. Her oral temperature is 38°C and her heart rate is 100/min. Physical findings include pale conjunctivae, borderline tachycardia, bilateral costovertebral tenderness, and several purpuric skin lesions. Her urine dipstick is strongly positive for hemoglobin, but negative for nitrites and leukocyte esterase. The test that will most likely reveal the correct diagnosis is:**

   a. Intravenous pyelogram.

   b. CBC with differential and peripheral smear.

   c. Complete urinalysis with microscopic examination.

   d. Blood cultures.

   e. Liver function tests.

   The answer is b. This patient exhibits classic signs and symptoms of thrombotic thrombocytopenic purpura (TTP), a microangiopathic hemolytic anemia (MAHA). TTP is a syndrome characterized by anemia, thrombocytopenia, fever, renal dysfunction, and a wide variety of neurologic symptoms including change in mental status, stroke, seizures, and coma. Once almost uniformly fatal, treatment has markedly improved mortality. Initial therapy includes steroids and antiplatelet agents. The use of gamma-globulin infusion, vincristine, plasma exchange (plasmapheresis), and surgical splenectomy in resistant cases has further reduced the mortality rate. Platelet transfusion should be avoided because platelets may cause additional thrombi in the microcirculation, though it may be necessary in cases of life-threatening hemorrhage. Most cases of TTP are idiopathic, but it has been associated with *E. coli* 0157:H7 infection and medications such as quinine. Clinically, TTP must be differentiated from other causes of MAHA such as: disseminated intravascular coagulation (DIC), the hemolytic uremic syndrome (HUS), and HELLP syndrome.

2.　**Which of the following statements is true regarding renal calculi?**

　　a.　There is no association between diet and the development of renal stones.

　　b.　The development of renal dysfunction is related to the size and location of renal stones.

　　c.　Female gender and an active lifestyle are known risk factors.

　　d.　The majority contain calcium.

　　e.　Recurrence is unusual.

The answer is d: Risk factors for the development of renal stones include age between 20 and 50 years, male gender, sedentary lifestyle, and family history. Stones form as a result of metabolic abnormalities including milk-alkali syndrome, sarcoidosis, Crohn disease, recurrent UTIs, and laxative abuse. They can be classified as calcium, struvite, uric acid, or cystine. The majority of stones are composed of either calcium oxalate alone or with calcium phosphate and hypercalciuria, due to excessive dietary intake, hyperparathyroidism, or peptic ulcer disease, is a major risk factor in the development of renal stones. The size and location of the stone are the major determinants of the severity of patient symptoms. Because of the urinary outflow obstruction and resultant urostasis, patients with renal stones are at increased risk of pyelonephritis, perinephric abscess, sepsis, and other severe urinary tract infections. The presence of comorbid urinary infection, rather than stone size or location, is the major cause of renal dysfunction.

3.　**A 48-year-old man complains of colicky, severe, "10/10" right flank pain that extends around his abdomen and radiates into the right groin. Although the pain waxes/wanes, it does not resolve totally between episodes. There have been no previous similar episodes. On examination, the patient is writhing in pain on the stretcher and seems unable to find a comfortable position. The patient has severe right CVA tenderness but a benign abdomen. You suspect renal calculi. A basic metabolic panel is still pending. Which of the following additional features is an indication to undergo a more extensive metabolic evaluation?**

　　a.　Persistent nausea and vomiting despite medication.

　　b.　An ultrasound shows right-sided hydronephrosis.

　　c.　A CT scan shows multiple small bilateral calculi.

　　d.　Finding a stone lodged in the calyx of the right kidney.

　　e.　The patient is 48 years of age.

The answer is c: Renal stones may affect up to 7% of the US population and patients with renal colic are commonly seen in the emergency department. For a patient with the initial diagnosis of an isolated renal stone, many sources advise the routine evaluation of serum electrolytes, creatinine, calcium, uric acid, and phosphorus. Indications for additional metabolic evaluation include residual calculi after lithotripsy or surgical treatment, an initial presentation with multiple calculi, significant family history, or more than a single stone in the past year. In these cases, evaluation is aimed at diagnosing less common conditions associated with renal stones including Crohn's disease, milk-alkali syndrome, hypernitraturia, hyperuricosuria, sarcoidosis, gout, renal tubular acidosis (type I), and chronic laxative abuse. Additionally, it is advisable to aggressively evaluate, diagnose, and treat patients who initially develop stones in their teens or twenties because this group is more likely to experience recurrent stone formation.

4. **You are treating a patient with a suspected Bartholin gland abscess. Which of the following statements regarding the diagnosis, evaluation, and management of this condition is true?**

   a. A Word catheter may be placed, but the preferred emergency treatment is marsupialization.

   b. The Bartholin glands are located superior and lateral to the vaginal introitus.

   c. The majority are caused by sexually transmitted diseases such as *N. gonorrhoeae* and *C. trachomatis*.

   d. Patients should follow up with their gynecologist or return to the ED in 2–3 days for a reexamination.

   e. In addition to drainage, the patient should be started on oral antibiotics.

   The answer is d: The Bartholin glands are located inferior and lateral to the vaginal introitus. When these glands become clogged, a painless simple cyst forms. However, an abscess will develop if this cyst becomes secondarily infected. Typically, this infection is polymicrobial and related to the vaginal flora, but sexually transmitted organisms cause a significant minority. Therefore, STD testing should be performed along with sending cultures from the abscess. Incision and drainage with placement of a Word catheter to allow for continued drainage is sufficient treatment in a majority of patients. Antibiotics may be indicated if an STD is suspected. Although the catheter is often left in place for 4–6 weeks, patients should be instructed to follow up with their gynecologist or return to the ED in 2–3 days for a reexamination to ensure adequate drainage. In patients with recurrent episodes, marsupialization may be required.

5. **A 40-year-old diabetic woman complaints of 3 days of fever, chills, dysuria, and flank pain. This morning, she noted some dizziness with standing and vomited once. In the ED, her rectal temperature is 38.8°C. You note her to be thin with dry lips. The remainder of the examination is unremarkable except for right costovertebral angle tenderness. Urinalysis shows trace ketones, numerous WBCs in clumps and casts, and 4+ bacteria. Her peripheral white blood cell count is 9.5 and her blood glucose is 220. She has no prior history of urinary infection. Your most appropriate treatment is to:**

   a. Infuse 2000 mL normal saline, administer a dose of intravenous ceftriaxone, and discharge home on oral antibiotics.

   b. Infuse 2000 mL normal saline, administer a dose of intravenous ceftriaxone, and admit to the hospital.

   c. Obtain renal ultrasound; if negative, proceed as in choice **b**.

   d. Give 4 units of regular insulin now, 2000 mL intravenous normal saline, administer a dose of intravenous ceftriaxone, order blood and urine cultures, and admit to the hospital.

   e. Insert a central venous catheter for central venous pressure monitoring, begin presumptive treatment with fluids, give intravenous steroids, start empiric antibiotics, and admit to the intensive care unit.

   The answer is d. This patient has acute pyelonephritis. In general, young patients with uncomplicated urinary tract infections or simple acute pyelonephritis do not require admission and can be treated as outpatients with oral antibiotics, antipyretics, and pain medications. However, patients with the following complicating conditions are at higher risk of severe complication and should be admitted: pregnancy, diabetes, cancer, immunosuppression, sickle cell anemia, organ transplant recipients, comorbid obstructing renal calculi, intractable nausea and vomiting, and azotemia. Debilitated patients or those unable to care for themselves should also be admitted. Complications of pyelonephritis include urosepsis and septic shock, emphysematous pyelonephritis, perinephric abscess, papillary necrosis, and renal failure. Because of her diabetes, this patient is also at risk of developing diabetic ketoacidosis and adequate fluid replacement and insulin therapy are particularly important.

6. **In the evaluation of hematuria:**

    a. Blood clots indicate a glomerular source.

    b. Red cell casts indicate a hematologic source.

    c. Smoke-colored urine usually has a renal source.

    d. Proteinuria indicates a postrenal source.

    e. Hematuria present throughout urination indicates a nonglomerular renal source.

    The answer is c. The amount of blood in the urine does not correlate with the severity of the condition that caused it. In fact, as little as 1 mL of blood in 1 L of urine can cause grossly appreciable hematuria. The causes of hematuria can be roughly divided into the following four groupings: (1) Hematologic (sickle cell disease, coagulopathies); (2) intrarenal–glomerular (systemic lupus, Wegener granulomatosis, Goodpasture syndrome); (3) intrarenal–nonglomerular (polycystic kidney disease, acute interstitial nephritis, trauma); and (4) postrenal (renal stone, cystitis, tumor, etc.) causes. Blood clots indicate a nonglomerular renal or postrenal source. Red cell casts and proteinuria indicate a renal source. Hematuria that is present throughout voiding is usually due to a bladder, ureter, or renal source.

7. **Fire rescue brings you a 55-year-old man with no known medical history for evaluation. His neighbor, who last saw him 4 days ago, found him on the floor. On arrival, he is somnolent but arousable. Examination shows an afebrile, ill-appearing man with a heart rate of 130/min and a blood pressure of 90/60 mm Hg. His urine is tea-colored and shows a large amount of blood on urine dipstick but the microscopy is negative for blood. Although his laboratory results are still pending, you suspect rhabdomyolysis and are concerned about acute renal failure. Which of the following is an indication to begin emergent hemodialysis?**

    a. A BUN of 76 mg/dL.

    b. A serum creatinine of 8.4 mg/dL.

    c. An oxygen requirement of 4 L by nasal cannula.

    d. An arterial pH of 7.02.

    e. A potassium level of 7.2 with hyperacute T waves on EKG.

    The answer is e. In patients with acute renal failure, indications for emergent dialysis include signs and symptoms of uremia (nausea, vomiting, depressed mental status), intractable volume overload, and life-threatening hyperkalemia. Many nephrologists will also initiate hemodialysis for patients with BUN levels above 100 mg/dL or serum creatinine levels above 10 mg/dL. In patients with chronic end-stage renal disease (ESRD), indications for emergent dialysis include pulmonary edema, severe uncontrollable hypertension, severe electrolyte (hyperkalemia, hypercalcemia, hypermagnesemia, etc.), or acid–base disturbances. Emergent hemodialysis is also indicated in certain poisonings such as the toxic alcohols, lithium, and other dialyzable toxins.

8. **A 22-year-old college student complains of penile pain and deformity. He states that 2 hours ago he was having intercourse when he noted a "snapping" sensation in his penis followed by localized pain and asymmetric swelling. You suspect a penile fracture. Which of the following statements is true?**

    a. The injury is due to a traumatic fracture of the corpus spongiosum and resulting hematoma formation.

    b. This injury is typically managed conservatively and rarely requires operative repair.

    c. A stat ultrasound should be obtained to evaluate the penile compartments.

    d. A Foley catheter should be immediately placed to prevent acute urinary retention.

    e. Of patients with this injury, a minority will experience a permanent deformity.

The answer is e. The penis consists of three main compartments: two corpora cavernosa and the corpus spongiosum. The corpora cavernosa comprise the main body of the penis while the corpus spongiosum lies on the ventral surface and contains the urethra and enlarges at the tip to form the glans penis. In a penile fracture, a traumatic tear of the tunica albuginea, most commonly during vigorous intercourse, leads to a subsequent rupture of the corpus cavernosum and penile hematoma. This injury is typically managed by operative hematoma evacuation, repair of the tunica albuginea, and placement of a pressure dressing. Up to 10% of all patients will experience permanent deformity, sexual dysfunction, and impaired erections. Nonsurgical treatment with bed rest, ice, and pressure dressing may be tried, but is associated with increased rates of complication. Patients will be able to void if there is no injury to the urethra.

9. **In evaluating a patient with clinical signs and symptoms of an uncomplicated lower urinary tract infection (UTI), you know that:**

   a. The specificity of the urine nitrite test for infection is low, but its sensitivity is high.

   b. The specificity of the leukocyte esterase test for infection is high, but its sensitivity is low.

   c. In an adult patient with pyuria and dysuria, penicillin VK is the antibiotic of choice.

   d. A 3-day treatment regimen is appropriate in a pregnant patient.

   e. Urine cultures should be obtained in the symptomatic patient with recurrent infections, as well as in children, men, and pregnant women.

The answer is e. The most commonly used screening tests to diagnose a urinary tract infection are the presence of nitrites and leukocyte esterase on the urine dipstick. *Nitrites* are produced from urinary *nitrates* by the enzyme nitrate reductase, which is found only in gram-negative bacteria. Therefore, specificity of the urine nitrite test for infection is high, but its sensitivity is low as it will be negative in gram-positive and other infections. Leukocyte esterase is an enzyme found in neutrophils. The specificity of the leukocyte esterase test for infection is low as it will be positive in many cases of pyuria such as renal stones, but its sensitivity is high. UTIs are one of the most common complications of pregnancy. Because of an increased risk of development of pyelonephritis, pregnant patients with an uncomplicated UTI require a 7- to 10-day course of antibiotics, rather than the 3-day course that is widely recommended. A wide range of bacteria have been implicated in UTIs including *E. coli, K. pneumoniae, Proteus enterobacter, Enterococcus, S. saprophyticus,* and group B *Streptococcus.* These organisms are sensitive to a wide variety of antibiotics, but penicillin VK is not generally recommended for treatment.

10. **A 15-year-old boy complains of sharp, radiating left testicular pain, which started while playing basketball 1 hour ago. He denies specific trauma, but tells you he first noted the pain while running. He also says that he was recently treated for epididymitis "with two antibiotics" but admits that he did not finish them. Physical examination reveals a tender, slightly enlarged left testicle lying in the horizontal plane. There is no cremasteric reflex on the left, but it is present on the right. When you look at his scrotum, you do not see a "blue dot" sign. Your next step is to:**

    a. Place him in the supine position, administer parenteral analgesics, and observe for changes.

    b. Hospitalize him for treatment with intravenous antibiotics.

    c. Counsel him on the importance of taking medications as prescribed and discharge him with scrotal elevation and oral antibiotics.

    d. Consult urology and obtain consent for surgery.

    e. Place ice packs on the area for 5 minutes out of every 20 minutes.

The answer is d. Although torsion may occur at any age, it is most common in the first year of life and at puberty. It is more common in undescended testis and should be considered in a patient with a painful inguinal mass and an empty scrotum. The onset is usually acute and frequently follows physical activity. The initial effect of torsion is venous engorgement, which leads to edema, pain, and tenderness. Depending on the extent of vascular compromise, it can progress to necrosis and infarction and attempts at detorsion should be made as soon as possible. Emergent urologic consultation should be obtained and manual detorsion can be attempted after appropriate analgesia. Even if successful, the patient still requires definitive surgical care. In cases where the diagnosis is in doubt, a testicular ultrasound with color Doppler flow is the test of choice at most institutions. The differential diagnosis of a young male patient with acute testicular pain is testicular torsion, infection, trauma, tumor with hemorrhage, and torsion of the appendices of the testis or epididymis. The last may be diagnosed clinically with reasonable certainty if a "blue dot" sign (indicative of venous engorgement) is seen through the scrotal skin.

11. **A woman brings her 19-month-old uncircumcised son to be evaluated for swelling and irritation of his penis. You see that the boy's penis and glans are edematous, erythematous, and excoriated. Retraction of the foreskin is painful and there is white cheesy material between foreskin and glans. No erosive lesions are present. There is no urethral discharge, pain with urination, or other urinary problems. He has had three prior similar episodes, all of which grew *Candida albicans*. The entity most commonly associated with this condition is:**

    a. Diabetes mellitus.

    b. Lymphoma.

    c. Asymptomatic chlamydial urethritis.

    d. Tuberculosis.

    e. Peyronie disease.

The answer is a. Balanitis is an inflammation of the glans penis only, while balanoposthitis refers to inflammation of the glans penis and foreskin. Both are caused primarily by infection that leads the glans and inner prepuce to become inflamed, tender, and excoriated. Etiologic agents include group A beta-hemolytic streptococci, *Neisseria gonorrhoeae*, and *Chlamydia trachomatis*. However, chemical irritation, trauma, and poor hygiene may also contribute to this condition. Diabetes mellitus is a common underlying cause and should be suspected in a patient presenting with recurrent episodes of this disorder, especially when *C. albicans* has been implicated. Treatment includes daily sitz baths, washing with mild soap, topical, and antibacterial or antifungal cream. A topical steroid cream may also be helpful if there is extensive inflammation. Circumcision should be considered for severe or recurrent disease. Oral antibiotics with streptococcal coverage should be prescribed for a secondary infection.

12. **In children, priapism is most commonly associated with:**

    a. Thrombocytopenia.

    b. Reactive arthritis syndrome.

    c. Kawasaki disease.

    d. Subarachnoid hemorrhage.

    e. Leukemia.

    The answer is e. In adults, common causes of priapism include sickle cell anemia, spinal cord lesions, medications (SSRIs, phenothiazines, antihypertensives, anticoagulants, etc.), drugs of abuse, sexual arousal, intercavernosal injections for impotence, phenothiazines, and other medications. In children, the most common causes of priapism are sickle cell anemia and leukemia. Rarely, priapism can also be seen in Kawasaki disease. Priapism, a prolonged erection, results from the engorgement of the dorsal corpora cavernosa while the corpus spongiosum and glans remain soft. There are two types: low-flow priapism is typically painful and results from decreased venous outflow; high-flow priapism is typically painless and results from increased arterial inflow associated with a penile laceration. Initial management for all causes includes terbutaline 0.25 mg SQ in the deltoid, a dorsal penile nerve block for pain control, and a urologic consultation. If refractory, additional treatment options include corporal aspiration, heparin irrigation, injection with phentolamine, phenylephrine, ephedrine or epinephrine, exchange transfusion, or shunt surgery. To avoid long-term dysfunction, interventions should be initiated within 12 hours.

13. **A 21-year-old man complains of leg and facial swelling. For the last 3 days he has noted dark-colored urine and he last voided 18 hours ago. Vital signs: heart rate 90/min; blood pressure 180/110 mm Hg. Physical examination shows puffy eyelids and bilateral pitting leg edema, and mild tachypnea. A catheterized urine specimen shows numerous red cells and red cell casts, 3+ protein, white blood cells, and no bacteria. Urine osmolality is 225 mOsm/L, urine sodium is 120 mOsm/L, BUN is 109 mg/dL, serum creatinine is 11 mg/dL, and urine creatinine is 115 mg/dL. In the evaluation of this patient:**

    a. Intravenous calcium chloride, 10 mL of a 10% solution, should be given immediately if cardiac arrest occurs.

    b. A renal biopsy is unlikely to yield useful information.

    c. A low calorie, low protein diet may help.

    d. 300 mg of intravenous push furosemide, repeated at hourly intervals for a maximum of three doses, should be used in an attempt to convert his oliguric renal failure to nonoliguric renal failure.

    e. Pericardial involvement is unlikely.

    The answer is a. This patient's clinical features (hematuria, azotemia, edema, hypertension, proteinuria, anuria) characterize rapidly progressive acute glomerulonephritis. This may be due to a primary renal process or secondary to a wide variety of diseases. Although the diagnosis is often made by renal biopsy, hematuria, proteinuria, and red cell casts, in particular, are strongly suggestive of glomerulonephritis as the cause of acute renal failure. The most common cause of cardiac arrest in uremic patients presenting to the ED is hyperkalemia, although uremic pericarditis may cause cardiac tamponade. General treatment measures include restricting protein, fluid, potassium, and sodium in the diet, and providing a high-caloric diet to prevent protein catabolism. However, emergent dialysis may be required to treat the complications of pericarditis, acidosis, hyperkalemia, hypertension, and fluid overload. Diuretics have limited benefit in the management of acute intrinsic renal failure. They rarely convert nonoliguric renal failure to an oliguric form. Mannitol may cause acute pulmonary edema.

14. **Renal failure can result from prerenal, renal, and postrenal pathophysiologic processes. An example of a postrenal cause of renal failure is:**

a. Pancreatitis.

b. Bacterial endocarditis.

c. Methysergide use.

d. Indomethacin use.

e. Ethylene glycol poisoning.

The answer is c. Acute renal failure may be divided into three categories: prerenal (due to renal hypoperfusion and azotemia); intrinsic (due to intrarenal vascular disease, glomerular disease, or tubulointerstitial dysfunction); and postrenal (due to obstruction at any level of the urinary tract). Pancreatitis and bacterial endocarditis are causes of prerenal acute renal failure. Indomethacin and ethylene glycol are associated with interstitial disease that leads to intrinsic acute renal failure. Ethylene glycol is metabolized to oxalic acid, which precipitates and obstructs the renal tubules. Methysergide is associated with retroperitoneal fibrosis, which can cause bilateral ureteral obstruction and postrenal acute renal failure.

15. **Concerning the evaluation of a fever in a renal transplant patient:**

a. Opportunistic infections are most common within the first month following transplant.

b. Although a wide variety of bacterial, mycobacterial, viral, and parasitic opportunistic infections are frequently seen within the first year following transplant, patients rarely develop fungal infections until more than 3 years posttransplant.

c. In contrast to HIV, cytomegalovirus infection is rare and typically follows a benign course.

d. Noninfectious causes of fever include atelectasis, acute rejection, and posttransplant lymphoma.

e. Rectal temperatures should never be obtained, regardless of the absolute neutrophil count (ANC), due to the risk of infection.

The answer is d. During the first posttransplant month, infections tend to be the usual postoperative infections seen in the general population (pneumonia, wound infection, catheter-related sepsis, etc.) and opportunistic infections are rare. The incidence of opportunistic infections is highest following the first month until months 6–12 when the incidence decreases. The initial evaluation of a febrile transplant patient should include a CBC, BUN, serum creatinine, urinalysis, and urine and blood cultures. Although noninfectious causes of fever including atelectasis, acute rejection, and posttransplant lymphoma are common, empiric antibiotics are often started due to the underlying immunosuppression. Patients who present within the first year following transplant generally require admission due to the frequency of opportunistic infection during this period.

16. **A 31-year-old man complains of nausea, vomiting, and headache 2 hours following hemodialysis. He is oriented to person only and appears confused, but states that he got a "full treatment". His past medical history includes malignant hypertension and he has recently started hemodialysis due to end-stage renal disease. His medications include captopril and meperidine tablets for pain. Vital signs: temperature 37.6°C, heart rate 80/min, blood pressure 195/100 mm Hg, respiratory rate 19/min. His blood glucose is 98. Other than the stigmata of chronic renal failure and his confusion, the remainder of his physical examination is unremarkable. His confusion is probably caused by:**

a. Dialysis disequilibrium syndrome.

b. An adverse reaction to meperidine.

c. Aseptic meningitis.

d. An acute stroke.

e. Azotemia.

The answer is a. Dialysis disequilibrium syndrome results from a sudden increase in intracranial pressure due to the acute fluid and electrolyte shifts that occur during dialysis; the change in the osmotic gradient shifts fluid from the blood into the CSF. It usually occurs in patients with elevated BUN and who have not been on dialysis for a long time. Dialysis disequilibrium syndrome is typified by the development of a headache, nausea, vomiting, and confusion within hours of hemodialysis. In severe cases, patients may develop a change in mental status, seizures, or coma. Symptoms generally slowly improve over several hours of observation as fluid and electrolytes are redistributed. Interestingly, dialysis disequilibrium syndrome is not seen following peritoneal dialysis, possibly because of the more gradual osmotic shifts.

17. **Choose the correct statement about renovascular hypertension:**

    a. The hypertension results from the underproduction of renin by the affected side.
    b. The response to surgery is unpredictable and rarely curative.
    c. It is the most common form of essential hypertension.
    d. Increased serum renin levels leads to a down-regulation of the angiotensin pathway.
    e. The condition is diagnosed when the renin level in the affected kidney is greater than 50% higher than the level in the unaffected kidney.

    The answer is e. The most common cause of hypertension is essential hypertension. However, all types of renal disease have been associated with the development of hypertension. Although the exact mechanism is not understood in many cases, in renovascular hypertension the overproduction of rennin due to decreased renal artery blood flow to one kidney leads to hyperactivation of the angiotensin pathway. Surgical removal of the affected kidney may cure the hypertension and may be predicted by determining rennin levels in selected renal veins. In patients with bilateral renovascular disease, angiotensin converting enzyme (ACE) inhibitors should not be used as they may precipitate renal failure.

18. **Choose the correct statement about contrast-induced nephropathy:**

    a. Pretreatment with intravenous steroids and diphenhydramine (Benadryl) may reduce the risk of developing nephropathy.
    b. Pretreatment with furosemide (Lasix) may reduce the risk of developing nephropathy.
    c. Pretreatment with intravenous fluids may reduce the risk of developing nephropathy.
    d. There is no association between the patient's age and the risk of developing contrast-induced nephropathy.
    e. Following contrast administration, serum creatinine levels typically peak at 14 days and resolve in 60–90 days.

    The answer is c. Contrast-induced nephropathy is defined by a 25% increase in serum creatinine levels after administration of IV contrast medium. This elevation is usually transient, peaking at 3 days and resolving within 10 days; however, dialysis and long-term renal dysfunction has been reported. Patients with increased baseline creatinine (greater than 1.5 mg/dL), heart failure (New York Heart Association class III or IV), diabetes, volume depletion, hypertension, concomitant use of NSAIDs, heart failure, liver failure, and age older than 75 years are at increased risk of developing contrast-induced nephropathy. Pretreatment with IV fluids is recommended to reduce the risk of developing contrast-induced nephropathy, although there is disagreement about the optimum regimen and amount. Initial studies with *N*-acetylcysteine (NAC) were encouraging, but further research is needed before its use becomes widely recommended. Forced diuresis with furosemide, mannitol, dopamine, or other agents has not been shown to be effective.

19.   **A 65-year-old man with chronic renal failure complains of chest pain, partially relieved by sitting up and leaning forward. Vitals signs: temperature 100.0°F, irregularly irregular heart rate 90/min, blood pressure 130/100 mm Hg. On examination, you hear muffled heart tones and find mild right upper quadrant tenderness. The patient's lungs are clear and you do not hear a rub. The EKG shows atrial fibrillation at a rate of 90/min. The chest radiograph shows clear lung fields. However there is massive cardiomegaly and a 4-mm lucent anterior pericardial stripe posterior to the dark line of the pericardial fat on the lateral film. In considering this patient you:**

a.   Give two 81-mg aspirin and 0.4 mg of sublingual nitroglycerin to relieve the pain.

b.   Recognize that the chest x-ray is highly characteristic of this disorder.

c.   Know that this complication is more common with peritoneal dialysis than with hemodialysis.

d.   Know that pericardiocentesis is the definitive treatment.

e.   Understand that corticosteroids may exacerbate the problem.

The answer is b. Pericarditis is a common complication of uremia. The mechanism is not known but may be related to the accumulation of toxic metabolites, an acquired bleeding diathesis, and/or infectious or immunologic processes. Uremic pericarditis typically presents with sharp chest pain that is relieved by sitting forward. Atrial arrhythmias, a low-grade fever, and signs of right ventricular failure, such as hepatomegaly and JVD, may be present. Unfortunately, a friction rub is not always heard, the EKG is often normal, and the characteristic chest x-ray finding of cardiomegaly with the separation of the peri- and epicardial fat is not sensitive. Echocardiography is diagnostic. Pericarditis without hemodynamic instability can be treated with intensive dialysis and systemic steroids. Pericardiocentesis should be limited to the treatment of tamponade. Relapses may be prevented by instilling steroids into the pericardium; however, the definitive treatment is a surgical pericardial window.

20.   **A 65-year-old man complains of generalized malaise, chills, low-back pain, and increased urinary frequency and dysuria. On digital rectal examination, you palpate a tender, boggy prostate. You suspect acute bacterial prostatitis. The appropriate treatment regimen is:**

a.   Ciprofloxacin 500 mg orally twice daily for 7–10 days.

b.   Ciprofloxacin 500 mg orally twice daily for 14–21 days.

c.   Ciprofloxacin 500 mg orally twice daily for 4–6 weeks.

d.   Doxycycline 100 mg orally twice daily for 7–10 days.

e.   Doxycycline 100 mg orally twice daily for 14–21 days.

The answer is b. Acute bacterial prostatitis is caused by infection of the prostate by gram-negative such as *E. coli*, *Klebsiella*, *Enterobacter*, and *Proteus*. The diagnosis of prostatitis is made clinically based on rectal examination and diagnostically based on the presence of pyuria/bacteriuria found only in the final 15 mL of urine, collected after prostatic massage in the course of obtaining a "three-cup specimen." However, manipulation of an inflamed prostate should be limited to avoid potential seeding and the development of bacteremia. For the same reason, urethral catheterization should be avoided and suprapubic aspiration or catheter placement is the preferred method of bladder drainage in patients with painful urinary retention. All patients should receive supportive therapy including stool softeners, analgesics, and adequate hydration. Nontoxic patients should be treated with prolonged antibiotics aimed at covering the enteric bacteria listed above. Toxic patients, or patients with acute urinary retention, should be hospitalized for IV antibiotics and urologic consultation.

21.   **In the diagnosis of vulvovaginitis:**

a. A pH less than 4.5 is suggestive of bacterial vaginitis.

b. Finding clue cells on wet mount is diagnostic of trichomonas.

c. A white, clumpy discharge indicates *Gardnerella vaginalis*.

d. Mycelia are pathognomonic for candida.

e. A pH greater than 4.5 is suggestive of vaginal candidiasis.

The answer is d. Vulvovaginitis is a heterogeneous group of disorders that commonly cause dyspareunia, vulvovaginal irritation, and vaginal discharge. The specific etiology is often identifiable based on the vaginal pH, appearance of the discharge, and microscopic features on wet mount. Bacterial vaginosis, the most common cause of foul-smelling vaginal discharge, is often caused by a polymicrobial overgrowth that includes *G. vaginalis*. It is diagnosed based on having a vaginal pH greater than 4.5, a gray/white milky malodorous discharge, and clue cells evident on wet mount. Trichomonas also has a pH greater than 4.5. Vulvovaginal candidiasis results in a pH less than 4.5 with a white cottage-cheese like discharge. Hyphae and mycelia are seen on wet mount and KOH prep.

22.   **Complicated urinary tract infection (UTI) and subclinical pyelonephritis are found most frequently in patients:**

a. With symptoms for 4 days before treatment.

b. Diagnosed in a rural emergency department.

c. With two previous episodes of UTI within the past year.

d. With two UTIs during adolescence.

e. Who relapse 1 week after adequate treatment for a UTI.

The answer is e. Although urinary tract infections in women are quite common and typically run a benign course, certain groups are at increased risk of complications and a malignant course. Urban emergency department setting, lower socioeconomic status, diabetes, sickle cell disease and trait, pregnancy, and immunosuppression are all risk factors for subclinical pyelonephritis, complicated UTI, or drug-resistant pathogens. In addition, patients with a recent history of multiple UTIs, a catheter-associated UTI or recent urinary tract instrumentation, a concomitant renal stone, or a delay in seeking treatment should be considered higher risk. In these patients, liberal admission criteria should be considered and a urine culture sent to help modify treatment as necessary.

23.   Regarding a patient with suspected traumatic urinary bladder rupture:

a. If there is not a pelvic fracture, grossly clear urine after catheterization virtually eliminates the possibility of bladder rupture.

b. Antegrade CT cystogram has a high sensitivity for the diagnosis.

c. Intraperitoneal bladder rupture typically heals spontaneously.

d. Extraperitoneal bladder rupture rarely heals spontaneously and requires surgical repair.

e. Retrograde cystogram is preferred to CT cystogram for the diagnosis of bladder injury.

The answer is a. The mechanism of injury that leads to bladder trauma is usually severe with multiple concomitant injuries. The vast majority of patients with a bladder rupture will have gross hematuria. Therefore, grossly clear urine after catheterization virtually eliminates the possibility of bladder rupture, unless there is an associated pelvic fracture. In a patient with suspected bladder injury, either retrograde conventional cystography or CT cystography is indicated. However, CT may be preferred as these patients are often being evaluated for other injuries. With superficial mucosal bladder lacerations, contusions, or hematomas, patients may have hematuria but will not extravasation on cystography. In cases of extraperitoneal bladder rupture, extravasation of contrast material will be seen near the pubic symphysis and pelvic outlet. These injuries will often heal spontaneously with conservative treatment and Foley catheter drainage for 7–10 days to allow for bladder decompression. In cases of intraperitoneal bladder rupture, extravasated contrast will be seen throughout the abdominal cavity. Intraperitoneal bladder perforations will not heal spontaneously and require surgical repair, although it may be delayed to address more pressing, life-threatening injuries.

24.   A 3-year-old uncircumcised boy is brought by his parents with concerns about pain and swelling at the tip of his penis. They state that they were bathing him this morning but were unable to return the foreskin to the original position. The child looks anxious, but is otherwise in no acute distress. On examination, you note a flaccid proximal penis with redness and edema distal to an edematous, retracted foreskin. Which of the following statements is true regarding the diagnosis and management of this condition?

a. This patient has a paraphimosis—immediate attempts at manual reduction should be undertaken.

b. This patient has a paraphimosis—he is at risk of acute urinary obstruction and needs an emergent ultrasound to evaluate for hydronephrosis.

c. This patient has a paraphimosis—he may be safely discharged without further evaluation.

d. This patient has a phimosis—steroids should be avoided due to the risk of superinfection.

e. This patient has a phimosis and will require emergent surgical intervention.

The answer is a. The distinction between phimosis and paraphimosis is often difficult to make. Phimosis refers to a constriction of the foreskin around the glans so that it is unable to be retracted. This is uncomfortable and may cover the meatus, resulting in urinary obstruction. In uncircumcised infants and newborns, most cases are physiologic, resolving as age increases, and do not require intervention. However, in severe cases, postrenal acute renal failure may result. These patients should have their renal function evaluated with laboratory tests (to assess the BUN and creatinine) and an ultrasound (to evaluate for hydronephrosis). They may require anti-inflammatory treatment with steroids (topical or oral), circumcision, or a dorsal slit procedure. Patients with minor symptoms, without evidence of infection or renal failure, may be safely discharged with urologic follow-up. Paraphimosis is the inability to reduce a retracted proximal foreskin back over the glans. It is a true urologic emergency and delay in reduction can result in arterial compromise, tissue ischemia, and necrosis. Attempts at manual reduction should be undertaken after a penile nerve block and/or systemic analgesia. Other reduction techniques include emerging the penis in cold water, applying circumferential pressure to the area, or draining the edematous foreskin with a needle puncture. If these fail, urology should be consulted and a dorsal slit procedure may be required.

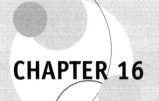

CHAPTER 16

Thoracic and Respiratory Emergencies

Colin M. Bucks, MD

1. A 37-year-old woman complains of chills, weakness, pleuritic chest pain, and a nonproductive cough for 5 days. She reports stopping her highly active antiretroviral therapy (HAART) medications 2 months ago due to the side effects. Her chest x-ray shows patchy, perihilar infiltrates. Her arterial blood gas shows a PaO₂ of 68 mm Hg. In order to blunt alveolar macrophage-induced proinflammatory cytokine release, you should give her:

    a. Ceftriaxone 2 g intravenously daily.

    b. Dapsone 100 mg orally daily.

    c. Prednisone 40 mg orally twice daily.

    d. Trimethoprim-sulfamethoxazole 15 mg/kg (TMP component) intravenously every 6 hours.

    e. Moxifloxacin 400 mg intravenously daily.

    The answer is c. This patient has *Pneumocystis jiroveci* (formerly *Pneumocystis carini*) pneumonia (PCP). TMP/SMX has been the primary antibiotic used in both the prophylaxis and treatment of PCP pneumonia. Dapsone is an antibiotic that is used for PCP treatment in patients with sulfa allergies. Ceftriaxone and moxifloxacin are antibiotics used to treat more common respiratory pathogens. Prednisone is utilized in the treatment of PCP pneumonia in patients with PaO₂ < 70 mm Hg. It is given prior to the administration of antibiotics in order to mediate a proinflammatory cytokine response triggered by components of the *P. jiroveci* cell wall.

2. **A 55-year-old man with a history of alcoholism complains of more than a month of malaise, low-grade fever, and a productive cough with greenish sputum tinged with blood. Examination shows periodontal disease with bad breath and clubbing of fingers. On chest x-ray, there is a 2 cm cavity with an air–fluid level in the posterior segment of the right upper lobe. Sputum smear shows many neutrophils and a variety of bacteria. Appropriate treatment includes:**

    a. Isolate the patient and initiate a four-drug antituberculosis treatment.

    b. Start intravenous administration of clindamycin.

    c. Refer the patient to a dentist for periodontal care.

    d. Schedule a bronchoscopy for the next day.

    e. Start administration of methicillin and tobramycin.

    The answer is b. The predisposing factors of alcoholism and periodontal disease, the duration of illness, the symptoms and signs, and the cavity in a dependent segment of the lung seen on CXR suggest an anaerobic lung abscess caused by aspiration of bacteria from the mouth. Clindamycin is the drug of choice. Tuberculosis is not as likely a diagnosis as anaerobic lung abscess. The patient should be isolated until tuberculosis can be ruled out, but empiric treatment without microscopic or culture evidence is not warranted in this chronically ill patient who is stable. Bronchoscopy prior to antibiotic treatment of a lung abscess carries a risk of dissemination and acute sepsis. Dental work without antibiotic coverage also carries a risk of sepsis. Staphylococcal and gram-negative antibiotics are not indicated.

3. **A 35-year-old woman who is generally healthy complains of fever and cough with sputum production. Vital signs: heart rate 115/min; respiratory rate 24/min; blood pressure 126/88 mm Hg; pulse oximetry, 97% on room air. You initially hear wheezing, but she improves with nebulized albuterol. Chest x-ray shows a right lower lobe infiltrate with effusion. The most appropriate next step is to:**

    a. Obtain decubitus films and begin intravenous ceftriaxone for possible empyema.

    b. Obtain CBC and sputum and blood cultures and begin intravenous ceftriaxone and intravenous azithromycin.

    c. Obtain urgent echocardiography to determine ejection fraction and evidence of pericardial effusion.

    d. Begin oral azithromycin and discharge home.

    e. Begin oral penicillin VK and discharge home.

    The answer is d. Criteria for hospital admission in healthy young patients include respiratory distress, hypoxemia, and dehydration as evidenced by BUN > 25. The treatment of choice is an oral macrolide.

4. **You choose to use intravenous magnesium sulfate to treat a patient with status asthmaticus, but know you must watch for signs of toxicity such as:**

    a. Respiratory depression.

    b. Diarrhea.

    c. Pruritus.

    d. Hyperreflexia.

    e. Dry mouth.

    The answer is a. Magnesium sulfate may be administered via intravenous infusion for the treatment of acute asthma exacerbations. It has a direct relaxing effect on bronchial smooth muscle. The mechanisms of action include inhibition of cholinergic neuromuscular transmission, calcium channel blockade, mast cell and T-lymphocyte stabilization, and stimulation of nitric oxide and prostacyclin. Clinical trials have demonstrated improved airflow and decreased hospitalization when magnesium is used as an adjunct for the treatment of severe asthma attacks.

The side effects include warmth, flushing, sweating, nausea and vomiting, muscle weakness and loss of deep tendon reflexes, hypotension, and respiratory depression. These side effects are typically dose-related and managed by slowing or stopping the infusion.

5. **You have chosen to use air medical evacuation to transport a patient to the tertiary care center 80 miles away. You recall from your college physics that, according to Boyle's Law:**

    a. Decreasing barometric pressure allows for lower supplemental oxygen supplies.

    b. The mass of gas absorbed by the blood stream will increase.

    c. Ambient temperature will decrease if the pilot pressurizes the cabin.

    d. As atmospheric pressures decrease a pneumothorax is more likely to convert to a tension pneumothorax.

    e. The effects of altitude-related hypoxia will develop over a predictable timeline and with readily apparent signs and symptoms.

    The answer is d. Boyle's law states that the volume of a unit of gas (a fixed number of molecules) is inversely proportional to the pressure on it. As altitude increases atmospheric pressure decreases, and molecules of gas become separated by greater distances. The volume of gas will expand as atmospheric pressure decreases on ascent. Air trapped within closed spaces will expand and exert increasing pressure on adjacent bony, neurovascular, and parenchymal structures. Other ascent injuries include barotitis media, barosinusitis, and rupture of hollow viscus by expansion of intestinal gas. Henry's law states that the mass of gas absorbed by a liquid is directly proportional to the partial pressure of the gas above the liquid. As atmospheric pressures decrease, the mass of gas absorbed will decrease, and increasing supplemental oxygen supplies will be necessary. Charles' law explains that ambient temperature decreases with increasing altitude because the gas molecules experience fewer collisions and generate less heat. The ambient temperature would decrease in an unpressurized cabin as altitude increased. The effects of hypoxia include headache, drowsiness, fatigue, unconsciousness, and death. The onset of these symptoms is variable depending on the individual and can be highly insidious.

6. **A 46-year-old asthmatic man complains of wheezing for 2 days despite regular use of his inhaled albuterol, ipratropium, fluticasone, and salmeterol. Yesterday he took 40 mg of prednisone on his family physician's phone advice. He now:**

    a. Needs a chest x-ray and arterial blood gas prior to hospitalization, as he has failed outpatient therapy.

    b. Should receive three more treatments of nebulized beta-agonist therapy, then be admitted if still not improving.

    c. Should be admitted to the hospital if, despite further therapy, his PEFR is 280 L/min.

    d. Is considered to have a "mild" asthma exacerbation with arterial blood gases: Pao_2 78, $Paco_2$ 38, pH 7.38.

    e. Requires arterial blood gas testing to determine degree of hypoxemia, especially if he appears clinically ill (i.e., deteriorating mental status, use of accessory muscles, and pulsus paradoxus).

    The answer is b. Physicians must determine the severity of an asthma attack and the response to treatment. Clinicians often underestimate the severity of obstruction. Mental status, respiratory rate, use of accessory muscles, and pulsus paradoxus are important signs. Objective measurements of obstruction of the airway are the forced expiratory volume in 1 second (FEV_1) and the peak expiratory flow rate (PEFR). Although absolute PFT measurements can be used, percentages of predicted performance values are preferable because they account for individual factors such as age, sex, and height. The ideal use of PFTs is when compared to the patient's established personal best to take response to therapy. A PEFR of 50–80% predicted or the patient's best effort is consistent with a moderate exacerbation. A PEFR value <50% of predicted or personal best is a severe exacerbation. Measurements of arterial blood gases (ABG) are used primarily to determine the $Paco_2$ and should be limited to the subset of patients with PFTs <30% of predicted. Hypoxemia with normocarbia or hypercarbia and a pH of <7.35 indicates severe asthma and impending respiratory failure.

7. **A 22-year-old man is brought to the emergency department after being found in distress by the family swimming pool shed. Family members report recent depression. The patient is alert but unable to provide history due to obvious physical discomfort and a severely hoarse voice. Vital signs: temperature 99.1°F, heart rate 117/min, blood pressure 95/62 mm Hg, respiratory rate 22/min, oxygen saturation 96%. A brief physical examination shows liquefactive necrosis in his oropharynx, subcutaneous emphysema on his chest and neck, and a systolic crunch. His lungs are clear, and his abdomen is soft. After you insert an endotracheal tube and begin fluid resuscitation, you order:**

    a. Emergent psychiatric consultation.
    b. Ewald tube placement and charcoal lavage.
    c. Methylprednisolone intravenous 125 mg.
    d. Induced emesis with 30 mL syrup of ipecac.
    e. Piperacillin-tazobactam intravenous 3.375 g.

    The answer is e. This patient has a perforated esophagus. The history of depression and presence of liquefactive necrosis in the oropharynx suggests an intentional ingestion of a strong alkali, likely a pool cleaning agent. Agents with a pH >12 cause liquefactive necrosis and are more likely to produce esophageal perforation than strong acids (pH <2), which cause coagulative necrosis. Esophageal perforation is strongly suggested by the physical examination findings of subcutaneous emphysema and a systolic crunch (Hamman crunch), a finding consistent with pneumomediastinum. It is essential to institute broad-spectrum antibiotics early in the course of esophageal perforation due to high likelihood of mediastinitis. Early surgical consultation is also necessary. Psychiatric consultation will likely be necessary but would contribute little to the emergent management. Ewald tube placement, charcoal lavage, and induced vomiting could dramatically complicate an esophageal perforation. Corticosteroids have been utilized for some circumferential or transmural burns, but have been shown to complicate the management of large alkali ingestions.

8. **A 64-year-old man with chronic obstructive pulmonary disease (COPD):**

    a. Is unlikely to benefit from bronchodilator and anti-inflammatory therapy during acute exacerbation.
    b. With elevated liver transaminases, leg and scrotal swelling probably has concomitant right heart failure.
    c. Should not be treated with oxygen if there is a history of hypercarbia.
    d. With acute exacerbation should be treated with oxygen therapy to maintain a PaO_2 of at least 65 mm Hg.
    e. Will, if intubated, require a tidal volume between 15 and 18 mL/kg to compensate for dead-space volume.

    The answer is b. Asthma can lead to COPD, especially if poorly controlled and accompanied by repeated infections. Right ventricular failure from cor pulmonale can cause liver congestion, elevation of hepatic enzymes, and proteinuria. Patients with COPD may depend on hypoxic drive for ventilation, although the clinical significance of this is uncertain. Even if this state is suspected, you should never withhold oxygen from a patient. It is not unusual for the $PaCO_2$ to rise slightly with appropriate oxygen therapy, and this is acceptable as long as the pH does not drop below 7.30 and the patient remains alert. Systemic steroids should be started immediately if a response to treatment has not occurred, since their beneficial effects (they restore response to beta-agonists and decrease inflammation) are not seen for several hours. If intubation is required, tidal volume should be much less than 15 mL/kg ideal body weight.

9. **Acute tension pneumothorax is commonly associated with:**

    a. Facial flushing.
    b. Hypotension and vagally mediated bradycardia.
    c. Ventricular fibrillation-induced cardiac arrest.
    d. Right axis deviation on electrocardiogram.
    e. Hyperresonance to percussion on the affected side.

The answer is e. Tension pneumothorax is characterized by dyspnea, hypotension, decreased venous return to the heart, midline shift of the trachea and mediastinal structures away from the side of tension, a hyperresonant percussion note, and tachycardia. Untreated tension pneumothorax can quickly deteriorate to cardiac arrest and pulseless electrical activity. Although sometimes clinically indistinguishable from tamponade, a tension pneumothorax is the more common occurrence and a clinical diagnosis is usually possible. Treatment is needle decompression followed by tube thoracostomy.

10. **Management of critically ill patients may be aided through monitoring pulmonary capillary wedge pressure (PCWP) and other parameters with a Swan-Ganz catheter. PCWP should be:**
    a. Kept as high as possible during the management of adult respiratory distress syndrome (ARDS) to maintain adequate coronary and systemic perfusion.
    b. Kept as low as possible when treating cardiogenic shock with the judicious use of diuretics and venodilators.
    c. Kept as high as possible when treating cardiogenic shock, to improve cardiac output by the Frank-Starling mechanism.
    d. Used in conjunction with cardiac output and systemic oxygen delivery and consumption measurements to determine the adequacy of peripheral perfusion.
    e. Avoided in patients with pulmonary hypertension.

The answer is d. In managing cardiogenic shock, the goal is to balance filling pressures and cardiac outputs against work done and oxygen consumption by the heart, usually by finding the lowest effective filling pressure that maximizes cardiac output. Reduction of afterload with vasodilators and reduction of preload with diuretics are both techniques to improve cardiac efficiency and improve oxygenation. Treatment of cardiogenic shock includes diuretics and vasodilators particularly arterial dilators that decrease afterload and promote forward flow. The goal is to minimize any additional hydrostatic gradients that would cause efflux of fluid from pulmonary capillaries into the alveoli in ARDS.

11. **A 67-year-old building contractor is brought to the ED by his wife. She says that he has become very confused and is suffering from watery diarrhea and a dry cough. The patient appears acutely ill, tachypneic, diaphoretic, and confused. His temperature is elevated at 38.9°C (102°F). You hear scattered, dry rales, but the remainder of the examination is unremarkable. WBC is 23,000/mm³ with a left shift; chest x-ray shows a patchy left upper lobe air-space infiltrate. Which of the following statements concerning the most likely cause of his illness is correct?**
    a. Transmission is generally person-to-person.
    b. The usual incubation period is in the range of weeks rather than days.
    c. Other complications include skin sloughing and mucosal ulcerations.
    d. Travel and work histories are important considerations when diagnosing this illness.
    e. Early empiric antibiotic therapy with intravenous Trimethoprim every 12 hours is necessary to reduce mortality, which is as high as 40% if the disease is untreated.

The answer is d. Many clinicians have been alerted to the possibility of Legionella infection by the characteristic and striking associations with intestinal complaints, diarrhea, and mental status changes in the setting of an atypical pneumonia. Myocarditis, pericarditis, and coma are other possible manifestations. Direct immunofluorescent sputum testing is helpful in the acute diagnosis. Indirect immunofluorescent antibody (IFA) testing is required for diagnosis. Person-to-person transmission probably does not occur, but outbreaks from point sources (water supplies, excavation work) are more common than isolated cases, making notification of health authorities important if the disease is suspected. Early empiric antibiotic therapy with intravenous erythromycin is necessary to reduce mortality, which is as high as 40% if the disease is untreated. Oral erythromycin is continued for 3 weeks to avoid relapse.

12.   Choose the correct statement concerning the diagnosis of an aspirated foreign body in children:

a. Fever should cause you to suspect another diagnosis.

b. A normal posteroanterior and lateral chest x-ray effectively rules out the diagnosis.

c. A 3-week history of cough, fever, and a left–lower-lobe pneumonia on chest x-ray effectively rules out the diagnosis.

d. An inspiratory posteroanterior chest x-ray that demonstrates hyperinflation on the right when wheezes were heard only on the left is more consistent with a vascular ring.

e. Bilateral decubitus chest x-rays may clinch the diagnosis; obstruction is heralded by a lack of dependent atelectasis on the side of the foreign body.

The answer is e. Eighty percent of aspirated foreign bodies occur in children younger than 6 years. Coughing and airway distress usually call attention to a problem immediately, but foreign bodies such as peanuts can cause a severe pneumonia for weeks or more. A normal inspiratory CXR does not exclude the diagnosis, and expiratory films, which demonstrate mediastinal shift or air trapping on the side of obstruction when compared with inspiratory films, are necessary. In uncooperative patients, decubitus chest films may be obtained and will show a lack of atelectasis of the dependent obstructed lung due to air trapping. Sixty percent of foreign bodies are found on the right, but a foreign body may "flip" to the other bronchus as a result of coughing. Bronchoscopy is diagnostic and therapeutic.

13.   A 72-year-old, 70-kg man presents in respiratory distress. He is barrel-chested and thin, with marked accessory muscle use and retractions. He complains, through pursed lips, that he cannot catch his breath and his inhaler does not help. Admission blood gases: pH 7.28, PaO_2 45 mm Hg, $PaCO_2$ 70 mm Hg. Despite therapy his mental status and respiratory rate deteriorate, and you intubate him. Chest x-ray confirms proper tube placement and no other acute problem. After 5 minutes of manual ventilation, the most appropriate initial ventilator settings are:

a. Pressure-cycled ventilator, FIO_2 60%, assist-control rate 18, tidal volume 600 mL.

b. Volume-cycled ventilator, FIO_2 70%, intermittent mandatory ventilation (IMV) rate 4, tidal volume 600 mL.

c. Volume-cycled ventilator, FIO_2 70%, PEEP 5 cm H_2O, assist-control rate 20, tidal volume 600 mL.

d. Volume-cycled ventilator, FIO_2 80%, assist-control rate 10, tidal volume 450 mL.

e. Volume-cycled ventilator, FIO_2 100%, IMV rate 20, tidal volume 450 mL.

The answer is d. Although you should make an effort to avoid intubating the patient with decompensated COPD, the deteriorating mental status and respiratory rate indicates worsening hypoxia, increasing hypercarbia, and fatigue. This patient has a chronic respiratory acidosis with a compensatory metabolic alkalosis, since a $PaCO_2$ of 65 would otherwise result in a pH of 7.16 (for every 10 mm Hg change in CO_2 from 40 mm Hg, pH changes by 0.08). If the patient is hyperventilated to a "normal" $PaCO_2$ he will become alkalotic (pH 7.52). Alkalosis shifts the oxygen dissociation curve to the left, decreases O_2 delivery, and may result in hypotension, arrhythmias, and seizures. A rule of thumb is that total minute ventilation for an adult is normally 10 L/min, and alveolar ventilation approximately 5 L/min. Dead-space ventilation for the average intubated patient is 50% of the total minute ventilation, or approximately 5 L/min (physiologic dead space + ventilator tubing). In general, doubling the minute ventilation halves the $PaCO_2$. Observations of the adverse effects of barotrauma and volutrauma have led to recommendations of lower tidal volumes than in years past (tidal volume = 5.0–10 mL/kg). An initial tidal volume of 5.0–8.0 mL/kg is indicated in the presence of obstructive airway disease and acute respiratory distress syndrome (ARDS). The goal is to adjust the TV so that plateau pressures are less than 35 cm H_2O. Assist control for the fatigued patient is probably preferable to IMV in the emergency department, although some patients may hyperventilate and require sedation. The initial FIO_2 should be high, but prolonged 100% O_2 may promote atelectasis, so a lower concentration should be used after resuscitation and adjusted according to blood gas results. Pressure-cycled ventilators and PEEP is not often indicated in the patient with decompensated COPD.

14. **Administration of isoniazid for the treatment of tuberculosis is associated with:**

    a. Hemolysis and thrombocytopenia.
    b. Central or peripheral loss of visual field.
    c. Muscle fasciculations and rhabdomyolysis.
    d. Photodermatitis.
    e. Hepatitis.

    The answer is e. Hepatitis is the most severe potential side effect of isoniazid and may be fatal. Its incidence increases in older patients. Peripheral neuropathy is the most common toxic reaction; vitamin B_6 is often given to ameliorate this effect. Skin reactions do occur, but photodermatitis is not particularly associated with isoniazid.

15. **It is generally agreed that tube thoracostomy is the best management of a nontraumatic spontaneous pneumothorax of greater than:**

    a. 10%.
    b. 20%.
    c. 30%.
    d. 40%.
    e. 50%.

    The answer is b. The decision to treat a nontraumatic spontaneous pneumothorax with aspiration by catheter, tube thoracostomy, or observation is based on the mechanism, underlying disease, and complicating factors. Any patient requiring general anesthesia or mechanical ventilation should have a tube thoracostomy. Aspiration by catheter may be successful in selected patients, but they should be watched for a period of time with repeat x-rays before being discharged. The possibility of the occurrence of a tension pneumothorax in association with any simple pneumothorax must be kept in mind. Most traumatic pneumothoraces require thoracostomy.

16. **In selecting empiric antibiotic therapy for bacterial pneumonia, it is helpful to remember that:**

    a. Pneumonia in seizure patients or alcoholics is seldom due to anaerobic or gram-negative bacteria.
    b. Intravenous nafcillin or vancomycin are better options than intravenous azithromycin for the treatment of bacterial pneumonia following influenza.
    c. A patient with chronic obstructive pulmonary disease who has a bulging interlobar fissure and a necrotizing pneumonia of the right upper lobe on chest x-ray should initially be treated with intravenous penicillin pending sputum culture and sensitivity studies.
    d. Acutely ill elderly patients who present with a patchy alveolar infiltrate and mild cough, in association with confusion, bradycardia, diarrhea, or myalgia, should be treated with intravenous ceftriaxone 1 g daily.
    e. A negative posteroanterior and lateral chest x-ray of adequate quality essentially excludes the diagnosis of pneumonia.

    The answer is b. Patients at risk for aspiration or debilitated patients with pneumonia require initial therapy to cover gram-negative and anaerobic organisms. Staphylococcal pneumonia only accounts for 1% of bacterial pneumonias, but should be considered in patients with the abrupt onset of chills, fever, and cough following a viral illness, especially measles and influenza. Legionella may present with unremarkable pulmonary symptoms but marked extrapulmonary findings: diarrhea, chills, headache, and myalgias. Untreated Legionella pneumonia has a mortality rate as high as 40%. A negative initial chest x-ray does not exclude the diagnosis of pneumonia, especially in elderly, neutropenic, or dehydrated patients. Some authorities maintain that "dry pneumonia" may become evident on chest x-ray after rehydration, although by this logic we should be able to give intravenous diuretic and make the pneumonia look better on radiograph.

17.   Choose the correct statement regarding the management of acute asthma attacks:

a. A patient's use of sternocleidomastoid muscles during inspiration is useful in judging the severity of the attack.

b. Oxygen supplementation to prevent hypoxemia facilitates the action of beta-adrenergic bronchodilator therapy.

c. Hypercarbia generally precedes hypoxemia with worsening asthma exacerbation.

d. Decreased wheezing after oxygen administration is a useful indicator of a positive response to treatment.

e. An improvement in the difference in systolic blood pressure between inspiration and expiration is useful to identify patients who can potentially be discharged after acute asthma exacerbation.

The answer is a. Use of the neck muscles usually indicates severe asthma and an FEV_1 of less than 1.0 L. Beta-agonists may transiently worsen hypoxemia during the early treatment of asthma by causing perfusion of poorly ventilated lung segments. Hypoxemia and hypocarbia are the most common findings in asthma; hypercarbia (and in some case normocarbia) indicates impending respiratory failure. Wheezing is a clinically useful sign when present, but bronchospasm may be so severe as to prevent sufficient airflow to allow wheezing. A pulsus paradoxus of >20 mm Hg indicates a severe attack.

18.   Aspiration pneumonia is a relatively common complication among debilitated patients. Choose the true statement regarding aspiration:

a. Early use of intravenous proton pump inhibitors (PPIs) greatly reduces the rate of ventilator-associated pneumonias (VAP).

b. High-dose steroids have been shown to be beneficial if administered to patients who have aspirated stomach contents with a pH of less than 2.5.

c. Early mechanical ventilation and positive end-expiratory pressure (PEEP) can reduce the mortality rate in severe aspiration pneumonia.

d. Aspiration of particulate stomach content is best treated by bronchoscopy and irrigation with large volumes of saline solution.

e. A properly placed nasogastric tube and manual syringe decompression of the stomach in the obtunded or postresuscitation patient will prevent aspiration.

The answer is c. In adults, a cuffed endotracheal tube is necessary for complete airway protection. An NG tube does not insure against the possibility of aspiration, since it may fail to remove all stomach material. Neither prophylactic steroids nor antibiotics have been shown to be of value after aspiration and should not be routinely used. If clinical evidence of infection develops, antibiotics effective against aerobes and anaerobes should be given. Oxygen should be given after aspiration, and endotracheal intubation may be needed to protect the airway from further aspiration as well as for treatment. Bronchoscopy is often indicated, but large-volume irrigation is to be avoided, since this may force particles deeper into the airway. Early mechanical ventilation and PEEP have been shown to reduce mortality.

19.   Choose the correct statement about Legionella pneumonia:

a. It is most commonly seen in the elderly in the winter.

b. It may result in multiple laboratory abnormalities including hypokalemia, elevations in pancreas function tests, and hematuria.

c. Clustered outbreaks are more common than sporadic cases.

d. The diagnosis can often be made by sputum Gram stain and should be used to guide antibiotic choice.

e. Person-to-person is the usual mode of transmission.

The answer is c. In patients proven to have legionellosis, sputum Gram stain shows few PMNs and no predominant organism. Direct immunofluorescence testing of the sputum has a high specificity but a low sensitivity. Risk factors include diabetes, smoking, living near excavation sites, and immunosuppression. The patients appear toxic. Tachypnea, diaphoresis, and a dry cough with diffuse inspiratory rales are the most common pulmonary signs. Typical chest x-ray findings are a unilateral, patchy air-space infiltrate, progressing to bilateral infiltrates and consolidation. Effusions are seen in 15–33% of patients. Extrapulmonary findings such as confusion, diarrhea, and coma are common. Other laboratory abnormalities include mild elevations in liver function tests and, inexplicably, microscopic hematuria in 10% of patients.

20. **Choose the correct statement concerning the treatment of asthma in pregnancy:**
    a. The use of subcutaneous epinephrine early in pregnancy has been associated with an increased risk of fetal malformations.
    b. Theophylline is associated with an increased incidence of premature labor.
    c. Parenteral beta-agonists given near-term promote uterine contractility and lead to premature delivery.
    d. Erythromycin stimulates cytochrome P450–mediated metabolism and decreases the serum concentration of theophylline.
    e. The dosage of corticosteroids must be reduced during pregnancy.

The answer is a. Parenteral epinephrine has been associated with fetal malformations during early pregnancy and should be avoided (pregnancy class C). The methylxanthines are not contraindicated during pregnancy. Tetracyclines are to be avoided during pregnancy, and iodide-containing mucolytic agents can result in fetal goiter and hypothyroidism. Erythromycin is safe, but it increases the serum levels of theophylline, therefore, levels should be monitored. Corticosteroids may be used in appropriate dosages.

21. **A multiparous woman presents in imminent labor with rupture of the membranes. You note greenish material on the infant's face as you deliver the head. The preferred sequence in the management of this infant would be:**
    a. Suction the nose and mouth immediately, then, after delivery, apply oxygen by bag-mask ventilation.
    b. Suction the nose and oropharynx, then immediately apply oxygen by bag-mask ventilation prior to complete delivery.
    c. Deliver the infant, suction the nose and oropharynx, and apply a continuous positive airway pressure (CPAP) mask with an oxygen concentration of 100%.
    d. Suction the nose and pharynx immediately, then after delivery intubate the infant and begin immediate positive-pressure ventilation with 100% oxygen.
    e. Suction the nose and pharynx immediately, then after delivery assess for vigor. Intubate the infant, suction the trachea, and begin assisted ventilation as necessary if signs of respiratory distress or lack of vigor.

The answer is e. Aspiration of meconium is anticipated when the amniotic fluid is meconium-stained. The meconium must be removed from the oropharynx and trachea prior to the infant's first inspiratory efforts or positive-pressure ventilation to avoid forcing the meconium from the airways into the lungs. Vigorous newborns exposed to meconium are not automatically intubated. They are monitored for signs of respiratory distress, provided supplemental oxygen via an oxygen hood, and intubated if signs of distress develop. Vigorous is defined as (1) strong respiratory effort, (2) good muscle tone, and (3) a heart rate >100/min. Nonvigorous newborns are intubated and suctioned prior to stimulation. Early transfer to a center with a neonatal intensive care unit is appropriate in either case.

22.   Choose the correct statement about viral pneumonia:

a. Respiratory syncytial virus (RSV) pneumonia is most often seen in patients with AIDS and older immunocompromised patients.

b. Varicella zoster and chickenpox may cause a fulminant viral pneumonia in adults.

c. Staphylococcal pneumonia following an influenza outbreak would be distinctly unusual and suggests a point source for the infection.

d. Amantadine is useful in reducing the clinical symptoms of influenza B infection if started within 48 hours of exposure.

e. Viral pneumonia rarely results in hypoxemic respiratory failure in the immunocompetent adult.

The answer is b. RSV is usually associated with children. While viral pneumonias are usually characterized by a moderate elevation in the white count, scant sputum production, and a benign clinical course, severe infections can occur even in the healthy adult. Staphylococcal pneumonia, though uncommon, has a peak incidence during influenza and measles epidemics. Amantadine is recommended for unvaccinated patients who are at high risk of complications from infections caused by influenza A.

23.   A 33-year-old man complains of fever, sore throat, mild cough, and tenderness with swelling over the left neck. Temperature 39.5°C (103.1°F); heart rate 110/min; respiratory rate 25/min. You note bulging in the left peritonsillar region and edema with tenderness anterior to the course of the left sternocleidomastoid muscle; he also has diffuse rales. White blood count is 27,000/mm^3 and soft tissue x-ray of the neck shows some swelling of the retropharyngeal space. Chest radiograph reveals multiple, bilateral, rounded air-space infiltrates, several of which have a central area of lucency within them. Choose the correct statement:

a. This condition may be associated with heart murmur or splinter hemorrhages.

b. Drainage of the peritonsillar abscess alone would be curative.

c. Blood cultures will probably be negative.

d. Chest radiographs are often negative or show only minor abnormalities; and CT confirmation is required prior to treatment.

e. The results of sputum cultures should be used over the results of blood cultures in choosing antibiotic therapy.

The answer is a. Multiple, rounded, patchy lung infiltrates with cavitation should suggest the diagnosis of septic pulmonary emboli. Tricuspid valve endocarditis, particularly in drug addicts, and septic thrombophlebitis as a result of infected indwelling venous catheters or hemodialysis catheters are the most common causes, and the organism isolated from blood culture is usually *Staphylococcus*. However, other infections may lead to septic thrombophlebitis. In this case, a peritonsillar abscess extended to cause septic thrombophlebitis of the internal jugular vein. Treatment consists of surgical drainage of the abscess, removal of the thrombosed infected vein, and administration of antibiotics. A mix of aerobic and anaerobic oropharyngeal flora usually causes peritonsillar abscesses. Therefore, penicillin is usually effective for infections arising from this source.

24.   A 59-year-old man with a history of COPD is having an acute exacerbation. You have given methylprednisolone intravenous 125 mg, supplemental oxygen, nebulized ipratropium, and several albuterol treatments. He is alert and cooperative, but he is using accessory muscles to support a respiratory rate of 27/min. The intervention most likely to prevent this patient from being intubated is:

a. BiPAP with iPAP at 10 cm H$_2$O, ePAP at 4 cm H$_2$O.

b. BiPAP with iPAP at 4 cm H$_2$O, ePAP at 10 cm H$_2$O.

c. Azithromycin intravenous 500 mg.

d. Doxapram 400 mg intravenous infusion.

e. Inhaled helium 30%/oxygen 70%.

The answer is a. Although helium/oxygen mixtures, antibiotics, and respiratory stimulants such as doxapram have been used in the management of COPD exacerbations, none of these interventions is likely to prevent the patient from being intubated. Of note, helium/oxygen has been shown to be of benefit in acute asthma exacerbations, but has not shown the same benefit in COPD. The inspiratory positive airway pressure must be set with a higher pressure than the expiratory positive airway pressure. Patients will often require fine adjustments of these pressures to find the optimal setting, and an experienced respiratory therapist can be useful ally in determining the most effective pressure settings and mask fit.

25. **Choose the correct statement regarding anticholinergic drug therapy in acute asthma:**
    a. The effects of anticholinergic and beta-agonists are additive.
    b. Atropine is more potent and longer acting than ipratropium bromide.
    c. Nebulized anticholinergics yield symptomatic improvement within minutes of administration.
    d. Aerosolized anticholinergic agents frequently cause systemic side effects such as tachycardia, urinary obstruction, blurred vision, and ileus.
    e. Nebulized atropine must be administered separate from beta-agonist medications in order to be effective.

The answer is a. The effects of anticholinergics and beta-agonists appear to be additive, primarily because the anticholinergics affect larger central airways while the beta-agonists act primarily on the smaller peripheral airways. Their delayed onset of action (60–90 minutes) is a disadvantage in treating acute attacks, but an advantage of their use is the relative lack of cardiac side effects. Systemic toxicity is low, particularly with the newer, long-acting agents. Atropine is associated with more side effects from its greater systemic absorption and is less potent and shorter acting than the newer agents.

26. **A 20-year-old previously healthy woman presents after a witnessed syncopal event. She takes a multivitamin and a monophasic oral contraceptive. She appears comfortable in the emergency department, and her physical examination provides no suggestion of acute illness. Urine pregnancy is negative, and EKG shows no signs of strain or dysrhythmia. The finding that would complete the evaluation for pulmonary embolism is:**
    a. Normal heart examination and lack of leg swelling.
    b. Pulse oximetry saturation >94%.
    c. Normal lung examination.
    d. Quantitative D-dimer less than 500 ng/mL.
    e. PA/lateral chest x-ray without infiltrate, effusion, or atelectasis.

The answer is d. The evaluation of venous thromboembolic disease and pulmonary embolism in the emergency department has been subject to ongoing evolution over the past two decades. Recommended algorithms begin with the clinician estimating the patient's pretest probability for pulmonary embolism (PE) prior to initiating any testing. This patient presents with a symptom associated with PE, one identified risk factor of thromboembolic disease, and no diagnosis that is immediately more apparent. Although the patient is not at high risk for PE, consideration of the pulmonary embolism rule-out criteria (PERC) suggests that additional evaluation is justified (use of estrogen does not allow us to use this rule). In low-risk patients, a negative quantitative D-dimer test may be used to exclude the diagnosis of PE. Additional imaging by ventilation–perfusion scintigraphy, CT angiography, or pulmonary arteriogram would not be necessary in this patient. None of the other answer options have been reliably incorporated into clinical decision-making algorithms in the diagnosis of PE.

27.   **A 56-year-old woman with a history of alcohol abuse has a 1-day history of fever, dry cough, and pleuritic left chest pain. Nine days ago she was admitted for a GI bleeding and received endoscopic sclerotherapy. Physical examination today is significant only for percussive dullness at the left lung base with "e to a" auscultatory changes and a temperature of 38.3°C (101°F). Chest x-ray shows a large left pleural effusion. You perform ultrasound-guided thoracentesis and obtain 300 mL of cloudy fluid: pH of 6.86; LDH 650 U/mL (serum level 200), glucose 42 mg/100 mL (serum level 140); protein 3.1 g/100 mL (serum protein 2.9); amylase 5000 U/100 mL. Gram stain shows mixed gram-negative and gram-positive organisms. The most likely diagnosis is:**

a.   Dissection of pancreatic pseudocyst into the chest.

b.   Parapneumonic effusion.

c.   Superinfected tuberculous effusion.

d.   Delayed rupture of the esophagus.

e.   Diaphragmatic hernia with incarcerated bowel and effusion.

The answer is d. A complication of sclerotherapy is rupture of ulcerative areas of the distal esophagus caused by the sclerosing agent. Such effusions are exudative, with a low pH and a high amylase (of salivary origin) in contrast to uncomplicated pancreatic pseudocysts, which generally exhibit the latter. Tuberculosis, malignancy, pneumonia, pulmonary emboli, collagen vascular diseases, and drugs are the most common causes of exudative effusions. A low pH suggests infection, and with the exception of rheumatoid effusions and some malignancies, so does a low glucose. Most purulent effusions and effusions with a pH of less than 7.3 should be drained by tube thoracostomy. Treatment in this case is surgical, with operative drainage and tube thoracostomy along with broad-spectrum antibiotics. The mortality is high, and early diagnosis is essential.

28.   **A 35-year-old aerobics instructor complains of severe, nonproductive cough, chills, fever, and malaise. He recounts a 10-day history of headache and myalgia. Physical examination shows mild dyspnea, a fever of 38.5°C (101.3°F), and bilateral scattered rales. Chest radiograph shows faint bilateral, patchy air-space infiltrates without effusion. Of the drugs regimens listed below, you should prescribe:**

a.   Amantadine 100 mg po bid for 10 days.

b.   Tetracycline 250 mg po bid for 10 days.

c.   Tetracycline 500 mg po bid for 10 days.

d.   Azithromycin 500 mg po today, and 250 mg po for 4 more days.

e.   A codeine-formulated antitussive for symptomatic relief, but no antibiotic.

The answer is d. Amantadine given in the first 24–48 hours of symptoms may shorten the course of influenza A and can be used as chemoprophylaxis during outbreaks. Its use is generally reserved for the elderly and higher risk patients. This patient appears to have a postviral pneumonia, probably mycoplasma pneumonia. A macrolide is usually considered the drug of choice in community-acquired pneumonia because of its activity against Legionella, Mycoplasma, and *Streptococcus pneumoniae*. Tetracycline is much less effective against pneumococcus and is not recommended. Penicillin has no activity against Mycoplasma or Legionella. Staphylococcal pneumonia is seen with an increased frequency as a complication of postviral pneumonia.

29. **A 47-year-old man is brought by ambulance from the scene of a bus bombing in respiratory distress. His examination is significant for many minor abrasions, partial thickness burns on the extremities, dyspnea, poor air movement, dullness to percussion bilaterally, and a superficial crackling sensation noted on palpation of the chest. His chest x-ray shows subcutaneous emphysema and bilateral patchy infiltrates in a butterfly pattern. After intubation, management of his pulmonary injuries should include:**

    a. Hyperbaric oxygen treatment.

    b. Aggressive positive end-tidal expiratory pressure for alveolar recruitment.

    c. Intravenous corticosteroids to reduce secondary inflammatory lung injury.

    d. Extracorporeal membrane oxygenation.

    e. Permissive hypercapnia with reduced tidal volumes and peak inspiratory pressures.

    The answer is e. The patient has sustained blast lung injury (BLI). BLI occurs as part of a spectrum of overpressure injuries of which the hollow, air-containing organs are especially susceptible. The traumatic process of compression and expansion disrupts alveolar membranes and interalveolar septa resulting in separation of lung parenchyma from the vascular structures. The subsequent hemorrhage from the distal vasculature tree results in ventilation–perfusion mismatch and reduced lung compliance. The clinical picture is not dissimilar to ARDS or pulmonary contusion. Additional complications, including hemopneumothorax, pneumomediastinum, subcutaneous emphysema, air emboli, and foreign body impaction often accompany and complicate BLI. Recent successes have been found by utilizing permissive hypercapnea and limiting peak inspiratory pressures. Additional treatment modalities include prophylactic bilateral chest tubes and early attempts to stimulate spontaneous breathing with intermittent mechanic ventilation and continuous positive airway pressure.

30. **PEEP is useful in the management of ARDS because it can:**

    a. Increase the production and effectiveness of pulmonary surfactant.

    b. Recruit additional alveolar air space, thereby reducing pulmonary ventilation–perfusion mismatch.

    c. Increase hydrostatic resistance to pulmonary capillary blood flow and thus reduce leakage of fluid and protein.

    d. Improve oxygen delivery across the thickened, dysfunctional alveolar membrane.

    e. Allow a higher F_{IO_2} to be used for patients in critical condition.

    The answer is b. PEEP acts to open up fluid-filled alveoli and make them available for gas exchange. This allows lower concentrations of inspired oxygen to be used. The use of PEEP is not without problems, since higher levels may impede venous return to the heart and result in decreased cardiac output and oxygen delivery. A Swan-Ganz catheter may be necessary when PEEP is used.

31. **In managing the patient with COPD, the measurement or finding which best corresponds with day-to-day function and long-term prognosis is the:**

    a. Forced expiratory volume in 1 second as a fraction of the forced vital capacity (FEV_1%).

    b. Arterial blood gas.

    c. Dead-space volume.

    d. Chest radiograph.

    e. Forced vital capacity.

    The answer is a. The FEV_1 (forced expiratory volume in 1 second) as a fraction of the FVC (forced vital capacity) correlates well with physiologic function. An increase in dead space is common in COPD but is poorly correlated with function or prognosis. CXR is often misleading in predicting performance, although it can rule out superimposed complications. A single blood gas is not predictive of long-term prognosis. A combination of physiologic and laboratory tests is necessary to accurately stage the severity of disease.

32.   **A 65-year-old man is seen for evaluation of progressive dyspnea. He has a 40-year smoking history. The spirometric value diagnostic of chronic obstructive pulmonary disease (COPD) is:**

a.   Forced vital capacity (FVC) 120% of predicted, forced expiratory volume in 1 second (FEV_1) 110% of predicted, and FEV_1/FVC 73%.

b.   FVC 90% of predicted, FEV_1 85% of predicted, and FEV_1/FVC 80%.

c.   FVC 75% of predicted, FEV_1/FVC 90%.

d.   FVC 85% of predicted, FEV_1/FVC 52%.

e. FEV_1/FVC is 60% of predicted, improves to 75% postbronchodilator therapy.

The answer is d. An obstructive spirometric pattern that does not normalize following bronchodilator administration is diagnostic of COPD (irreversible airflow obstruction).

33.   **A 70-year-old man with a history of chronic obstructive pulmonary disease is brought to the hospital with confusion, fever, chills, productive cough, and severe dyspnea. He is tachycardic, tachypneic, and hypotensive. His chest radiograph reveals bilateral infiltrates and he requires intubation and admission to the intensive care unit (ICU). His sputum is purulent, green, and has a smell you associate with *Pseudomonas aeruginosa*. An appropriate antibiotic regimen would be:**

a.   Ceftriaxone and azithromycin.

b.   Levofloxacin and metronidazole.

c.   Cefuroxime.

d.   Cefuroxime and azithromycin.

e.   Amikacin and piperacillin/tazobactam.

The answer is e. Pneumonia resulting from pseudomonal infection may develop in patients with chronic lung disease or congestive heart failure. Pneumonia results from the aspiration of upper tract secretions, which is more likely in patients with cerebrovascular accident. Pneumonia may present as an acute life-threatening infection. Early antibiotic treatment should be instituted. When pseudomonal pneumonia is suspected, antibiotics with antipseudomonal activity are used, including aminoglycosides, select third-generation cephalosporins (e.g., ceftazidime, cefoperazone), select extended-spectrum penicillins, carbapenems (imipenem, meropenem), aztreonam, and fluoroquinolones.

34.   **For the severe asthmatic patient who is not responsive to aggressive beta-agonist and steroid therapy, there may be an indication for using Heliox (helium–oxygen mixture):**

a.   This will make arterial blood gas measurements useless, since the Heliox displaces oxygen on the hemoglobin molecule and causes falsely low Po_2 readings.

b.   Originally used as a gas mixture for deep dives, Heliox triggers the mammalian diving reflex, which protects the brain from hypoxia.

c.   The addition of helium to the breathing mixture lowers alveolar Pco_2, thereby reducing the work of respiration.

d.   The Heliox mixture directly causes bronchial smooth muscle relaxation.

e.   The Heliox mixture is less dense than air, allowing increased flow and less work of respiration.

The answer is e. Heliox (a mixture of 60–80% helium and 20–40% oxygen) improves PEFR and ABG results in nonintubated asthmatics and decreases peak airway pressures in ventilated asthmatics. Helium is an inert gas with one-eighth the density of nitrogen. When helium is blended with oxygen, the resulting gas mixture has a threefold reduction in density compared to air. Heliox reduces the resistance associated with gas flow through airways with nonlaminar flow (the upper and more proximal airways). This reduces respiratory muscle work and possibly improves gas exchange by improving ventilation–perfusion relationships or distal gas mixing and diffusion. Constant monitoring of oxygen saturation and frequent blood gas monitoring are recommended for patients receiving Heliox.

35. **Cor pulmonale:**

   a. Is an early sign of COPD and will respond to bronchodilator therapy.
   b. Is more commonly seen in patients in whom emphysema predominates.
   c. Produces a left bundle-branch pattern on the ECG.
   d. Results from chronic hypoxia inducing pulmonary hypertension.
   e. Results from the cardiac toxicity of inhaled bronchodilators.

   The answer is d. Pulmonary dysfunction causing hypoxia reduces myocardial oxygen supply while increasing cardiac output demand by perfusing all tissues with suboptimally oxygenated blood. Hypoxia leads to pulmonary arteriolar vasoconstriction, and along with various destructive processes such as emphysema and pulmonary fibrosis, which reduces lung vascular bed area, causes elevation of pulmonary artery pressures. Chronic increases in pulmonary arterial pressure lead to right ventricular hypertrophy and dilation. When compensatory mechanisms fail, the patient develops clinical evidence of right heart failure (cor pulmonale), usually with left ventricular output preserved, at least at rest.

36. **A 37-year-old woman arrives by fire rescue in status epilepticus. The medics have given both intravenous and intramuscular benzodiazepines, but the patient continues to seize. You notice a Medic-Alert bracelet that states "ASTHMA." The cardiac monitor shows a heart rate of 154/min. In addition to an arterial blood gas, you should also check a:**

   a. Serum calcium.
   b. Serum magnesium.
   c. Serum potassium.
   d. Serum sodium.
   e. Theophylline level.

   The answer is e. The most common side effects of theophylline are nervousness, nausea, vomiting, anorexia, and headache. At plasma levels greater than 30 mg/mL, there is a risk of seizures and cardiac dysrhythmias.

37. **A 24-year-old man complains of fever, rigors, and productive cough. He is HIV positive, but does not know his CD4 count or viral load. His chest x-ray shows bilateral lobar infiltrates. You should treat for the most common bacterial pathogen, which is:**

   a. *Legionella.*
   b. *Pneumococcus.*
   c. *Chlamydia.*
   d. *Staphylococcus.*
   e. Tuberculosis.

   The answer is b. Respiratory infections are the most common type of opportunistic infection in patients with AIDS. *Pneumocystis jiroveci* is a common cause of pneumonia in patients with AIDS, but there is also an increased incidence of pneumonia caused by *M. tuberculosis* and common bacterial pathogens such as *S. pneumoniae* and *H. influenzae.* In fact, the incidence of pneumococcal pneumonia is 7–10 times higher in HIV-infected persons, and the incidence of *H. influenzae* pneumonia is approximately 100 times higher than in non–HIV-infected individuals.

38. **A 78-year-old man with cancer of the left lung presents with massive hemoptysis and is in danger of aspirating. While arranging for emergency bronchoscopy, you instruct the nurse to place the patient:**

   a. Left chest down.

   b. In reverse Trendelenburg position.

   c. Right chest down.

   d. In Trendelenburg position.

   e. In the upright or semi-upright position.

   The answer is a. Massive hemoptysis is defined as at least 600 mL of blood in 24 hours. Exsanguination rarely occurs, but the major morbidity is due to asphyxiation from aspirated blood. It takes as little as 150 mL (5 oz) of blood to completely fill the tracheobronchial tree. You should secure the airway with a large diameter (8 mm) endotracheal tube (ETT) that can accommodate fiberoptic bronchoscopy. You should position the patient with the bleeding lung in a dependent position in order to avoid soiling of the unaffected side. The ETT may be positioned above the carina or in the case of bleeding from the right lung into the left mainstem bronchus. Placement into the right mainstem bronchus is not recommended because of the risk of occluding the right upper lobe bronchus. These patients require emergent consultations for bronchoscopy, surgical resection, or angiography with selective embolization.

39. **A patient underwent emergent subclavian central line placement 3 days ago. She subsequently developed difficulty breathing and a nonproductive cough. Chest x-ray demonstrates a large pleural effusion. Thoracentesis produces a milky white fluid with high fat and lymphocyte count and 4 g/dL of protein. The structure inadvertently injured during the procedure was the:**

   a. Lung parenchyma.

   b. Thoracic duct.

   c. Subclavian artery.

   d. Esophagus.

   e. Thymus gland.

   The answer is b. The thoracic duct is the largest lymphatic vessel in the body. It terminates in the left subclavian vein just distal to the junction with the left internal jugular vein. In this case, the thoracentesis demonstrates a chylothorax, an accumulation of lymphatic fluid in the thorax that has slowly accumulated in the pleural cavity. Disruption of the thoracic duct can result from central line misadventure, chest trauma, or intraoperative injury. Management includes repeated thoracentesis or tube thoracostomy and parenteral alimentation.

40. **A 71-year-old patient with end-stage COPD complains of severe breathlessness and cough. He is breathing 36 times a minute and his pulse oximetry reading is 84%. You are able to easily intubate him without using induction agents or paralytics. You place him on what you feel to believe appropriate ventilator settings, but know you must scrupulously avoid:**

   a. Hypoxemia, which can lead to brain damage if the patient is hyponatremic.

   b. Alkalosis, which can lead to seizures, especially if the patient is hypokalemic.

   c. Hypercarbia, which can cause myocardial ischemia if the patient is hypocalcemic.

   d. Acidosis, which can lead to fulminant liver failure if the patient is hyperkalemic.

   e. Hypocarbia, which is irreversible if the patient is hypomagnesemic.

   The answer is b. After intubating a patient, draw an arterial blood gas after 15–20 minutes to ensure that ventilation is appropriate. Hyperventilation alkalosis must be scrupulously avoided, particularly because patients may have preexisting chronic metabolic alkalosis. This alkalosis can result in seizures and dysrhythmias, especially with coexisting hypokalemia.

41. **When tuberculosis spreads to bone, the most common site is the:**
    a. Hip.
    b. Pelvis.
    c. Skull
    d. Sternum.
    e. Spine.

    The answer is e. Generally spinal TB (Pott's disease) accounts for 50–70% of the reported cases of bone tuberculosis; the hip or knee is involved in 15–20% of cases; and the ankle, elbow, wrists, and shoulders and other bones and joints account for 15–20% of cases.

42. **The most common cause of pneumonia is:**
    a. Pneumococcus.
    b. Viral.
    c. Atypical bacteria, such as mycoplasma and chlamydia.
    d. Unknown.
    e. Community-associated MRSA.

    The answer is d. While *Streptococcus pneumoniae* is the most commonly identified organism, the majority of patients with pneumonia never have a specific pathogen identified.

43. **An 82-year-old man is sent from the local nursing home for evaluation of "cough and fever." His chest radiograph shows cavitation and pneumatocoele formation. The most likely etiologic agent is:**
    a. *Klebsiella pneumoniae.*
    b. More likely during epidemics of influenza.
    c. Commonly associated with end-stage liver disease.
    d. Anaerobic pathogens from aspiration.
    e. Noninfectious.

    The answer is b. Necrotizing pneumonia is most often staphylococcal, which frequently occurs as a complication of influenza pneumonia. It may be associated with endocarditis.

44. **A 30-year-old man has had a week's worsening of low-grade fever and nonproductive cough. You hear scattered rales and rhonchi, but the patient is not toxic. You know that:**
    a. Atypical pneumonia cannot be differentiated from typical pneumonia on clinical grounds.
    b. Atypical pneumonia can be caused by *H. influenzae* and other gram-negative organisms.
    c. A nonproductive cough is more often associated with atypical pneumonia.
    d. The finding of bullous myringitis would suggest chlamydial pneumonia.
    e. Pleurisy is rarely seen with atypical pneumonia.

    The answer is a. Atypical pneumonia cannot reliably be differentiated from typical, pyogenic pneumonia on clinical grounds. Either type of pneumonia may present in a gradual fashion with nonproductive cough and low-grade fever, with or without pleuritic pain. Bullous myringitis is an unusual finding but is sometimes seen with mycoplasma infection.

45. **A 30-year-old woman complains of cough and fever. She is not toxic-appearing. When you listen to her lungs, you hear right basilar rales. Her chest x-ray shows a right lower lobe infiltrate with bilateral hilar adenopathy:**

    a. Young, healthy adults who will be treated as outpatients always require a chest x-ray.

    b. Hilar adenopathy suggests the presence of tuberculosis or fungal disease.

    c. Radiographic findings will generally suggest the specific infectious etiology.

    d. The absence of radiographic abnormality would preclude the diagnosis of pneumonia.

    e. This patient is unlikely to have an underlying noninfectious illness.

The answer is b. Hilar adenopathy suggests an unusual infection, such as tuberculosis or fungal disease, or a noninfectious etiology, such as sarcoid or a malignancy. Young adults with findings suggestive of clinically mild pneumonia may be treated initially with an x-ray. Radiographic findings are nonspecific for specific infectious etiology of pneumonia.

46. **Blood cultures are routinely ordered for patients hospitalized with pneumonia. You know that:**

    a. Blood cultures are true-positive less than 5% of the time.

    b. When positive, blood cultures will usually lead to a change in therapy.

    c. Blood cultures correlate well with severity of illness.

    d. Blood cultures cannot be drawn if antibiotic therapy has already been initiated.

    e. Blood cultures are proven to be cost-effective.

The answer is a. Blood cultures are most likely to be positive with pneumococcal pneumonia, but overall are only positive 3–4% of the time. When positive, they rarely lead to a change in therapy. Cultures have not been found to correlate with severity of pneumonia. While it is recommended that cultures be drawn prior to initiating antibiotics, it is clearly recommended that therapy not be delayed in order to obtain cultures. Cultures are not cost-effective, but they nevertheless have significant value in tracking community patterns of resistance.

47. **You have just diagnosed lobar pneumonia in an otherwise healthy 40-year-old nonsmoking man:**

    a. A third- or fourth-generation fluoroquinolone is the recommended first-line therapy.

    b. In the oral formulations, macrolides and fluoroquinolones have similar bioavailability.

    c. The Infectious Disease Society of America recommends doxycycline as first-line treatment for young adults.

    d. It is not accepted therapy to give a first-dose intravenous antibiotic in the emergency department and discharge the patients with a prescription for a less expensive antibiotic.

    e. The Pneumonia Severity Index predicts a mortality rate of 2% for class II patients.

The answer is c. Fluoroquinolones are recommended for outpatient treatment of pneumonia in elderly patients but are not first-line treatment for young, healthy adults. Fluoroquinolones have greater than 90% bioavailability in oral form, whereas macrolides have less than 50% bioavailability. The IDSA recommends either doxycycline or a macrolide for this patient. Initial ED treatment with one dose of an intravenous antibiotic is accepted therapy. The Pneumonia Severity Index, which guides admissions decisions but is only a predictive measure of mortality, predicts mortality of less than 0.4% in this patient.

48. **Antibiotic resistance in community-acquired pneumonia is increasing:**
    a. There has been little change in resistance to fluoroquinolones.
    b. Risk factors for penicillin-resistant pneumococcus include exposure to a child at a daycare center.
    c. Resistance of pneumococcus to beta-lactam antibiotics is not dose-related.
    d. Clinical studies consistently demonstrate worsened clinical outcomes when drug-resistant pneumococcus is present.
    e. *H. influenzae* and *M. catarrhalis* show significant resistance to advanced-generation cephalosporins.

    The answer is b. There is an increasing resistance of pneumococcus and other organisms to fluoroquinolones, though the resistance is less to beta-lactams and macrolides. There are numerous risk factors for drug-resistant pneumococcus, including exposure to a child who goes to a daycare center, age older than 65 years, alcoholism, and use of a beta-lactam antibiotic in the previous 3 months. Resistance to beta-lactams is dose-related, that is, it can be overcome with increasing dosages. Studies have not consistently demonstrated poorer outcomes when drug-resistant pneumococcus is found. *H. influenzae* and *M. catarrhalis* continue to be highly sensitive to beta-lactams.

49. **Acute respiratory distress syndrome (ARDS) is respiratory failure in association with noncardiogenic pulmonary edema. Which of the following statement about ARDS is correct?**
    a. Outcome may be improved by the use of increased tidal volumes by ventilator.
    b. Inflammatory mediators from nonpulmonary sites often cause the lung injury.
    c. Treatment often includes aggressive fluid resuscitation.
    d. Ventilation is more effective with prolonged expiratory times.
    e. Survivors of ARDS rarely recover normal or near-normal respiratory function.

    The answer is b. Endothelial disruption that leads to ARDS is caused by inflammatory mediators that often arise from nonpulmonary sites. Lung injury may be lessened by use of small tidal volumes on the ventilator. Aggressive fluid resuscitation may increase pulmonary edema. Ventilation is more effective with prolonged inspiratory times to expand alveoli and decrease alveolar fluid accumulation. Mortality is high in ARDS, but survivors usually recover lung function.

50. **A 50-year-old man is hospitalized with community-acquired pneumonia:**
    a. Respiratory isolation is probably required.
    b. Respiratory isolation is not necessary if the x-ray suggests typical pneumonia.
    c. Respiratory isolation may be needed if viral pneumonia is suspected.
    d. Social factors should not determine the need for respiratory isolation.
    e. Reverse isolation is necessary if tuberculosis is suspected.

    The answer is c. Most patients with pneumonia do not need isolation. Patients with an infection that could be dangerous and transmissible include those with influenza and tuberculosis. Radiographic findings suggestive of pyogenic pneumonia do not exclude the possibility of viral or tuberculosis pneumonia. Neutropenic patients require reverse isolation.

51.   **Septic shock:**

   a. Is associated with reduced cardiac output.

   b. Leads to decreased net oxygen consumption.

   c. Is associated with increased vascular resistance.

   d. Results in localized tissue edema due to endothelial disruption.

   e. Is associated with hypotension responsive to fluid resuscitation.

The answer is d. Septic shock, at outset, is associated with a hyperdynamic cardiac response, with increased output. While there are effects of hypoxia at the cellular level, there is overall increased oxygen delivery and increased net consumption. Septic shock is associated with decreased vascular tone/resistance and marked disruption of the endothelial barrier. By definition, septic shock is differentiated from severe sepsis by lack of response to fluid resuscitation.

52.   **Severe sepsis and septic shock are recognized by the presence of acute organ dysfunction (AOD):**

   a. AOD leads to permanent organ damage in survivors.

   b. AOD is highly correlated with mortality.

   c. Systemic Inflammatory Response Score directly correlates with AOD score.

   d. AOD is seen in moderate sepsis.

   e. AOD is seen in mild sepsis.

The answer is b. Increased number of acutely damaged organ systems is directly associated with increased mortality. SIRS score does not have a clear relationship to mortality rate or AOD. Survivors of sepsis generally have resolution of acute organ dysfunction. AOD, by definition, is only seen with severe sepsis or shock.

53.   **An elderly man with change in mental status has no fever or cough but is found to have a left lower lobe infiltrate on chest x-ray:**

   a. The mortality rate for patients older than 65 years is approximately 20%.

   b. Less than half of elderly patients will have a nonclassical presentation of pneumonia, i.e., without respiratory symptoms.

   c. The mortality rate is higher for those with classical symptoms (fever, cough, shortness of breath).

   d. The elderly are more at risk for drug-resistant *S. pneumoniae*.

   e. Elderly patients rarely present with purely functional complaints, i.e., falls, decreased appetite, confusion.

The answer is d. The mortality rate for patients older than 65 years hospitalized with pneumonia is at least 20%. Age is a specific risk factor for drug-resistant *S. pneumonia*e. More than half of elderly patients will have a nonclassical presentation of pneumonia, with functional complaints rather than cough, fever, or respiratory distress. The mortality rate is greater for those with nonclassical presentations, probably reflecting poorer underlying functional status.

54.   **In selecting antibiotic regimen for treating inpatients with pneumonia, you should remember that:**

   a. Elderly patients rarely have pneumonia caused by atypical organisms.

   b. Fluoroquinolones are significantly more effective in parenteral form.

   c. Patients admitted to the intensive care unit generally need antibiotic coverage for *Pseudomonas* and *Staphylococcus*.

   d. Moxifloxacin is the most active fluoroquinolone against *Pseudomonas*.

   e. Azithromycin is acceptable monotherapy for in-patients likely to have atypical pneumonia.

The answer is c. Consensus guidelines recommend coverage for *Staphylococcus* and *Pseudomonas* in the ICU. It is not known with what frequency elderly patients are infected with atypical agents, but outcomes clearly improve when appropriate antibiotic coverage is provided for these agents. Fluoroquinolones are as effective in oral form as in parenteral. Moxifloxacin is an effective respiratory fluoroquinolone, but is specifically less effective against *Pseudomonas* than other fluoroquinolones. Azithromycin is highly effective against atypical organisms. It is not recommended as monotherapy because pyogenic pneumonia cannot be excluded on initial evaluation.

55. **The transition from systemic inflammatory response syndrome (SIRS) to severe sepsis and septic shock:**

   a. Is a gradual, predictable process.
   b. Results in global tissue hypoxia.
   c. Is best corrected by aggressive therapy begun in the intensive care unit.
   d. Needs to be monitored by pulmonary artery (mixed venous) oxygen saturation rather than by right atrium or superior vena cava (central venous) oxygen saturation.
   e. Results in death more often from sudden vascular collapse rather than multiple organ failure.

   The answer is b. Severe sepsis leads to tissue hypoxia, with release of a cascade of inflammatory mediators that lead to septic shock. Clinical deterioration can be abrupt. Early goal-directed therapy indicates that aggressive treatment is more effective when begun prior to ICU placement. Oxygen uptake/extraction is monitored by central venous oxygen saturation. While a substantial number of septic patients succumb to sudden cardiovascular collapse, the more common cause of mortality is multiple organ failure.

56. **The PORT study that justified the use of blood cultures in patients with pneumonia:**

   a. Demonstrated improved survival when blood cultures were drawn prior to administering antibiotics.
   b. Was a prospective clinical trial.
   c. Has been cited as level A evidence by the guidelines of the Infectious Disease Society of America.
   d. Meticulously eliminated confounding factors.
   e. May have shown results that were a marker of overall more aggressive care.

   The answer is e. The PORT study was retrospective chart review. It did not show a benefit to pretreatment blood cultures. There was an attempt to stratify patients according to risk (per Pneumonia Severity Index), but confounding factors could not be eliminated from a study consisting of chart reviews from hundreds of different hospital sites.

57. **In discharging patients treated in the ED for asthma, you must remember that:**

   a. Airway inflammation and edema usually takes 6–12 hours to resolve.
   b. Patients receiving systemic corticosteroids should continue this medication for at least 10 days.
   c. The relapse rate of those discharged is less than 10%.
   d. It is not the responsibility of the emergency physician to initiate controller medications.
   e. Those who require ED treatment are likely to have less asthma management skills than the average asthmatic patient.

   The answer is e. Airway inflammation often takes 3–4 days to resolve. Oral steroid medication should not be prescribed for more than 5 days, though the primary physician may determine that a longer course is needed. More than 10% of ED-treated asthmatic patients return to the ED with a relapse. Studies have shown that ED physicians rarely prescribe controller medications, in spite of obvious potential benefit for this population of patients with frequent relapses. Asthmatic patients in the ED are not representative of the general population of asthmatics. They either have more severe asthma, or they have not learned how to properly manage their disease.

58.   **Your asthmatic patient is deteriorating in spite of steroid treatment and multiple doses of nebulized beta-agonist therapy. In preparing for intubation and mechanical ventilation:**

a. Succinylcholine is contraindicated.

b. Ketamine is the preferred induction agent.

c. Ventilator settings should attempt to achieve mild hypocapnia.

d. Neuromuscular blocking agents increase oxygen consumption.

e. Hypotension while on the ventilator should be managed with pressor agents.

The answer is b. Ketamine is an effective induction agent that has bronchodilator properties. The asthmatic patient will do better with permissive hypercapnia. Neuromuscular agents decrease oxygen consumption. Hyotension in this setting is most likely caused by decreased venous return from increased intrathoracic pressure and should be managed with smaller tidal volume.

59.   **Patients who succumb to fatal asthma:**

a. Tend to be older.

b. Usually have a gradually progressive course of symptoms over several days.

c. Are more likely to have serious psychiatric disease or social problems.

d. Cannot be identified by history of severe asthmatic attacks.

e. Are more likely to have had previous intubation than patients with near-fatal asthma.

The answer is c. Fatal asthma attacks tend to occur in younger patients, who often have a history of psychiatric disease, drug use, or homelessness. They usually have a history of previous severe attacks, although cases of near-fatal asthma are more likely to have been previously intubated than fatal attacks.

CHAPTER 17 Toxicologic Emergencies

Jane M. Prosser, MD

1. A 54-year-old man with past medical history of HIV, hypertension, and tuberculosis is brought to the emergency department by a family friend after he is found seizing on the floor of his living room. The seizures persist despite the administration of appropriate doses of benzodiazepines. Serum glucose is normal. The next agent you should give is:

   a. Phenytoin.
   b. Barbiturates.
   c. Pyridoxine.
   d. Etomidate.
   e. Propofol.

   The answer is c. All of the agents listed are useful in treating seizures. In patients with a history of tuberculosis, status epilepticus should be considered secondary to isoniazid toxicity until proven otherwise. In overdose, isoniazid causes confusion, agitation, seizures, and acidosis. It depletes the body of vitamin B_6 (pyridoxine) leading to a reduction of gamma-aminobutyric acid (GABA) in the central nervous system. GABA acts as an important inhibitory neurotransmitter, therefore depletion leads to unopposed CNS excitation. The treatment of an acute INH overdose in an adult is 5 g of pyridoxine given intravenously. The dose in children is 70 mg/kg. One dose of pyridoxine has virtually no risk of toxicity and should be given empirically in the setting of status epilepticus when there is any possibility of an INH exposure.

2. **A 35-year-old man complains of chest pain, which began following the use of cocaine 30 minutes prior to arrival. The patient describes severe substernal chest pressure, radiating to the left arm and jaw. It is associated with shortness of breath. Initial vital signs: temperature 100.4°F, heart rate 120/min, respiratory rate 20/min, blood pressure 185/100 mm Hg, pulse oximetry 98% on room air. An ECG is consistent with acute myocardial infarction. A drug which is contraindicated is:**

    a. Oxygen.

    b. Aspirin.

    c. Lorazepam.

    d. Metoprolol.

    e. Morphine.

    The answer is d. Cocaine-associated chest pain and cocaine-induced myocardial infarction are treated identically to non–cocaine-associated acute coronary syndromes with one important exception: beta-blockers are contraindicated in patients who have taken cocaine. The use of cocaine leads to increased neurotransmitter release into the neuronal synapse. It also inhibits the reuptake of both norepinephrine and epinephrine. This leads to increased adrenergic tone causing tachycardia, hypertension, and hyperthermia. Cocaine has been shown to both accelerate atherosclerosis and cause vasoconstriction of the coronary arteries. Use of beta-blockers in the setting of cocaine use can lead to unopposed alpha-agonism, which can increase the toxic effects by worsening tachycardia, hypertension, and vasoconstriction.

3. **A 19-year-old woman is brought to the emergency department by her roommate, who reports the patient is "not acting right." She has a history of depression for which she is prescribed fluoxetine. Her friend reports that she was well and without complaints until a few hours prior to arrival when she took some ecstasy. Vital signs: temperature 105°F, heart rate 125/min, respiratory rate 20/min, blood pressure 140/80 mm Hg, and pulse oximetry of 99% on room air. Her physical examination is notable for diaphoresis, confusion, and disorientation. She also has lower extremity hypertonicity and clonus. Appropriate treatment includes administration of:**

    a. Charcoal.

    b. Acetaminophen.

    c. Glucose.

    d. Dantrolene and benzodiazepines.

    e. Cyproheptadine and benzodiazepines.

    The answer is e. This is a classic presentation of serotonin syndrome. Serotonin syndrome is caused by an excess of serotonin in the central nervous system (CNS). The list of medications that increase serotonin is large. Selective serotonin reuptake inhibitors (SSRI) and methylenedioxymethamphetamine (MDMA, or Ecstasy) both work by increasing serotonin. Antidepressants such as monoamine oxidase inhibitors (MAOI) and tricyclic antidepressants (TCA), analgesics such as meperidine and fentanyl, serotonin 5-HT blockers (triptans), dextromethorphan, LSD, and lithium can also increase serum serotonin levels. The symptoms are a spectrum beginning with mild tremor and agitation, then increasing in severity to altered mentation, hypertonicity, and hyperthermia. Emergency department management begins with removal of all serotonergic agents and supportive care. There is no role for centrally acting antipyretics such as acetaminophen because the hyperthermia comes from increased muscular activity. Cyproheptadine (Periactin) is a serotonin antagonist and is used to counter the effects of serotonin. It can only be given orally and its efficacy has been questioned by some experts, but it remains the standard of care. Benzodiazepines should be used to decrease muscular tone and agitation. In severe cases, paralytics may be necessary to reduce muscle tone. Activated charcoal is contraindicated in patients with an altered mental status or those who are at risk for aspiration. Given orally, charcoal is very safe; however, when aspirated into the lungs, it can be lethal. Dantrolene is indicated for the treatment of malignant hyperthermia, which is a genetic disorder of calcium reuptake into the sarcoplasmic reticulum of the muscle cell. Dantrolene is a drug that blocks calcium release from the sarcoplasmic reticulum. It has not been proven to be beneficial in serotonin syndrome.

4. **A 65-year-old man with past medical history of schizophrenia complains of vomiting for the past 24 hours. He reports feeling very hot for several days, but denies other symptoms including abdominal pain, chest pain, and shortness of breath. You are unable to obtain further details as he is having trouble hearing the questions. Vital signs: temperature 101°F, heart rate 130/min, respiratory rate 35/min, blood pressure 120/80 mm Hg, pulse oximetry 100% on room air. You would also expect this patient to have:**

   a. A respiratory alkalosis with a metabolic acidosis.

   b. A respiratory acidosis with metabolic alkalosis.

   c. A 40-degree right axis deviation manifested by a terminal r wave in AVR on ECG.

   d. An intracranial hemorrhage on CT scan of the brain.

   e. An elevated lithium level.

   The answer is a. Aspirin intoxication caused a mixed acid base disturbance. Stimulation of the central respiratory center in the medulla leads to a respiratory alkalosis. Metabolic acidosis can be severe and is caused via several mechanisms. Uncoupling of oxidative phosphorylation leads to an increase in oxygen use and CO_2 production. Pyruvate and lactate are by-products of anaerobic respiration. Increased CO_2 increases the respiratory rate further. It also causes the kidneys to increase excretion of bicarbonate causing a metabolic acidosis. Additionally the Krebs cycle is disrupted leading to increased lipolysis and gluconeogenesis. The by-product of these pathways is increased ketone production, which contributes to the acidosis. Of note, children typically do not develop respiratory alkalosis with salicylate intoxication: they usually present with only a metabolic acidosis. Treatment should be aggressive. Charcoal is indicated in a patient with an adequate mental status. Avoid intubation if possible, as deaths have resulted from inadequate ventilation. Treat dehydration with a bolus of 1–2 L of normal saline. Use intravenous bicarbonate to alkalinize the urine; potassium repletion is important, as a psuedohypokalemia will develop. Closely monitor both serum and urine pH. Hemodialysis is indicated for a salicylate level greater than 100 mg/dL in an acute ingestion, or >60 mg/dL in a chronic ingestion, volume overload (pulmonary edema, renal failure, CHF), altered mental status, severe academia, or lack of improvement with IV fluids and bicarbonate. A 40-degree right axis deviation manifested by a terminal r wave in AVR on ECG is seen in tricyclic antidepressant overdoses. Lithium toxicity is manifested by tremor, vomiting, diarrhea, lethargy, and seizures. It is not usually associated with fever and tachypnea. Increased intracranial pressure causes hypertension and bradycardia via the Cushing reflex.

5. **A 21-year-old woman is brought to the emergency department from a rave party after having a witnessed seizure. She is currently complaining of generalized weakness, but denies all other symptoms. She denies past medical history and medication use. She says that she took ecstasy at the rave. The most likely cause of her seizure is:**

   a. Epilepsy.

   b. Hyponatremia.

   c. Hypomagnesaemia.

   d. Hypocalcaemia.

   e. Hypercalcemia.

   The answer is b. Use of ecstasy (MDMA) is associated with profound hyponatremia, which can cause seizures, coma, and death. While the association is well described, the mechanism is less clear. The two most likely causes are either MDMA release of antidiuretic hormone (ADH) or excessive free water intake by MDMA users trying to avoid dehydration. Treatment of mild hyponatremia can be accomplished with water restriction. Treatment of moderate and severe hyponatremia can be treated with isotonic or hypertonic saline.

6. **A 76-year-old man with a past medical history of hypertension, diabetes, and congestive heart failure complains of nausea, vomiting, and diarrhea. Routine laboratory results show an elevated anion gap, elevated creatinine, and a lactic acidosis. Blood glucose is normal. The offending agent is most likely to be:**

    a. Metoprolol.

    b. Furosemide.

    c. Glyburide.

    d. Rosiglitazone.

    e. Metformin.

    The answer is e. Metformin is associated with a lactic acidosis in the setting of overdose or renal failure. It does not cause hypoglycemia. The other medications are not associated with a lactic acidosis. Metformin is metabolized by the kidney and renal insufficiency is a contraindication to use. It does not stimulate the release of insulin but works to increase insulin receptor binding and decrease glucose production and absorption. Metformin causes increased lactic acid via decreased gluconeogenesis and accumulation of lactic acid. Accumulation of metformin itself also leads to lactic acidosis. Symptoms of metformin overdose are nonspecific and include lethargy, abdominal pain, nausea, and vomiting. Bicarbonate should be given for a pH of less than 7.1. For refractory cases, hemodialysis may be necessary as it will treat acidemia and will remove metformin from the blood.

7. **Inhalant abusers ("huffers" and "baggers") are at risk for:**

    a. Ventricular dysrhythmias.

    b. Acute lung injury.

    c. Hypoglycemia.

    d. Acidosis.

    e. Kidney failure.

    The answer is a. Inhalants are volatile hydrocarbons that are used by huffing, bagging, and sniffing methods. Huffing refers to pouring the substance onto a rag then placing the rag over the mouth and inhaling. Bagging refers to placing the substance into a bag then breathing into the bag. This method places users at risk for hypoxia and subsequent respiratory failure. Unless the hydrocarbon is aspirated into the lungs, no direct pulmonary toxicity occurs. Sniffing is inhaling the vapors from a container such as rubber cement or glue. Sudden sniffing death has been reported since the 1960s. The typical scenario is an adolescent who has been abusing inhalants who is discovered by parents or police then experiences sudden cardiac arrest. Research suggests that hydrocarbons sensitize the myocardium to dysrhythmia by blocking the inward rectifier potassium channels and prolonging repolarization. The stimulus for dysrhythmias is a catecholamine surge that occurs in the setting of stress or surprise, which leads to ventricular fibrillation and death. The treatment of sudden sniffing death is electrical defibrillation with the addition of beta-blockade, which has been shown in several case reports to be beneficial.

8. **A 37-year-old man is found to have tachycardia, hypertension, mydriasis, agitation, and hyperthermia. This presentation is consistent with:**

    a. Cholinergic toxicity.

    b. Anticholinergic toxicity.

    c. Sympathomimetic toxicity.

    d. Sedative-hypnotic toxicity.

    e. Both sympathomimetic and anticholinergic toxicity.

The answer is e. Both anticholinergic and sympathomimetic toxidromes cause the symptoms listed above. One significant difference between the two is the presence or absence of diaphoresis and sweating. Patients who have an anticholinergic overdose are "dry as a bone" while patients with a sympathomimetic overdose are typically diaphoretic. A mnemonic for remembering symptoms of an anticholinergic overdose is "red as a beet, hot as a hare, dry as a bone, mad as a hen, and blind as a bat." A mnemonic for cholinergic overdose is SLUDGE and the triple Bs for salivation, lacrimation, urination, defecation, GI hypermotility, emesis, bronchorrhea, bronchospasm, and bradycardia. A sedative–hypnotic overdose often presents with depressed mental status, hypotension, bradycardia, and lowered respiratory rate.

9. **A 40-year-old man is unresponsive on arrival after having been found at a house fire. He is unconscious, hypotensive, and tachycardic with agonal respirations. You quickly secure the airway while the nurse establishes two large-bore intravenous lines. After placing the patient on 100% oxygen, you send an arterial blood gas: pH 7.01, P_{CO_2} 21, P_{O_2} 575, COHb level 20%, and blood lactate 12 mmol/L. You should now administer:**

   a. Intravenous bicarbonate.

   b. Intravenous sodium thiosulfate.

   c. Inhaled amyl nitrate.

   d. Broad-spectrum antibiotics.

   e. Intravenous methylene blue.

   The answer is b. This patient needs to be emergently treated for cyanide toxicity. Cyanide poisoning can occur during a house fire secondary to combustion of materials such as silk, wool, and polyurethane. A lactate greater than 10 mmol/L in a patient who has been exposed to a fire is highly suggestive of concomitant cyanide poisoning. There are three steps in using the cyanide kit commonly found in United States emergency departments. The first recommended step is inhalation of amyl nitrate ampoules prior to establishing intravenous access (also known as "poppers" when abused). An unconscious patient will not be able to inhale amyl nitrate, and intravenous access has already been obtained. The second recommended step is administration of intravenous sodium nitrite, but this step is unnecessary and potentially harmful in a patient with a methemoglobin level greater than 10%, which would be expected in a patient suffering from smoke inhalation. Sodium nitrite works by increasing methemoglobin concentrations in red blood cells causing methemoglobin to combine with cyanide forming cyanomethemoglobin. The third and final step is critical in this patient: administration of sodium thiosulfate, which acts as a substrate for the conversion of cyanomethemoglobin into thiocyanate, which can be excreted in the urine. After initiation of treatment for cyanide toxicity, hyperbaric oxygen, and other appropriate therapies can be considered.

10. **A 32-year-old man complains of nausea and vomiting after ingesting some wild mushrooms that he picked himself. The information you need to determine prognosis and disposition is:**

   a. Liver function tests.

   b. Vital signs.

   c. Time since ingestion.

   d. The patient's level of experience with mushroom gathering.

   e. Concomitant alcohol ingestion.

   The answer is c. Determining the potential toxicity of mushroom ingestion in the emergency department can be difficult. Most species of mushrooms in the United States have no toxicity or mild toxicity in the form of gastrointestinal upset. However, ingestion of Amanita species can be deadly. The emergency physician must identify which patients are most at risk for Amanita poisoning. If the patient has brought the mushrooms attempts may be made to identify the species, but this can be difficult and may require the expertise of a mycologist. Experienced mushroom foragers may make mistakes when identifying mushrooms as many species have similar appearances. The most important criteria in determining the need for admission is the time of onset of symptoms after ingesting the mushrooms. If the onset of symptoms occurs less than 3 hours after ingestion and the patient improves with supportive care it is reasonable to discharge the patient with close outpatient follow-up as the likelihood of ingestion of an Amanita species is low. If the symptoms occur more than 5 hours after ingestion, then the likelihood of Amanita ingestion is much higher and the patient should be admitted for further workup and evaluation. This algorithm may not be applicable in the Pacific Northwest, as *Amanita smithiana* poisoning can cause early symptoms; it should be used with caution in all settings. Patients with Amanita poisoning exhibit three stages of poisoning. Stage I consists of severe nausea, vomiting, and diarrhea that begins 5–24 hours postingestion. During stage II, 12–36 hours after ingestion, the patient will have transient improvement in symptoms. Stage III begins 2–6 days after ingestion and consists of renal and hepatic failure. It is at this point the elevations of ALT and AST are present. For this reason, liver enzymes taken immediately after ingestion will not be helpful. Treatment of Amanita poisoning is controversial and difficult, as no therapies have been definitively proven. At this time, multidose activated charcoal remains the mainstay of therapy. Milk thistle and *N*-acetylcysteine may be helpful but have not yet been proven. Liver transplantation may be necessary.

11. **A 63-year-old man brought to the emergency department by EMS confused, agitated, and tremulous. Rectal temperature 100.8°F, heart rate 125/min, respiratory rate 20/min, blood pressure 170/80 mm Hg, and pulse oximetry 96% on room air. He gives a history of ingesting six beers every day, but denies illicit drug use. You give him 2 mg of intravenous lorazepam, but there is no change in his symptoms. You should now give him:**

   a. Intravenous vitamin C.

   b. Intravenous antibiotics.

   c. Intramuscular haloperidol.

   d. More intravenous lorazepam.

   e. Oral charcoal.

The answer is d. This patient has delirium tremens (DTs) from alcohol withdrawal and needs to be treated aggressively with benzodiazepines such as lorazepam or diazepam to prevent further complications. Alcohol withdrawal begins as early as 6 hours after a decreased level of ethanol intake. Serum ethanol levels do not have to fall to zero before withdrawal begins: can begin with a decreased alcohol intake in a heavy drinker. The first stage of alcohol withdrawal is hallucinosis, manifested by hallucinations with an otherwise clear sensorium. Approximately 12 hours after cessation or decreased alcohol intake, the patient may have alcohol withdrawal seizures. Delirium tremens is the most serious complication of withdrawal and classically begins 48–96 hours later. It is characterized by autonomic instability and mental status changes. The treatment of DTs and withdrawal is administration of alcohol or benzodiazepines. Benzodiazepines are titrated to effect; ideally the patient should be sedated but breathing. Use persistent tachycardia and hypertension as indicators of inadequate treatment. In this patient, 2 mg of lorazepam are not enough. Case reports of patients given diazepam for DTs have reported the need for 1–2 g to achieve adequate treatment. Haloperidol should not be given to those in alcohol withdrawal as it may mask the symptoms leading to inadequate benzodiazepine administration. It is important to look for underlying sources of infection in patients with alcohol withdrawal. Alcoholics often stop drinking because they are too sick to drink. Infection, trauma, liver failure, GI bleeding, and other physiologic stressors can all precipitate DTs. A chest x-ray and antibiotics may be indicated in this patient, but he should be stabilized and treated for DTs prior to an extensive evaluation.

12. **You are evaluating a 2-year-old girl whose parents brought her to the emergency department after she ingested one pill. After setting up your safety net, you observe her for 6 hours; she is playful and eating normally. It would be safe to discharge her if she ingested:**

    a. Methadone.

    b. A sulfonylurea.

    c. Citalopram.

    d. Iron.

    e. Diphenoxylate/atropine (Lomotil).

    The answer is d. It is important to know the medications that could be toxic in small quantities (such as one pill or a few drops) in a child. If a child has ingested one of these medications or even if clinical suspicion is high that the child may have ingested one of these medications, the patient must be admitted for 24 hours of observation. Opioids, especially long-acting preparations like methadone, can lead to lethal respiratory depression and apnea if a small child ingests one pill. Ingestion of one tablet of sustained release calcium channel and beta-blockers has caused death in children. Long-acting preparations require observation as the onset of symptoms may be delayed. Sulfonylureas, oral hypoglycemic agents, may cause severe life-threatening hypoglycemia. Evaluation includes frequent blood glucose monitoring for 24 hours. Citalopram and escitalopram in sustained release preparations have been reported to cause seizures, QT prolongation, and torsades de pointes. Children who have ingested one pill need to be monitored for 24 hours. Other substances that are potentially lethal in very small doses include cyclic antidepressants, benzocaine, clonidine, phenothiazines, and theophylline. A few drops of oil of wintergreen (methyl salicylate), methanol, or ethylene glycol can also be lethal in a child. Lomotil is a combination of an opioid and atropine; while the respiratory depression from diphenoxylate can be treated with naloxone, there are numerous case reports of delayed onset of symptoms even after an extended period of symptom-free observation. Children may also exhibit delayed onset of atropine intoxication, and death has been reported with ingestion of one pill. Iron overdose can be life threatening, but most poison centers do not make hospital referrals until the ingested dose is greater than 20–60 mg/kg. The amount of iron in vitamins and other preparation varies, but a typical prenatal vitamin contains 65 mg of iron. Iron toxicity is often described in five stages. Stage 1 is the initial symptoms of acute iron poisoning including nausea, vomiting, abdominal pain, and diarrhea. This is followed by the latent stage lasting 6–24 hours. The third stage is the "shock" stage and occurs typically 12–24 hours later. The fourth stage is hepatotoxicity. The fifth stage includes delayed sequelae and includes gastric outlet obstruction and strictures. If a child presents to the hospital and has no symptoms of iron poisoning, then it is safe to discharge the patient home after 6 hours of observation.

13.   **A 44-year-old man complains of nausea, vomiting, diarrhea, and a wobbly gait. Vital signs: heart rate 42/min, respiratory rate 20/min, blood pressure 95/60 mm Hg. Pertinent findings include disorientation, slurred speech, muscle fasciculations, and hand tremors. His wife states that he has bipolar disease and has taken lithium for several years without problems; recently he was started on furosemide for signs of water retention. A serum lithium level is 2.6 mEq/L. An EKG shows sinus bradycardia. Serum creatinine is 2.4 mg/dL. In order to treat him appropriately, you know that:**

   a. Intravenous normal saline and a loop diuretic will help promote lithium diuresis.

   b. Alkalinization of urine with intravenous bicarbonate will significantly lower his lithium level.

   c. Activated charcoal effectively adsorbs lithium.

   d. Intravascular fluid replacement with normal saline and hemodialysis are indicated for this patient.

   e. The most common significant cardiac dysfunction in lithium toxicity is ventricular dysrhythmias.

   The answer is d. Lithium toxicity can be acute or chronic, with the clinical difference often only a matter of degree. CNS or neuromuscular symptoms of toxicity (confusion, ataxia, dysarthria, seizures, tremors, fasciculations) predominate. Gastrointestinal (nausea, vomiting) and cardiovascular (bradycardia, PVCs, hypotension) findings are also common. The most common cardiac dysfunction is sinus node dysfunction. Lithium causes renal tubular dysfunction and sodium loss even in therapeutic doses, causing a compensatory increase in lithium reabsorption. Natriuretic diuretics (furosemide) will thus tend to increase serum levels. In general, clinical findings are more important in judging lithium toxicity, since "toxic" levels of >2 mEq/L are occasionally therapeutic, and "therapeutic" levels (<2 mEq/L) toxic. Volume replacement with normal saline to create euvolemia is essential. Hemodialysis is indicated in the acute ingestion when the serum lithium level is >4.0 mEq/L and in the chronic ingestion when the lithium level is >2.5 mEq/L. Hemodialysis is also indicated in the patient with renal failure, or in the patient with neurologic dysfunction including an altered mental status. Hypothyroidism and nephrogenic diabetes insipidus are other complications of lithium therapy.

14.   **Which of the following statements about poisoning from alcohol or glycol is true?**

   a. In both methanol and ethylene glycol poisoning, elevation of the osmolar gap occurs after the development of a wide anion gap.

   b. A major route of elimination of methanol is the lungs.

   c. When you find a large anion gap metabolic acidosis and a large osmolar gap, you should immediately start treatment with intravenous ethanol or fomepizole.

   d. Treatment of methanol poisoning also includes intravenous thiamine and pyridoxine.

   e. Serum levels of ethylene glycol are readily available and should be used to determine which patients should be treated with hemodialysis.

   The answer is c. Ethanol and fomepizole are used to competitively inhibit the metabolism of both methanol and ethylene glycol by alcohol dehydrogenase. Formic acid is the major toxic product of methanol metabolism. Glyoxylate and oxalate are the major toxic metabolite of ethylene glycol. In both types of poisoning CNS symptoms resemble those of ethanol intoxication. An increase in the osmolar gap is followed by an increased anion gap as metabolism occurs, then the development of a metabolic acidosis. Large quantities of intravenous bicarbonate may be needed to maintain a blood pH above 7.2. Ethanol or fomepizole should be given as soon as either diagnosis is suspected based on an increased anion or osmolar gap. Serum levels of ethylene glycol are not readily available. Thiamine and pyridoxine are cofactors in the metabolism of ethylene glycol to nontoxic metabolites. Folic acid is metabolized to the active cofactor folinic acid (leukovorin). Folinic acid is a cofactor used in the metabolism of methanol to inactive metabolites.

15. **Which of the following clinical syndromes is correctly identified?**
    a. Tachycardia, mydriasis, urinary retention, diaphoresis → cholinergic toxicity.
    b. Tachycardia, hypertension, diaphoresis, urinary incontinence → sympathomimetic syndrome.
    c. Pinpoint pupils, bradycardia, hypotension → alpha₂-agonist syndrome.
    d. Insomnia, diarrhea, hallucinosis, tachycardia, hypotension → opioid withdrawal syndrome.

    The answer is d. The anticholinergic poisoning syndrome can be remembered as: hot as a hare, blind as a bat, dry as a bone, red as a beet, mad as a hen. Clinically the anticholinergic poisoning syndrome presents with altered mental status, tachycardia, mydriasis, decreased bowel sounds, urinary retention, and dry axilla. The cholinergic poisoning syndrome can be remembered by the mnemonic SLUDGE (Salivation, Lacrimation, Urination, Defecation, GI hypermotility, and Emesis). The sympathomimetic syndrome includes tachycardia, hypertension, mydriasis, and diaphoresis. Urinary retention can also be found in the patient poisoned with sympathomimetics secondary to alpha-receptor agonism on the sphincter muscle of the bladder. Alpha₂-receptor agonism essentially produces a sympatholytic syndrome. Clonidine and other imidazoles are alpha₂-agonists that act presynaptically to inhibit sympathetic outflow from the CNS. Alpha₂-agonists therefore produce miosis, bradycardia, and hypotension. Alpha₂-agonist poisoning also produces a depressed mental status, respiratory depression, and coma. Alpha₂-agonist poisoning can be confused with opiate poisoning. Opiate poisoning usually does not result in significant bradycardia or hypotension. Withdrawal syndrome produces insomnia, diarrhea, hallucinosis, tachycardia, diaphoresis, and hypertension.

16. **A 30-year-old migrant worker drank from a soda can that had been filled with an unknown farm chemical. He is awake, but had to be carried in by his friends. Physical examination is remarkable for pinpoint pupils, wheezing, salivation, dysarthria, and marked generalized muscle weakness. Choose the correct statement:**
    a. The patient is demonstrating a sympatholytic syndrome of poisoning.
    b. You should administer atropine in a dose of 2 mg intravenously every 15 minutes to a maximum total dose of 6 mg or until mydriasis occurs.
    c. Urinary alkalinization will increase the elimination of the poison.
    d. You should administer pralidoxime (2-PAM) intravenously with a loading dose of 1 g over 15 minutes then at 0.5 g/h.
    e. Sinus tachycardia should prompt you to decrease the rate of an atropine infusion.

    The answer is d. The patient described is exhibiting cholinergic toxicity probably from the ingestion of an organophosphate or carbamate. The first rule in management of organophosphate poisoning is to maintain a patent airway. Upper airway obstruction from vomitus and copious secretions may occur. Increased airway resistance from bronchospasm may prove to exceed the respiratory capacity of the weakened muscles of respiration. Hypoxia rapidly ensues from bronchospasm and increased bronchial secretions. Early intubation is paramount in treating the poisoning. The most common cause of treatment failure in severe organophosphate poisoning is inadequate atropinization. The end-point of atropine administration is when drying of secretions occur. Tachycardia after organophosphate poisoning may be secondary to excessive atropinization necessitating a lower infusion rate. Hypoxia caused by increased pulmonary secretions may also produce tachycardia necessitating a higher infusion rate of atropine. 2-PAM should be given early based on the suspicion of cholinesterase poisoning. It is effective in reversing muscle weakness (nicotinic effects) but only if given within 36 hours of exposure. 2-PAM will reactivate acetylcholinesterase by displacing the organophosphate. Because true cholinesterase regenerates at a rate of only 1% a day, it can take months for symptoms to resolve if cholinesterase is not regenerated with 2-PAM.

17. **The physical factor that best correlates with mortality in intoxications with pure petroleum distillates is its:**

a. Viscosity.

b. Lipid solubility.

c. Flash point.

d. Surface tension.

e. Boiling point.

The answer is a. Pulmonary toxicity is the major cause of morbidity and mortality in ingestion of petroleum distillates. Distillates with a viscosity less than 60 SSU (Saybolt Seconds Universal) are the most likely to enter and deeply penetrate into the tracheobronchial tree. As little as 0.2 mL of a distillate with an SSU less than 60 can result in pneumonitis if it enters the trachea. Substances with an SSU greater than 100 (motor oils, petroleum jelly) are unlikely to be aspirated, but if aspirated, the result is a chronic lipoid pneumonia. Surface tension, boiling points, and the length of the molecule are of somewhat lesser importance. The short-chain distillates are more likely to irritate the lung, which can result in bronchospasm; and distillates with a low boiling point may vaporize at body temperature and displace air, resulting in more severe atelectasis or hypoxia.

18. **A 2-year-old, 20-kg boy ingested at least five and perhaps as many as fifteen 500-mg acetaminophen (APAP) tablets more than 2 hours ago. The mother states she found out about it only when he vomited 30 minutes prior to arrival in the ED. On examination, the child is awake, alert, and in no apparent distress. The laboratory calls and explains that the test for acetaminophen levels will need to be sent out; the results will be back in 24 hours. At this point you should:**

a. Administer syrup of ipecac to complete gastric emptying.

b. Perform gastric lavage and then administer activated charcoal.

c. Immediately send out an acetaminophen level.

d. Begin protocol treatment with *N*-acetylcysteine (NAC).

e. Consult the Done nomogram to determine the potential for APAP toxicity.

The answer is d. The Rumack-Matthew nomogram allows you to predict if the serum acetaminophen (APAP) levels are within the range of probable or possible hepatic toxicity. APAP levels should be drawn at least 4 hours after ingestion to allow absorption and tissue distribution to take place. The nomogram stops after 24 hours because NAC treatment after this is not predictive. Patients who fall in the range of possible toxicity should be treated. If the time since ingestion or the amount taken is unknown, NAC treatment should be started if the APAP level exceeds 8 mg/mL, and a second level drawn 4 hours later. If the second level is greater than one-half the initial level, NAC treatment should be continued. The patient in the question potentially ingested from 125–375 mg/kg of APAP. Patients who ingest more than 140 mg/kg or more than 7.5 g over a 24-hour period or less should be treated with NAC if plasma acetaminophen levels are not immediately available. NAC can be stopped if the levels are shown to be nontoxic. The Done nomogram is used for salicylate poisoning.

19. **A 2-year-old girl is brought to the ED for evaluation after she was seen chewing on her grandmother's discarded clonidine skin patch. You would expect to find:**

a. Hyperventilation.

b. Mydriasis.

c. Hypotension followed by hypertension.

d. Bronchospasm.

e. Bradycardia.

The answer is e. Clonidine is an alpha$_2$-agonist that produces its hypotensive effects by reducing central sympathetic outflow. It also possesses some peripheral alpha$_1$-agonist activity, which explains why hypertension may precede hypotension in accidental overdoses. Children are susceptible to even low doses of the drug, and neurologic symptoms ranging from drowsiness to coma may be the presenting signs. Bradycardia and AV blocks are treated with atropine, and hypotension with IV fluids and dopamine if necessary.

20. **Choose the true statement regarding cholinesterase intoxication with organophosphates or carbamates:**

    a. Low plasma cholinesterase activity is pathognomonic for organophosphate intoxication.
    b. Carbamate poisoning is typically less severe than organophosphate poisoning but presents with marked CNS symptoms.
    c. Clinical relapses from organophosphate poisoning may occur for months after an apparent recovery from an acute episode.
    d. Bradycardia is a universal finding in clinically important organophosphate poisoning; its absence should prompt an alternative diagnosis.
    e. The most common cause of death is cardiac failure.

    The answer is c. Symptoms in organophosphate poisoning may persist for weeks to months as a result of the slow regeneration time for cholinesterase and intermittent mobilization of tissue stores of these lipophilic toxins. Carbamate poisoning is less severe and CNS symptoms are uncommon because, unlike the organophosphates, these agents do not cross the blood–brain barrier. Cholinergic effects do not always predominate, since organophosphates also have nicotinic effects. The typical pattern following intoxication is tachycardia, followed by bradycardia, AV blocks, and a prolonged QT interval. The most common cause of death is respiratory failure. Low plasma (pseudo) cholinesterase activity is found in a variety of other conditions besides cholinesterase poisoning, including malnutrition, infections, and liver disease. RBC (true) cholinesterase is a more specific but less sensitive measure of poisoning.

21. **In the typical patient who is poisoned by iron:**

    a. Hypoglycemia initially occurs then hyperglycemia secondary to pancreatitis.
    b. Gastrointestinal hemorrhage is commonly seen secondary to liver dysfunction and coagulation abnormalities.
    c. Lactic acidosis is rarely seen in the toxic patient.
    d. Strictures may develop late in poisoning causing gastric outlet obstruction or bowel obstruction.
    e. The iron accumulates in the bone and may cause pathologic fractures.

    The answer is d. Direct caustic effects on the bowel by iron can result in early gastric and small bowel hemorrhage, which can result in hypovolemia and shock. Late strictures may present as gastric outlet or bowel obstruction. As toxic amounts of iron enter the mitochondria and disrupt oxidative phosphorylation, lactic acidosis occurs. Hyperglycemia is often seen early, but later hepatic failure results in hypoglycemia. Iron does not accumulate in the bone.

22.   **A 70-kg patient is being treated for acute salicylate overdose. After infusing 2 L of lactated Ringer solution to correct hypovolemia, you give a 50-mEq bolus of sodium bicarbonate, then change the intravenous fluid to 1 L of 5% dextrose plus 150 mEq of sodium bicarbonate and 40 mEq of KCl at 150 mL/h. The urine pH is 7.0, the serum pH is 7.45, and the serum potassium is 4.7 mEq/L. Urine output is 200 mL/h. Ninety minutes later the urine pH is 6.9, serum pH is 7.49, and serum potassium is 3.2 mEq/L. The urine output is unchanged, as is the patient's condition. Your next step in the management of this patient would be to:**

a. Give additional boluses of sodium bicarbonate until the urine becomes alkaline.

b. Add acetazolamide to the treatment protocol to increase urine pH.

c. Make no change in the therapy.

d. Give additional boluses of potassium chloride.

e. Consult for hemodialysis.

The answer is d. Large quantities of potassium often need to be given along with the sodium bicarbonate if the urine is to be successfully alkalinized. If urine output is good, the serum pH kept above 7.4 (to prevent tissue accumulation of salicylate), and if the urine is acidic, more potassium is needed. If the serum pH is less than 7.4 with a normal potassium and acidic urine, more bicarbonate should also be given. Acetazolamide should not be used to alkalinize the urine. If the patient deteriorates and no alkaline urine can be produced using KCl and bicarbonate, then hemodialysis is needed. Furosemide is used in patients who would be expected to develop problems from the large sodium loads given with bicarbonate.

23.   **Which of the following statements about gut decontamination is true?**

a. Ipecac-induced emesis reduces absorption of toxic compounds by 70%.

b. Activated charcoal may reduce absorption of toxins by 80%.

c. Administration of activated charcoal prior to lavage is never appropriate.

d. Activated charcoal effectively reduces the serum half-life of certain absorbed toxins.

e. Gastric lavage should be performed in most acetaminophen overdoses.

The answer is d. Emesis induced by syrup of ipecac reduces absorption by about 30%. One disadvantage of its use is that it prevents the use of activated charcoal, which reduces absorption of most toxins by approximately 50%. Giving activated charcoal prior to gastric lavage should be considered, particularly in prehospital management. Multidose charcoal enhances the elimination of drugs that undergo enterohepatic circulation. Gastric lavage should be reserved for the patient who took a life-threatening quantity of a drug. Gastric lavage is rarely indicated in the acetaminophen-poisoned patient as the drug is readily absorbed, binds well to charcoal, and an effective antidote exists.

24.   **The serum half-life of naloxone is:**

a. 15 minutes.

b. 60 minutes.

c. 90 minutes.

d. 120 minutes.

e. 240 minutes.

The answer is b. Since the half-life of naloxone is significantly shorter than that of many opioids, patients can slip back into coma after its use. Its serum half-life is approximately 45–75 minutes, while its duration of action is 2–3 hours. Precipitating withdrawal is another complication of naloxone use.

25.   Which of the following poisonings is correctly paired with the antidote?

a. Carbamates → pralidoxime.

b. Lead → deferoxamine.

c. Cyanide → methylene blue.

d. Isoniazid → thiamine.

e. Ethylene glycol → fomepizole (4-MP).

The answer is e. Carbamates do not irreversibly bind to the acetylcholinesterase molecule therefore pralidoxime is not necessary. In the unknown patient suspected of a pesticide poisoning with cholinergic symptoms, pralidoxime should be administered before determining the causative agent. Calcium EDTA and BAL are used to treat lead poisoning. Chemet (DMSA) has largely replaced Calcium EDTA and BAL in the treatment of lead toxicity. Antidotes for cyanide include sodium thiosulfate and sodium nitrites. Methylene blue is used in the treatment of methemoglobinemia. The treatment for isoniazid poisoning is pyridoxine (vitamin B_6). 4-MP is an alcohol dehydrogenase competitive inhibitor used in the treatment of methanol and ethylene glycol poisonings.

26.   A 19-year-old woman presents to the ED in coma. You note a fruity odor to her breath and deep, slow respirations. Significant laboratory findings include a blood pH of 7.39, bicarbonate 23 mEq/L, glucose 180 mg/dL, sodium 134 mEq/L, chloride 103 mEq/L, BUN 28 mg/dL, creatinine 1.2 mg/dL, and serum ketones. A large amount of urine is present with a specific gravity of 1.025 and the only abnormality on urinalysis is 4+ ketones. The measured osmolality is 318 mOsm/L. A serum ethanol level is negative. Which of the following statements is true?

a. The estimated osmolar gap is 40.

b. Since all alcohols cross-react in laboratory analysis and her measured ethanol is 0, poisoning from all alcohols can be eliminated.

c. The anion gap should be much larger.

d. Hemorrhagic gastritis is a major complication.

e. Hemodialysis is unlikely to be needed.

The answer is d. Laboratory assays for alcohol do not cross-react with methanol, isopropyl alcohol, or ethylene glycol. Ketosis, osmolar gap without an anion gap, and conversion of the alcohol to acetone are the major findings in ingestion of isopropyl alcohol. The major differential diagnosis is between alcoholic ketoacidosis and diabetic ketoacidosis. Intoxication and coma readily occur, but fatalities are uncommon. Hemorrhagic gastritis is usually the most significant physical complication. Treatment is to empty the stomach, protect the airway, and provide supportive care. Hemodialysis is not needed except for severe intoxications. Approximately 20% of the absorbed dose is converted to acetone. Very high acetone levels can interfere with the laboratory test for creatinine.

27. **You are evaluating a 3-year-old boy whose mother found him playing with an open bottle of liquid drain cleaner. He had spilled some on his clothing, which the mother immediately removed; she also washed him off in the sink. The child is crying; but you see no burns on the face or mouth, but note some mild erythema on his chest and abdomen, which has a slippery feeling. Which of the following is true regarding alkali ingestions?**

a. Alkali injury to the skin should be irrigated with a dilute hydrogen chloride in order to neutralize the toxin.

b. Check each eye and a conjunctival pH for evidence of an occult eye splash and irrigate if the pH is greater than 7.0 until consultation with an ophthalmologist is made.

c. The child should be encouraged to drink milk.

d. Place a nasogastric tube and irrigate the stomach.

e. Administer 1 g/kg of charcoal.

The answer is b. Eight thousand accidental ingestions of lye a year occur in children younger than 5 years. Oral burns are not always present in cases of ingestion of lye, and if the possibility cannot be excluded on clinical grounds, esophageal endoscopy is necessary. Diluents are used only in cases of ingestion of solid lye; their use after ingestion of liquid lye is ineffective in reducing tissue injury and increases the risk of vomiting. Milk and water are the only diluents that should be used for ingestion of solid lye. Acid solutions cause an exothermic reaction, which increases tissue injury. The child in the question could by crying for a number of reasons, not the least of which would be an occult splash in the eye. Careful examination is mandatory; a conjunctival pH may be helpful but falsely low because of crying, and irrigation is necessary if there is any question. The immediate treatment for alkali skin burns is copious irrigation with water.

28. **Choose the correct association:**

a. Inhalation of leaded gasoline → treatment with deferoxamine.

b. Ingestion of nitrobenzene → treatment with sodium thiosulfate.

c. Ingestion of methylene chloride → increased carboxyhemoglobin.

d. Inhalation of typewriter correction fluid → ARDS.

e. Administration of corticosteroids after petroleum aspiration → decreased incidence of pneumatoceles.

The answer is c. Pneumatoceles are common following aspirations of petroleum distillates. They require no therapy and their incidence is not changed with the use of corticosteroids. Inhalation of gasoline may directly cause sudden death from arrhythmias but more commonly causes progressive intoxication and respiratory depression leading to death. Secondary toxicity results from inorganic lead poisoning with resultant polyneuropathies, cerebellar dysfunction, and encephalopathy. Benzene is also a component of gasoline. Ingestion of nitrobenzene causes methemoglobinemia, which is reversible by giving IV methylene blue. Methylene chloride is a paint remover. After exposure it is stored in body fat and partially degraded to carbon monoxide in the body. 1,1,1-Trichloroethane and trichloroethylene are solvents used for cleaning and degreasing. They are also used in typewriter correction fluid, which is often deliberately inhaled and has resulted in a number of deaths. Both agents cause CNS depression and cardiac arrhythmias; the latter can also cause neuropathy, blindness, and hepatic or renal necrosis in larger amounts.

29.   **A 34-year-old intravenous drug user complains of right-sided neck and chest pain. You see swelling at the base of his neck, and he admits to hiring the services of a "street doc" to shoot into his deep neck veins. Which of the following statements regarding "pocket shots" is true?**

a.   Sternoclavicular septic arthritis has not been described as a potential complication.

b.   Aneurysms have resulted from this practice.

c.   These patients can be safely discharged on antibiotics after emergency department incision and drainage.

d.   Ischemic necrosis of the sternocleidomastoid muscle secondary to compartment syndrome has been described.

e.   Tracheal deviation away from the swelling should prompt treatment of a contralateral pneumothorax.

The answer is b. The sternoclavicular joint and spine are frequent sites of skeletal infection in addicts, often by *Pseudomonas* and other uncommon causes of septic arthritis. Deep neck abscesses are not uncommon in these patients, but mycotic aneurysm must be excluded as a cause of a mass located near major vessels. A compartment syndrome would not occur in the sternocleidomastoid muscle because it is not in a fascial compartment. Thrombophlebitis is an obvious complication of intravenous drug use. Septic emboli from tricuspid valve endocarditis causes chest pain, but if there is associated neck swelling and tenderness, septic thrombophlebitis are also likely. Pneumothorax is commonly seen in neck shooters. Tension pneumothorax results in tracheal deviation away from the affected side. In addicts less adept at self-administration, bilateral tension pneumothoraces is possible. These patients may present in respiratory or cardiovascular distress.

30.   **A 23-year-old heroin addict is brought to the ED after being found unconscious in an alley. The paramedics gave intravenous naloxone and he immediately awakened. He complains of severe pain in his left lower leg, but denies a groin injection. Physical examination shows that he is unable to dorsiflex his left big toe, and he has anterior tibial pain when you passively plantar flex. Sensation and both patellar and Achilles reflexes are equal bilaterally, and bilateral posterior tibial pulses are intact. Nonpitting leg edema consistent with chronic venous stasis disease involves both legs. You should now:**

a.   Consult orthopedic surgery for emergency management.

b.   Consult radiology for an arteriogram.

c.   Consult neurology for management of neuropathy.

d.   Obtain lumbar spine films to rule out an epidural abscess.

e.   Obtain a bilateral venogram to rule out DVT.

The answer is a. A compartment syndrome should be suspected in this patient with loss of muscle function of the anterior tibial compartment (extensor hallucis longus), pain with passive flexion of the muscles, and a history of being unconscious. Drug abusers may assume positions that lead to compromised blood flow and schema-induced muscle swelling. Pedal pulses are not necessarily affected. The findings are not compatible with a cord lesion. Acute DVT in this patient is unlikely and would not account for the muscle weakness. A "woody" consistency to the leg may be present, but is difficult to appreciate in patients with chronic venous insufficiency. Prompt diagnosis and surgical fasciotomy are essential to prevent muscle necrosis. Associated signs of infection would indicate a possible necrotizing fasciitis.

31.   **Which of the following statements concerning cocaine is true?**

a. Cocaine-induced seizures should be treated with phenytoin.

b. Cocaine acts to prevent reuptake of choline at nerve terminals.

c. Cocaine-induced myocardial ischemia should initially be treated identically to myocardial ischemia from coronary artery disease with aspirin, nitrates, and beta-blockers.

d. Cocaine may induce myocardial infarction in a young casual user with normal coronary arteries.

e. Cocaine psychosis is best managed with a high-potency phenothiazine.

The answer is d. Cocaine blocks the reuptake of catecholamines at the nerve terminal. Cocaine may cause fatal dysrhythmias, hypertension, psychosis, paranoia, and fatal hyperpyrexia. Cocaine use should be suspected in any young person presenting with myocardial infarction-type symptoms or cardiac dysrhythmias. Myocardial infarction may occur in the young, casual cocaine user who has normal coronary arteries secondary to vasospasm. Benzodiazepines and barbiturates are used to treat cocaine-induced seizures. In theory, beta blockade could result in unopposed alpha-adrenergic stimulation resulted in hypertension. Phenothiazines lower the seizure threshold; therefore, benzodiazepines are preferred for sedation.

32.   **Regarding phenytoin poisoning which of the following statements is true?**

a. Seizures exclude the diagnosis.

b. Nystagmus is a late finding.

c. Cardiac toxicity is common after an oral overdose.

d. Phenytoin is primarily eliminated renally.

e. Intravenous phenytoin produces hypotension secondary to the diluent.

The answer is e. Although serum levels roughly correlate with phenytoin toxicity, clinical features are more important in guiding therapy and estimating toxicity, which may sometimes occur even at "therapeutic" levels of 10–20 mg/mL. At 20–30 mg/mL, lateral gaze nystagmus is prominent. At 30–40 mg/mL, lateral nystagmus increases and vertical nystagmus and ataxia are seen. At greater than 40 mg/mL psychosis, seizures, dysarthria, and confusion occur. The increased incidence of seizures secondary to phenytoin toxicity is not understood. Cardiac toxicity after oral overdose is exceedingly rare. Phenytoin is highly bound to albumin. Phenytoin levels should be corrected for serum albumin concentrations. Phenytoin infusions result in hypotension secondary to the propylene glycol diluent.

33.   **A 35-year-old patient enters the ED and loudly proclaims he took 50 imipramine tablets approximately an hour ago. Physical examination reveals an alert and oriented thin patient in no apparent distress. His heart rate is 110/min, blood pressure is 120/60 mm Hg, and his pupils are dilated but reactive. The remainder of his examination is normal. In managing this patient, you should know:**

a. He should immediately receive oral syrup of ipecac, be placed on a cardiac monitor, and have an intravenous line established.

b. Less than 5% of patients who die of antidepressant overdose are awake and alert at the time of first medical contact.

c. A short QT interval with a normal QRS duration and nonspecific ST-T wave changes should be expected on the EKG.

d. The amount of drug ingested is clinically irrelevant in initially managing the treatment.

e. Arterial blood gases should be drawn at the first sign of cardiovascular toxicity.

The answer is d. Twenty-five percent of fatal antidepressant overdoses are in people who are awake at the time of initial presentation. The amount taken is not useful in predicting the clinical outcome or guiding the initial management of overdose because of differences in sensitivity between patients. Gastric lavage should not be used for decontamination because of the risk of rapid deterioration. Ipecac delays the use of activated charcoal. Cardiovascular complications are dependent on pH. ABG measurements are indicated with any CNS changes, and blood pH should be kept above 7.4. Tachycardia, prolonged QRS duration, and conduction abnormalities are common, but death is often the result of profound myocardial depression.

34. **Choose the true statement regarding the management of barbiturate intoxication:**
    a. Hemodialysis or charcoal hemoperfusion are usually necessary in moderate and severe overdose cases.
    b. The use of repeated doses of activated charcoal has not been found to be of value.
    c. Hypotension unresponsive to saline infusion or intravenous pressor support is an indication for hemodialysis.
    d. Forced diuresis and alkalization of urine is universally successful in increasing the excretion of barbiturates.
    e. Major symptoms of barbiturate withdrawal typically occur within 24 hours of cessation.

    The answer is c. Phenobarbital is a long-acting barbiturate and excretion can be enhanced tenfold by increasing the urine pH to >7.5. Alkalinization and diuresis is not effective in enhancing excretion of short- and intermediate-acting barbiturates. Administration of multiple doses of activated charcoal (every 6 hours for six doses) is known to be effective in removing phenobarbital in overdoses. Hemodialysis is far more effective in removing barbiturates than is alkaline diuresis, and charcoal hemoperfusion is most effective of all. These methods are indicated only if clinical evidence of severe poisoning is present or if there is significant renal or hepatic failure. Barbiturates directly depress the myocardium and cardiovascular depression is the most common cause of early deaths. Late deaths are usually from respiratory complications. Minor symptoms of withdrawal are seen within 24 hours, but the major complications of withdrawal (seizures, hyperpyrexia, hallucinations, death) usually occur 2–3 days after the last dose.

CHAPTER 18   Traumatic Emergencies

Jeffrey Barrett, MD, FAAEM

1. **A 5-year-old, 23-kg boy was thrown from a sled while riding it down a steep hill approximately 4 hours ago. He complains of generalized abdominal pain and is diaphoretic and pale. Bedside ultrasound is not available. Vital signs: heart rate 120/min; respiratory rate 30/min; blood pressure is not measurable, and femoral pulse is weakly palpable. After two 20 mL/kg boluses of lactated Ringer solution, his condition is unchanged. Your next action is to:**

    a. Give a third crystalloid fluid bolus.

    b. Infuse 230 mL 5% albumin.

    c. Perform diagnostic peritoneal lavage.

    d. Infuse 460 mL type-specific whole blood or 230 mL O negative packed red blood cells.

    e. Infuse 690 mL type-specific whole blood or 345 mL O negative packed red blood cells.

    The answer is d. Pediatric patients presenting in shock from trauma should receive an initial 20 mL/kg bolus of isotonic crystalloid. This may be repeated once, but if no improvement in the hemodynamic status occurs, immediate transfusion with packed red blood cells, 10 mL/kg, should be performed while preparing for emergent surgery.

2. **The most important radiographs used in evaluating an adult trauma patient are:**

    a. Chest, lateral cervical spine, abdomen.

    b. Pelvis, abdomen, lateral and anteroposterior cervical spine.

    c. Lateral cervical spine, chest, pelvis.

    d. Abdomen, chest, lateral and anteroposterior cervical spine.

    e. Abdomen, chest, lateral cervical spine, pelvis

    The answer is c. Radiographs of the anteroposterior chest, pelvis, and lateral cervical spine are the standard initial radiographs obtained in most patients with significant blunt trauma. A pelvic film can identify pelvic fractures, which can cause massive blood loss. If a patient with blunt injuries has persistent hypotension despite normal chest and pelvic radiographs, the most likely causes of the hypotension are intraperitoneal hemorrhage or cardiac tamponade.

3.   Loss of cerebral autoregulation leads to:

a. Cerebral blood flow which varies with arterial pressure.

b. Compensatory hyperventilation.

c. Drastically decreased intracranial pressure.

d. Epidural hematoma.

e. Profound constriction of cerebral resistance vessels.

The answer is a. With the loss of autoregulation, massive cerebral vasodilation occurs. Systemic pressure is transmitted to the capillaries, and the outpouring of fluids into the extravascular space can contribute to vasogenic edema and thus further increase ICP.

4.   The Glasgow Coma Scale (GCS) includes:

a. Oculomotor response, best verbal response, best motor response, light touch.

b. Eye opening, best motor response.

c. Best verbal response, best motor response, eye opening.

d. Best verbal response, best motor response, oculomotor response.

e. Pupillary response, best verbal response, best motor response.

The answer is c. Total GCS = Best Motor Response (1–6) + Best Verbal Response (1–5) + Eye Opening (1–4) = 3–15. The score ranges from 3 (no response) to 15 (best response). There are helpful mnemonics; the letter "E" (for eye) has four straight lines, and Eye Opening has a maximum score of 4. "Verbal" begins with the letter "V," which is also the Roman numeral for "5," and Best Verbal Response has a maximum score of 5. The value of this system is the ability to rapidly quantify a patient's level of consciousness (LOC) with an easily repoduced system. The LOC is the most important factor in the assessment of the head injured patient. This examination is reproducible by all levels of health care providers. The motor response is the most important and reproducible component of the examination. Severe injury is defined as a score of 8 or less persisting for at least 6 hours. Moderate injury is defined as a score of 9–12. A patient with a score of 8 or below (in the setting of head trauma) should be intubated for airway protection.

5.   Choose the true statement about initial management of the patient with possible spinal injury:

a. In patients with suspected cervical spine injury, immobilization with a properly applied rigid cervical collar is not sufficient to protect the patient from further injury.

b. Because obtaining adequate views of the spine is necessary for complete examination, the physician rather than the radiologic technician should be available to carefully move the patient's neck in order to optimize the examination.

c. Patients walking at the scene of an accident or arriving in the ED under their own power are not at risk for cervical spine or cord injuries.

d. The absence of an anal reflex is synonymous with a complete transection of the lumbar cord.

e. MAST garments should not be used in patients with a lumbar or low thoracic spinal injury because of the displacement caused by compartment inflation.

The answer is a. No cervical collar completely immobilizes the cervical spine, especially at the level of C1-C2. They are of greater value when used in conjunction with a spinal board, sandbagging, and tape. Patients with a suspected cervical spine injury who are awake and have normal lateral x-rays of the cervical spine or at least no evidence of an unstable injury may be supervised by the physician and position themselves for additional views, but under no circumstance should the physician actively move the patient's neck or force the motion beyond the limits of pain. Ambulation at the trauma scene does not exclude a C-spine injury. Spinal cord integrity includes the presence of the anal reflex. Absence of this reflex implies severe cord injury or transection at any level.

6. **Choose the correct statement concerning cervical spine injury:**

    a. The most common mechanism for cervical spine injuries is falls.
    b. Fractures of the odontoid are rare in children aged 8 years and younger.
    c. Pseudosubluxation is rare in children.
    d. The older the patient, the lower the fracture.
    e. Management of nerve root injuries includes methylprednisolone.

    The answer is d. Pediatric cervical spine injuries differ from adult injuries because of a child's proportionately larger head, the presence of epiphyseal plates, and greater ligamentous laxity. Odontoid fractures are less common in adults (10%), but are the most common pediatric cervical fracture (up to 8 years of age). Most pediatric odontoid fractures occur at the epiphyseal plate. Physiologic ligamentous laxity results in pseudosubluxation of C2 on C3 and C3 on C4 (40% of children younger than 7 years have this finding). Those older than 12 years tend to have lower anatomical cervical injuries. Approximately 40% of patients with a cervical spine fracture have associated neurologic injury. Treatment of cord injuries may include methylprednisolone 30 mg/kg loading dose, followed by 5.4 mg/kg/h for 23 hours.

7. **In a patient with penetrating neck trauma, you should:**

    a. Control bleeding with direct pressure and avoid blind clamping of vessels.
    b. Not attempt rapid sequence intubation, as these patients invariably require a surgical airway.
    c. Recognize Zone II injuries as occurring between the angle of the mandible and the thyroid cartilage.
    d. Order fiberoptic esophagoscopy, which if negative excludes a significant esophageal injury.
    e. Order a Gastrografin swallow, which if negative excludes a significant esophageal injury.

    The answer is a. Up to 25% of patients with esophageal injuries have negative Gastrografin studies. A barium upper GI series may improve sensitivity. Fiberoptic esophagoscopy has up to a 20% false-negative rate. Posterior triangle injuries may include subclavian vessel and vertebral artery lacerations; thus, subclavian venous access should be avoided. Complications of penetrating injuries to the posterior triangle includes hemothorax and tension pneumothorax. The best initial method to control vascular hemorrhage in the neck is direct pressure. Blind attempts to clamp vessels can result in serious injury to associated structures. The management of neck injuries has been aided by dividing the neck into three zones and the availability of arteriography. Zone III injuries occur above the angle of the mandible and the cricoid. Zone II injuries occur between the mandible and the cricoid. Zone I injuries occur below the cricoid cartilage and above the clavicle.

8. **Isolated knee meniscus injuries are most commonly associated with:**

    a. An audible pop at the time of injury.
    b. Hemarthrosis with fat globules.
    c. Delayed onset of pain.
    d. A history of "locking" on flexion or extension
    e. Positive anterior drawer sign.

    The answer is a. A joint effusion may develop with a meniscal injury. Hemarthrosis with fat globules indicates a fracture involving marrow. Solitary hemarthrosis may result form skeletal, ligamentous, or cartilaginous injuries. If the cartilage interposes in the intercondylar notch, the joint will lock.

9.   **A 22-year-old woman complains of several days of progressive knee pain after sustaining a twisting injury. Her knee is stable to valgus and varus stress and you find no laxity and no soft end point on anterior drawer testing. There is, however, an effusion and tenderness of the medial joint line and anterior joint space. She probably has:**

a. An anterior cruciate ligament tear.

b. A posterior cruciate ligament tear.

c. Chondromalacia patella.

d. Osteochondritis dessicans.

e. A medial meniscal tear.

The answer is e. Valgus stress tests the medial collateral ligament, while the anterior drawer test is for assessing integrity of the anterior cruciate ligament. Meniscal injuries are typically caused by twisting injuries, and sometimes cause effusions. Chondromalacia patella is an overuse syndrome of the articular cartilage of the patella. Osteochondritis dessicans is a rare condition of unknown etiology commonly found in adolescents where the articular cartilage and subchondral bone become separated from the underlying bone.

10.   **A workman falls from a height of 10 ft and lands on his feet. He complains of severe left foot pain and has diffuse swelling. You know that:**

a. The most commonly fractured tarsal bone is the talus.

b. Bohler's angle should normally be 20 degrees or less.

c. An abnormal Bohler angle indicates a talus fracture.

d. Avascular necrosis is a complication of a talar fracture.

e. Lisfranc's fracture is treated with a weight-bearing cast.

The answer is d. Bohler's angle, normally 20–40 degrees, determines the presence of depression in calcaneal fractures. The calcaneus is the most frequently fractured tarsal bone. The mechanism of injury is usually compression. Associated injuries with a calcaneus fracture are injuries to the lumbar spine, pelvis, hip, and knee. Often, the only radiographic signs are the disruption of the trabecular pattern and an abnormal Bohler's angle (the angle formed by the axis of the subtalar joint and the superior surface of the tuberosity). Talar fractures are uncommon, although they are the second most common foot fracture. Because the blood supply to the talus is poor, avascular necrosis of the bone may result. Fracture/dislocations of the tarsal–metatarsal joint (Lisfranc's joint) are uncommon. A fracture through the base of the second metatarsal is almost pathognomonic of a disrupted joint. Separation between the base of the first and second metatarsals suggests separation or subluxation. Comparison views with the opposite foot are helpful. Treatment may require open reduction and internal fixation. (Some sources refer to Böehler's angle.)

11.   **Using the Young classification system, acetabular fractures are associated with which type of pelvic fracture?**

a. Type I.

b. Type II.

c. Type III.

d. Type IV.

e. Type V.

The answer is d. Pelvic fractures are divided into four anatomic types. Type IV fractures constitute approximately 20% of pelvic fractures and involve the acetabulum. The mechanism of injury is a force applied to the flexed hip. Type I fractures are stable pelvic fractures with no break in the pelvic ring, for example, a transverse sacral fracture. Type II fractures have a single break in the pelvic ring, such as a vertical fracture of the ileum parallel to the sacroiliac (SI) joint. Both type I and type II are stable fractures. Type III fractures (double break in the pelvic ring) are severe, unstable, and are associated with concomitant injuries. A Malgaigne fracture is a fracture of the ilium and a symphyseal dislocation.

12. **Choose the correct association:**

    a. Nondisplaced transverse ulnar fracture from a direct blow: nightstick fracture.
    b. Midshaft fracture of the radius and radioulnar dislocation: Monteggia fracture-dislocation.
    c. Fracture of the proximal third of the ulna and dislocation of the radial head: Galeazzi fracture-dislocation.
    d. Infant pulled by the arm, elbow pain, negative elbow x-rays: elbow sprain.
    e. Anterior shoulder dislocation with deltoid paresthesias: radial nerve palsy.

    The answer is a. A nightstick fracture is an isolated nondisplaced fracture of the midshaft of the ulna. Treatment is immobilization in a long arm cast. A Monteggia fracture-dislocation is a diaphyseal fracture of the proximal third of the ulna with an anterior dislocation of the radial head. A Galeazzi fracture is an isolated radial shaft fracture with a dislocation of the radioulnar joint. Nursemaid elbow is a frequent pediatric injury caused by subluxation of the radial head. Treatment requires passive supination and flexion. Function of the axillary nerve (innervation of the skin over the deltoid muscle) should be assessed in shoulder dislocations.

13. **Choose the correct answer about comparing diagnostic peritoneal lavage (DPL) to computerized axial tomography (CT) in the evaluation of blunt abdominal trauma:**

    a. CT is easier to interpret.
    b. CT is more specific.
    c. CT is more time consuming.
    d. DPL is more expensive.
    e. DPL requires contrast for optimal results.

    The answer is b. CT is more specific than DPL. CT scan for blunt abdominal trauma can reduce the rate of noninterventional laparotomy rates. Solid organ injuries (hepatic or splenic hematomas) in the hemodynamically stable patient may be managed nonoperatively. CT is less sensitive in identifying hollow viscous bowel injuries.

14. **An 8-year-old girl falls off the top of a slide and severely twists her ankle. You know that:**

    a. The ankle is the joint most commonly fractured in pediatrics.
    b. Significant ligamentous injuries of the ankle are uncommon in children.
    c. Most fractures involve the bone shaft; Salter-Harris ankle fractures are uncommon.
    d. The most commonly injured ankle ligament is the calcaneofibular ligament.
    e. As in adults, the medial malleolus is involved less than 10% of the time.

    The answer is b. Ankle fractures constitute 7% of pediatric fractures; the wrist and forearm is more commonly injured. Fifty percent of ankle fractures involve the medial malleolus. Patients with open growth plates rarely sustain ligamentous injuries, but more commonly sustain physeal-epiphyseal-metaphyseal injuries. Comparison views may be helpful. Fortunately, growth disturbances following these injuries are relatively uncommon.

15. **A 32-year-old man sustains a gunshot wound to the left midanterior chest. The carotid pulses are weak despite 2 L of crystalloid and one unit of blood. Clinical examination shows jugular venous distention and absent breath sounds on the left hemithorax. The patient is bradycardic and hypotensive. He has a transient improvement after a left chest tube thoracostomy. The subxiphoid pericardiocentesis is negative. Your next immediate step is:**

    a. Measure arterial blood gases.

    b. Administer atropine 1 mg IV push.

    c. Begin chest compressions.

    d. Perform femoral or saphenous venous cannulation and continue aggressive volume resuscitation.

    e. Perform left thoracostomy or emergent pericardial window.

    The answer is e. Up to 80% of patients with acute tamponade will have a false-negative pericardiocentesis. This patient has a high likelihood of cardiac injury based on the anatomical site of injury. External cardiac compressions and pharmacologic therapy provide no therapeutic benefit. Emergency left thoracotomy or emergent pericardial window should be performed to relieve the cardiac tamponade.

16. **A patient has traumatic intrabronchial bleeding. You know that:**

    a. A major complication is hypovolemic shock.

    b. Fiberoptic intubation is contraindicated.

    c. The patient should be positioned with the injured side down.

    d. Fresh frozen plasma is frequently therapeutic.

    e. Vigorous ventilation and high airway pressures should be started early.

    The answer is c. The most serious complication of intrabronchial bleeding is hypoxia; bleeding is generally not a problem, as the bronchial tubes are relatively avascular and the entire tracheobronchial tree can only hold approximately 150 mL of fluid. Treatment involves using a double-lumen endotracheal (Carlen) tube or fiberoptic bronchoscopic placement of an endotracheal tube into the bleeding main stem bronchus. Definitive treatment is surgery. Placing the bleeding side down helps prevent soiling of the uncontaminated lung.

17. **Stress fracture of the leg:**

    a. Usually involve the distal tibia in adults.

    b. Usually involve the proximal tibia in children.

    c. Generally have early radiographic signs of medullary sclerosis and periosteal callus.

    d. Should not undergo radionuclide bone scan until at least 1 week after symptoms begin.

    e. Are imperative to diagnose, since long-term prognosis is poor.

    The answer is b. Stress fractures result from bone fatigue secondary to repetitive stress. Initial x-ray findings are usually negative. A fracture line or new bone deposition may appear weeks after the initial symptoms. Bone scans are positive within 72 hours of the injury. Treatment of most stress fractures is symptomatic.

18. **Immediate complications of spinal cord transection include:**

    a. Tachycardia.

    b. Renal shutdown.

    c. Hypothermia.

    d. Hypertension.

    e. Hyperreflexia.

The answer is c. Severe injury to the spinal cord may cause spinal shock. The patient presents with flaccid paraplegia or quadriplegia and areflexia. Typically, within 24 hours the patient develops a spastic paralysis. There is loss of sympathetic tone. Despite severe hypotension, the patient has vasodilation (warm skin), paradoxical bradycardia, and good urine output. Priapism may also occur. Autonomic nervous system dysfunction signs include urinary retention, paralytic ileus, gastric distension, fecal incontinence, and hypothermia. Patients require a Foley catheter and a nasogastric tube.

19. **A 47-year-old woman is brought by a basic life support unit after her car collided with a bridge abutment. She complained of neck pain at the scene and was appropriately immobilized with long board, hard collar, and sandbags to prevent head and neck movement. You order a portable cross-table cervical spine radiograph, knowing that:**

    a. Initial radiographs required to exclude a cervical spine injury are lateral (C1-T1), PA, and Waters views.

    b. The widest area of the predental space in pediatric patients should measure no more than 6 mm with the neck held in gentle flexion.

    c. The lateral radiograph will reveal 70–80% of significant injuries.

    d. Anterior displacement of C3 and C4 by 20% or greater is an unstable injury.

    e. Prevertebral soft tissue swelling is a normal variant and carries no diagnostic value.

    The answer is c. A lateral view must include all cervical vertebrae and the upper margin of T1. The lateral view shows 70–80% of injuries. The odontoid and AP views reveal 10% and 1% respectively of significant injuries. Additional views include the pillar view (for lateral mass fractures) and oblique views (for facet, foramen, and pedicle). Indications for tomography and CT scan are inadequate radiographs, any patient with a neurologic deficit, fracture of the posterior arch, and burst fractures with bony fragments in the spinal canal. Injuries that appear stable may be evaluated by careful flexion/extension views or CT scan. The patient can slowly flex/extend the neck only is the absence of pain or neurologic symptoms (unimpaired level of consciousness or distracting injuries). In such cases, a neurosurgeon should review the radiographs and examine the patient. Prevertebral soft-tissue swelling (>5 mm down to C4) suggests a hematoma secondary to fracture.

20. **A 23-year-old patient sustains a gunshot wound to the left fourth intercostal space, midclavicular line. He had a palpable radial pulse at the scene. Bilateral breath sounds are present. After rapid infusion of 2000 mL of a crystalloid solution, he has only an intermittent, thready radial pulse. His neck veins are flat. The monitor shows a sinus tachycardia. This patient now requires:**

    a. Immediate portable chest radiograph.

    b. Cricothyrotomy or tracheostomy.

    c. Central line placement.

    d. Left tube thoracostomy.

    e. Nasotracheal intubation.

    The answer is d. Patients with refractory hypotension following 2 L of crystalloid infusion should receive blood (type specific or type O negative). Most patients with penetrating chest trauma require ventilatory–circulatory support and a tube thoracostomy. Approximately 10–20% of patients require a thoracotomy. The patient described in the question may be hypotensive from a tension pneumothorax or cardiac tamponade (flat neck veins may present if the patient is hypovolemic). This patient requires immediate intubation and a left tube thoracostomy. A thoracotomy is indicated if these measures prove unsuccessful.

21. **A 22-year-old man walks into your emergency department. He is covered in blood and pointing to his throat, where you see a large laceration and a hematoma that is displacing his trachea. His voice is hoarse and stridulous. You must immediately:**

    a. Consult ENT for emergent tracheostomy.

    b. Do a cricothyrotomy.

    c. Insert a laryngeal mask airway (LMA).

    d. Perform nasotracheal intubation.

    e. Perform rapid sequence intubation.

    The answer is e. Recent literature supports orotracheal RSI in trauma patients with blunt or penetrating neck injuries, and it should be considered the first-line airway technique unless contraindications exist. Concerns over sedative-induced muscle relaxation leading to airway distortion, although possible, have not been validated. Orotracheal RSI is often successful even after neck trauma with airway distortion. RSI also has been shown to be superior to intubation without paralytics. If the cervical spine must remain immobilized, an assistant should maintain in-line stabilization of the head and neck.

22. **A 32-year-old man struck his chest on the dashboard during a rapid deceleration motor vehicle collision. He has a displaced sternal fracture. You know that:**

    a. The diagnosis of myocardial contusion can reliably be made on the basis of the initial EKG and serum cardiac biomarker levels.

    b. Most displaced sternal fractures requires open fixation.

    c. Traumatic pericardial tamponade may occur days after the initial injury.

    d. He will require admission to a monitored bed.

    e. Opioid pain relievers are contraindicated.

    The answer is c. EKG and CPK-MB changes are initially absent in patients with myocardial contusion. Patients with persistent tachycardia following blunt chest trauma or a history consistent with significant blunt chest trauma are admitted for monitoring, serial EKG and isoenzyme determinations, and echocardiography. Echocardiography is a valuable diagnostic study for the evaluation of cardiac injury. Ventricular aneurysm is a late complication of myocardial contusion. Traumatic pericardial effusions may develop acutely or may develop days after injury. Constrictive pericarditis is a late complication of hemopericardium. Other complications following blunt cardiac injury include ventricular septal rupture, valvular injury, and aortic dissection.

23. **A patient sustains a comminuted fracture of the proximal fibula. The neurologic finding which would be most likely is:**

    a. Isolated paralysis of the extensor digitorum brevis muscle.

    b. Loss of dorsiflexion of the foot and loss of sensation over the dorsal surface.

    c. Isolated sensory loss over the lateral plantar surface.

    d. Loss of sensation over the lateral plantar surface and inability to invert the foot.

    e. Loss of sensation over the medial plantar surface and inability to evert the foot.

    The answer is b. The common peroneal nerve winds around the fibular head. This nerve divides into the superficial and deep peroneal nerves in the lateral compartment of the leg. The deep peroneal nerve innervates the dorsal webspace of the first and second toes and provides innervation to the anterior compartment muscles (dorsiflexion). The superficial peroneal nerve innervates the skin of the remainder of the dorsum of the foot and provides motor fibers to the peroneus longus and brevis (eversion) of the lateral compartment.

24. **The recommended diagnostic peritoneal lavage (DPL) technique for a patient with a severe pelvic fracture is:**

    a. Four quadrant abdominal tap.
    b. Infraumbilical open peritoneal cutdown.
    c. Infraumbilical Seldinger technique.
    d. Supraumbilical open peritoneal cutdown.
    e. Supraumbilical Seldinger technique.

    The answer is d. DPL has sensitivity greater than 95%. Indications for DPL include equivocal abdominal examination, inability to perform serial examinations, and questionable penetration of peritoneum. The only absolute contraindication is an indication for a laparotomy (intraperitoneal bladder rupture, pneumoperitoneum). The DPL does not evaluate the retroperitoneum. Pelvic fractures are associated with pelvic hematomas. A supraumbilical open technique limits complications and the incidence of false-positive results.

25. **Choose the correct statement about knee pain in children:**

    a. The most common cause of nontraumatic knee pain in adolescents is chondromalacia patella.
    b. Osgood-Schlatter disease is more common in boys than in girls.
    c. The medial collateral ligament is the most common ligamentous knee injury.
    d. Patellar dislocation implies severe internal derangement and carries a grim prognosis.
    e. Osteochondritis dissecans can occur following minor trauma.

    The answer is c. Osgood-Schlatter disease is frequently a bilateral tibial apophysitis seen in adolescents. Once thought more common in adolescent boys, it is now known to have no sexual predilection. Leg extension exacerbates the pain of Osgood-Schlatter disease. Epiphyseal plate/bony injuries are more common than ligamentous and cartilaginous injuries in the pediatric age group. Circumferential knee pain may indicate an epiphyseal injury. Stress views and comparison views may be necessary to diagnosis an epiphyseal fracture. Osteochondritis dessicans is usually idiopathic—no injury is reported in a majority of patients.

26. **Choose the correct statement about pediatric trauma:**

    a. Blunt thoracic trauma may cause pulmonary injury despite the absence of thoracic rib fractures.
    b. Space-occupying hematomas are the most common sequelae of closed head injury.
    c. Hypoxia occurs less rapidly than in adults.
    d. Intraosseous infusion is not recommended for fluid resuscitation.
    e. Fractures of the pelvic bone are relatively uncommon in children with blunt trauma.

    The answer is a. The general principles of adult and pediatric trauma management are identical. However, age modifies injury patterns and physiologic responses. A pediatric thorax is more pliable than an adult thorax. The pediatric chest may absorb significant force without sustaining rib fractures. Pulmonary contusions, hematomas, and cardiac contusions may exhibit minimal external stigmata. Children have less inspiratory reserve and have higher basal oxygen consumption than adults. Thus hypoxia occurs faster in the pediatric patient than in an adult. Cerebral edema occurs readily in children who have suffered blunt head trauma as compared with adults who are more likely to sustain intracranial hematomas. Specific measures to decrease intracranial pressure include hyperventilation, elevation of the head, diuretics, and mannitol. An intraosseous line may be used for fluid resuscitation.

27. **Choose the correct statement about lung trauma:**
    a. Respiratory distress in patients cannot be used as a prognostic sign.
    b. Chest tubes are out of position in 60–75% of patients.
    c. Bronchial or tracheal ruptures occur secondary to blunt injury in 14% of patients.
    d. Approximately 50% of bronchial injuries occur at the carina.
    e. Persistent pneumothorax despite multiple appropriately placed chest tubes should make the clinician suspect bronchial fracture.

    The answer is e. Respiratory distress is ominous. Approximately 50% of trauma patients presenting to the emergency department in respiratory distress die. If both respiratory distress and shock are present, 75% die. Chest tubes are out of place 5–10% of the time. More than 80% of bronchial fractures occur within 2.5 cm of the carina.

28. **Which of the following statements regarding imaging of thoracic trauma is true?**
    a. All patients with blunt thoracic trauma should undergo CT because chest x-ray has low sensitivity.
    b. CT is preferred for suspected diaphragmatic rupture, and CT may show of diaphragmatic injury despite a normal chest x-ray.
    c. Ultrasonography has no role in evaluating thoracic trauma.
    d. Lung contusion appears as an area of consolidation beneath an area of impact, and it appears within hours of the injury as an air bronchogram.
    e. The incidence of sternal fractures is higher in seat-belt users than nonusers.

    The answer is e. Seat-belt injuries related to a 3-point restraint may cause bruises in the subcutaneous tissues and fat of the anterior chest wall, which may be identified on CT scans. Seat-belt injuries severe enough to cause skin abrasions are associated with significant internal injuries in 30% of patients. Thus, the identification of seat-belt bruises on CT scans should prompt a careful search for the following: fractures of the sternum, ribs, clavicles, transverse processes of C7 or T1; aortic transection; cardiac contusions or ventricular rupture; vascular injuries to the subclavian artery or superior vena cava; tracheal or laryngeal tears; and diaphragmatic rupture. The incidence of sternal fractures is actually higher in seat-belt users than in nonusers, and most fractures occur within 2 cm of the manubrial–sternal junction.

29. **A 22-year-old man is brought by ambulance from the scene of a major motor vehicle crash. He is initially awake and alert, but somewhat combative. His prehospital hypotension and tachycardia have responded to 2 L of intravenous crystalloid. A cervical spine series is normal. Suddenly he vomits and loses consciousness. Your attempts to clear the airway are hampered by a malfunctioning suction apparatus and his pulse oximetry readings begin to plummet. Of the choices listed, your next move should be:**
    a. Transtracheal ventilation.
    b. Paralysis by pancuronium, bag-mask ventilation, obtain new suction device.
    c. Paralysis by succinylcholine and placement of a nasogastric tube.
    d. Emergent tracheostomy.
    e. Nasotracheal intubation.

    The answer is a. This patient has a multifactorial etiology for his altered level of consciousness: hypoxemia, alcohol, hypovolemia, and head injury. Transtracheal ventilation is a useful temporizing measure to provide oxygen until the upper airway is cleared. Muscle paralysis is frequently necessary in agitated patients to allow intubation. Succinylcholine has a faster onset of action and a shorter duration of action than that of pancuronium. Cricothyroidotomy is an alternative method for the difficult airway. Emergency tracheostomy is rarely required.

30. **The best definition of shock is:**

    a. Blood pressure below the fifth percentile for age.

    b. Altered level of consciousness associated with a falling blood pressure.

    c. Inadequate organ and tissue perfusion.

    d. Progressive lethargy with a fast heart rate.

    e. Mottling of the skin.

    The answer is c. Shock is defined as inadequate delivery of oxygen and nutrients to meet the metabolic needs of the tissues and organs. A state of shock may exist without hypotension or alterations in mental status. Shock may also exist with signs of brisk skin perfusion when distributive mechanisms, such as sepsis or anaphylaxis, are present.

31. **The most common Salter-Harris fracture is:**

    a. Type I.

    b. Type II.

    c. Type III.

    d. Type IV.

    e. Type V.

    The answer is b. The most common type of Salter-Harris fracture is type II, which is a fracture through the physis and metaphysis, although the epiphysis is not involved in the injury. This may be related to the mechanism that causes this injury. These fractures may cause minimal shortening; however, the injuries rarely result in functional limitations. This type of fracture has an excellent prognosis.

32. **A 7-year-old girl complains of wrist pain that has persisted for 1 week after a fall on her outstretched hand. The initial x-ray obtained on the day of the injury was read as normal. A repeat x-ray:**

    a. Should be obtained now.

    b. Should be obtained only if specific bone pain is present.

    c. After another week.

    d. Is not indicated.

    e. Should not be obtained at this time; however, if pain continues over the next few days, repeat x-ray may be warranted.

    The answer is a. Type I and type V Salter-Harris fractures may not be visible on initial x-rays. Type I fracture can cause pain that continues after injury. An x-ray obtained 7–10 days after injury often shows an abnormal finding in the growth plate. Type V fracture results from a compression injury. This type of fracture also causes continued pain; its correct diagnosis is important as the fracture can result in functional disability.

33.   **A 25-year-old man was assaulted with an aluminum baseball bat and received a blow to the forehead. Upon arrival to the ED, his vital signs are stable and the patient is alert and oriented. He complains of severe pain to the forehead. Physical examination reveals swelling and crepitus over the supraorbital rims. The most likely fracture is:**

a.   Frontal sinus fracture.

b.   LeFort I fracture.

c.   Zygomaticomaxillary complex fracture.

d.   LeFort III fracture.

e.   Mandibular fracture.

The answer is a. In a presentation like this, fractures of the anterior and posterior tables of the frontal sinus occur. The CT scan will show the fracture and fluid in the sinus. In this case, the posterior table was removed by the neurosurgeons, and the anterior table of the comminuted frontal bone was repaired by the oral and maxillofacial surgeons. The other fracture choices shown occur with more lateral face trauma versus the midline trauma described in this case.

34.   **The most common error made in initial evaluation of a burn victim is:**

a.   Overestimation of burn depth.

b.   Underestimation of burn depth.

c.   Underappreciation of early infection.

d.   Wrong choice of topical membrane.

e.   Wrong choice of topical medication.

The answer is b. The depth of partial-thickness burns is routinely underestimated in the outpatient setting. Nonviable tissues may appear viable for several days, and progressive microvascular thrombosis may occur to some extent. Importantly, allow for this possibility when planning follow-up visits. In addition the likelihood of infection is greater with a deeper versus a more superficial burn.

35.   **A 37-year-old man was brought to your ED approximately 3 hours after a major motor vehicle crash, which required prolonged extrication. He is awake and alert, and his right leg is fixed in a traction splint. The finding that most indicates the need for further resuscitation is:**

a.   Urine output of 40 cc/h.

b.   Serum lactate of 1.9 mmol/L.

c.   Blood pressure of 158/82 mm Hg.

d.   A heart rate of 105/min.

e.   Respiratory rate of 28/min.

The answer is e. A urine output of 40 cc/h represents greater than 0.5 cc/kg/h for this patient, which is acceptable. A serum lactate of less than 2.0 mmol/L and a mild degree of sinus tachycardia in a patient with painful injuries who is awake are normal. A respiratory rate greater than 24–25/min should raise concern for possible metabolic acidosis or undetected thoracic injuries. Systolic hypertension is not an indication for further resuscitation.

36. **Operative intervention for neurotrauma is absolutely indicated for:**
    a. Subarachnoid hemorrhage.
    b. Glasgow Coma Score of less than 8.
    c. Significantly depressed skull fractures.
    d. Intracerebral bleed.
    e. Unexplained prolonged comatose state.

    The answer is c. Significantly depressed skull fractures require elevation to prevent future complications. The other injuries described may selectively require neurosurgical intervention. Any penetrating head trauma carries a significant risk of infection and thus prophylactic antibiotic treatment is indicated in these patients.

37. **Medics bring you a 27-year-old, 70-kg man after he sustains a single gunshot wound to the leg. The medics tell you there was "a lot" of blood at the scene. Vital signs: heart rate 110/min, blood pressure 120/90 mm Hg, respiratory rate 16/min. You estimate the blood loss at a minimum of:**
    a. 250 cc.
    b. 500 cc.
    c. 1 L.
    d. 1.5 L.
    e. 2 L.

    The correct answer is c. The loss of up to 15% of the typical person's blood volume will not cause any change in pulse or systolic blood pressure, although it may manifest as a narrowed pulse pressure. The loss of 15–30% of one's blood volume will cause a mild tachycardia and a narrowed pulse pressure. Once a loss of 30–40% of one's blood volume is reached, there will be a drop in the systolic blood pressure, as well as a more prominent tachycardic response. This patient was noted to have a slight tachycardia and a slightly narrowed pulse pressure, so one can estimate his blood loss at 15–30%. Since the typical 70-kg man has a blood volume of 5 L, this corresponds to a blood loss of 750–1500 cc.

38. **A 23-year-old man with a history of seizures complains of left shoulder pain after he seized at a local shopping mall. You know that you must think about posterior glenohumeral dislocation and suspect he may have this condition because he holds his arm:**
    a. Adducted and externally rotated.
    b. Adducted internally rotated.
    c. Abducted and externally rotated.
    d. Abducted and internally rotated.
    e. Over his head.

    The answer is b. Posterior glenohumeral dislocations are relatively rare, but are typically caused by forceful internal rotation and adduction of the arm, which might occur with a generalized seizure or electric shock. Upon presentation, patients with posterior glenohumeral dislocations typically hold the affected limb in an adducted and internally rotated position. Anterior glenohumeral dislocations tend to present with the arm abducted and externally rotated.

39.   **A 32-year-old man sustained an electric shock while working on a high-voltage power line. He is awake, alert, and oriented and has normal vital signs but complains of paresthesias in the affected arm. Your management includes:**

   a.   Symptomatic treatment, discharge.

   b.   Analgesia, observation for 6 hours, discharge.

   c.   Analgesia, observation for 6 hours on a cardiac monitor, discharge.

   d.   Analgesia, observation for 6 hours on a cardiac monitor, check urine for myoglobin, discharge.

   e.   Analgesia, cardiac monitoring, CBC, basic metabolic panel, total CK, EKG, admission to a monitored bed.

   The answer is e. High-voltage can be defined as greater than 600 V. Patients with low-voltage injuries and evidence of complications such as rhabdomyolysis should be admitted. Those with high-voltage injuries are at risk for serious and sometimes delayed complications such as cardiac arrhythmias, arterial thrombosis, compartment syndromes, rhabdomyolysis, and nerve damage. Because of these risks, all patients with high-voltage injuries should be admitted to the hospital.

40.   **Which patient listed below should be prioritized to prompt operative intervention?**

   a.   22-year-old man with mild traumatic brain injury and frontal traumatic subarachnoid hemorrhage.

   b.   70-year-old man with moderate traumatic brain injury and an acute parietal subdural hematoma.

   c.   50-year-old man with severe traumatic brain injury and a frontal contusion.

   d.   19-year-old woman with mild traumatic brain injury, no CT abnormalities, but total global amnesia.

   e.   3-year-old comatose girl with basilar skull fracture and CSF otorrhea.

   The answer is b. Subdural hematomas are collections of blood in the subdural space. They are more likely to occur in those with substantial atrophy (e.g., elderly patients and alcoholics). Subdural hematomas are amenable to operative decompression, but the mortality increases substantially with delays >4 hours.

41.   **A 37-year-old man was involved in a high-speed, head-on collision with a truck. He was restrained driver and did not lose consciousness, but his left knee struck the dashboard. He now complains of severe left hip pain. Vital signs: heart rate 118/min; blood pressure 200/100 mm Hg. You note some lower cervical spine tenderness, a systolic murmur best heard between the scapulae, and a left hip that is adducted, internally rotated, and resistant to minimal range of motion. You prioritize his care, knowing the most important injury to consider emergently is:**

   a.   Cervical spine injury.

   b.   Hypertensive emergency.

   c.   Splenic rupture.

   d.   Traumatic aortic rupture.

   e.   Posterior dislocation of the hip leading to avascular necrosis.

   The answer is d. Traumatic rupture of the aorta typically occurs with deceleration mechanisms and occurs at the level of the ligamentum arteriosum. Associated physical findings can include upper extremity hypertension and a harsh systolic murmur heard best in the interscapular space. Patients often have associated injuries that dominate the clinical presentation, and this patient, in all likelihood, probably does have a posterior hip dislocation. The potential lethality of an aortic rupture makes it a more important diagnostic consideration however.

42. **Which of the following is a "hard sign" of peripheral vascular injury?**
    a. Injury to an anatomically associated nerve.
    b. Hypotension.
    c. Associated fracture.
    d. A palpable thrill.
    e. Proximity to a major vessel.

    The answer is d. Hard signs of peripheral vascular injury include: a pulse deficit, pulsatile bleeding, an expanding hematoma, an audible bruit, a palpable thrill, or distal ischemia. Soft signs include a stable hematoma, injury to an anatomically related nerve, unexplained hypotension, a history of hemorrhage, proximity to a major vascular structure, or a complex fracture.

43. **The organ most susceptible to injury from the temporary cavitation caused by a high-velocity missile is the:**
    a. Lung.
    b. Muscle.
    c. Bladder.
    d. Liver.
    e. Spinal cord.

    The answer is d. Faster, lighter bullets tend to produce greater temporary cavitation when they pass through tissue. Tissue that is close to water density and less elastic tends to sustain the greatest damage from this temporary cavity. More elastic tissue, such as lung, is less likely to be damaged when a temporary cavity forms within it.

44. **An 18-year-old man was involved in a fight. He tells you that he was punched once with a fist and had brief loss of consciousness. You find right-sided periorbital ecchymosis, diplopia with upward gaze, and ipsilateral infraorbital hypoesthesia. The most likely diagnosis is:**
    a. Left parietal subdural hematoma.
    b. Right temporal epidural hematoma.
    c. Traumatic subarachnoid hemorrhage.
    d. Cerebral contusion.
    e. Right orbital floor fracture.

    The answer is e. The orbital floor is the weakest part of the orbit and typically is the first to break in the setting of orbital trauma. Potential complications of such fractures include entrapment of the inferior rectus muscle, which manifests as diplopia on upward gaze on examination. Another common finding is infraorbital hypoesthesia that results from injury to the infraorbital nerve.

45. **The immediate treatment protocol for a patient with tension pneumothorax is:**

    a. Immediate drainage of blood from the chest.

    b. Immediate decompression of air from the affected side.

    c. Emergent endotracheal intubation with positive-pressure ventilation.

    d. Emergent thoracotomy on the affected side.

    e. Rapid infusion of isotonic fluid to maintain adequate cerebral perfusion pressure.

The answer is b. Tension pneumothorax may prove fatal unless immediately diagnosed and managed. Normal negative intrapleural pressure is reversed to positive pressure, leading to impedance of flow to the heart and decreased preload. The clinical characteristics are respiratory distress, tracheal deviation away from the affected side, absence of breath sounds on the affected side, and distended neck veins. Treatment is immediate decompression followed by tube thoracostomy. You can decompress by inserting a large-bore cannula (e.g., 14-gauge angiocath) in the midclavicular line, second intercostal space, on the affected side. You can drain the hemithorax by inserting a chest tube in the fourth or fifth intercostal space between the midclavicular line and the anterior axillary line.

46. **In the majority of patients, the best treatment for flail chest is:**

    a. Intubation and mechanical ventilation.

    b. Operative fixation of both ends of the rib fractures.

    c. Pain control and medical management of respiratory insufficiency.

    d. Towel clips around rib segments with weighted traction over pulleys.

    e. Negative-pressure ventilation in old-style iron lung ventilators.

The answer is c. Medical management of chest wall injury and underlying pulmonary contusion continues to be the standard of care. Intubation, mechanical ventilation, and operative stabilization are adjuncts in the overall care but are not always necessary. The way to remember the presentation of flail chest is that a flail segment presents in the opposite way to inhalation and exhalation as you would expect.

47. **The respiratory failure frequently observed with flail chest is mainly caused by:**

    a. Underlying pulmonary contusion.

    b. Decreased tidal volume due to pain.

    c. Decreased tidal volume due to paradoxical motion of chest wall.

    d. Preexisting smoking history.

    e. Alveolar collapse due to decreased negative intrathoracic pressure.

The answer is a. Severity of the underlying pulmonary contusion continues to be the most common cause of respiratory insufficiency and the need for mechanical ventilation, above all other factors. Pulmonary contusions are significantly under diagnosed which can result in significant repercussions.

48. **The leading cause of head injury in older adults in the United States is:**

    a. Fall.

    b. Assault.

    c. Sport-related.

    d. Road traffic accidents.

    e. Industrial accidents.

The answer is a. The leading causes of traumatic brain injuries vary according to age. Falls are the leading cause of traumatic brain injuries among persons aged 65 years and older, whereas transportation injuries leads among persons aged 5–64 years. Firearms surpassed motor vehicles as the largest single cause of death associated with traumatic brain injury in the United States in 1990. Nearly 50% of all trauma-related deaths are the result of head trauma.

49. **The most urgent maneuver in the initial management of a patient with a possible head injury is:**

    a. Perform a CT scan and transfer to a neurosurgical unit.

    b. Intravenous mannitol and hyperventilation.

    c. Emergency exploratory burr holes.

    d. Airway management.

    e. Spine stabilization.

The answer is d. Management of any obvious or potential CNS injury should be part of the overall patient stabilization and preparation at the scene of the injury, before transfer to the hospital. The circumstances of the accident or injury should be assessed quickly, and any potential risk of CNS injury should be identified alongside the rest of the injuries in order to guide appropriate care. Avoid moving the patient if at all possible; this can be dangerous, especially after high-velocity injuries. The most important immediate protective maneuvers for any CNS injury are securing and preserving the airway, maintaining and supporting breathing, and maintaining effective circulation. Protecting the spine (especially, but not exclusively, the cervical spine) should also be among the first priorities of the person providing care. The patient's neck should not be hyperextended, hyperflexed, or rotated, which is especially difficult to avoid while trying to maintain the airway. Ideally, this can be achieved with appropriate cervical immobilization devices (e.g., hard collar and tape). If these are not immediately available, sandbags or rolled up pieces of clothing can be used as a temporary support until a paramedic crew arrives. The use of spinal boards is very important because they offer a very effective and easy-to-use means of transferring trauma patients. Mannitol, an osmotic diuretic, can be useful in the management of cerebral edema and increased ICP associated with head trauma, but should not be first-line therapy.

50. **The physical finding most likely to differentiate cardiac tamponade from tension pneumothorax is:**

    a. Absent breath sounds.

    b. Agitation.

    c. Distended neck veins.

    d. Hypotension.

    e. Cyanosis.

The answer is a. Beck's triad for pericardial tamponade (hypotension, distended neck veins, and, rarely, distant or muffled heart tones) is sometimes difficult to demonstrate clinically, especially in the midst of a major resuscitation with concomitant hypovolemia. The most reliable signs of pericardial tamponade are a central venous pressure (CVP) elevated to 15 cm H_2O or higher associated with hypotension and tachycardia. Pulsus paradoxus may also be present. As with any patient in shock, the physical findings can include dyspnea, agitation, restlessness, cyanosis, tachycardia, hypotension, and decreasing mental activity. The cardinal signs of tension pneumothorax are tachycardia, jugular venous distention, and absent breath sounds on the ipsilateral side. These patients can also be dyspneic, agitated, restless, cyanotic, tachycardic, hypotensive, and confused. Absent breath sounds are the key to clinically differentiating these two conditions.

51.   Which statement is correct concerning pediatric head trauma?

a. Sutures provide pliability to the pediatric skull that protects not only the skull, but also the brain parenchyma from injury.

b. The pediatric brain is well myelinated.

c. Seizures that occur later (longer than 20 minutes after the insult) portend the greater possibility of both internal injury and the development of seizures at a later date.

d. Impact seizures are associated with intracranial parenchymal injury.

e. Subdural hematomas in children are almost always associated with the presence of overlying fractures.

The answer is c. Head injury is the most frequent cause of trauma death in children older than 1 year. There are some important anatomical differences between children and adults that play a role. The child's cranial vault is larger and heavier in proportion to the total body mass. This predisposes the child to high degrees of torque generated by any forces along the cervical spine. The sutures in the child's skull are both protective and detrimental regarding head injury in these patients. The cranium is more pliable and resistant to skull fractures, but forces are generated internally that can damage the brain parenchyma without fracturing the skull. The pediatric brain is less myelinated, predisposing it to shearing forces and further injury. A brief seizure that occurs immediately after the insult (with rapid return of normal level of consciousness) is commonly called an impact seizure and is unassociated with intracranial parenchymal injury. However, seizures that occur longer than 20 minutes after the insult indicate greater possibility of both internal injury and the development of seizures at a later date.

52.   A modification of the Glasgow Coma Score for children is called the AVPU system. The correct matching for the AVPU system is:

a. A—the child is able to Ask for something.

b. V—the child is able to Visually track the questioner.

c. P—the child is able to Point to specific people.

d. P—the child responds to Painful stimuli.

e. U—the child is Uncooperative when asked to move an extremity.

The answer is d. In the AVPU system, the child's consciousness is rated as: Alert, responds to Verbal stimuli, responds to Painful stimuli, or Unresponsive.

53.   Referral to a pediatric burn center is mandatory for a:

a. 12-year-old girl with chemical burns of her chest.

b. 10-year-old boy with second-degree circumferential burns of his left thigh.

c. 6-year-old boy with first-degree burns of his hands, feet, or genitalia.

d. 10-year-old girl with 8% TBSA second-degree burns.

e. 12-year-old boy with 3% TBSA third-degree burns of his arm.

The answer is b. Pediatric burn center referral criteria include the following:

- Third-degree burns greater than 5% BSA (body surface area).
- Second- and third-degree burns greater than 10% BSA of patients younger than 10 years.
- Second- and third-degree burns greater than 20%.
- Second- and third-degree burns which involve the face, hands, feet, genitalia, perineum, and major joints.
- Electrical burns, including lightning injury.
- Chemical burns with serious threat to functional or cosmetic impairment.
- Inhalation injury.
- Burn injury in patients with preexisting medical disorders that could complicate management, prolong recovery, or affect mortality.
- Hospitals without qualified personnel or equipment for pediatric care should transfer burned children to a burn center with these capabilities.
- Burn injury in patients who require special social, emotional, and/or long-term rehabilitative support, including child abuse, substance abuse, etc.

54. **Of the listed studies on a pregnant woman, the one giving greatest radiation exposure to a viable fetus is:**

   a. Plain abdominal x-ray.

   b. Cervical spine x-ray.

   c. Head CT scan.

   d. Lumbar spine x-ray.

   e. Pelvis x-ray.

   The answer is d. Radiation exposure from various procedures:

- X-ray lumbar spine: 204–1260 mrad
- X-ray abdomen and pelvis: 190–357 mrad
- X-ray cervical spine: <1 mrad
- CT head (1 cm slices): <50 mrad

55. **Choose the true statement about skull fractures:**

   a. A depressed skull fracture is a frequent physical finding in isolated basilar skull fractures.

   b. An occipital skull fracture extending through the foramen magnum is often associated with frontal lobe injuries.

   c. X-ray is superior in diagnosing basal skull fractures, but CT scan is superior in diagnosing linear fractures of the cranial vault.

   d. An oblique linear skull fracture seen on plain radiographs of the skull extending from just posterior to the mastoid to the junction of the occipital and sagittal sutures is not an indication for CT scan.

   e. Skull x-rays are generally necessary in patients with head trauma.

   The answer is b. Basal skull fractures most commonly involve the petrous portion of the temporal bone. Clinical findings of a basal skull fracture include Battle sign, rhinorrhea or otorrhea, hemotympanum, periorbital ecchymosis (raccoon eyes), and CN I, II, VII, and VIII nerve deficits. CT scan has better sensitivity than skull radiographs. Palpable depressions are not a feature of basal fractures. Indications for skull x-rays include penetrating trauma, a severe closed head injury (CHI), and depressed skull fractures. Most patients with a history of head trauma require no radiologic tests. The CT scan is the diagnostic study of choice to determine the presence/absence of an intracranial injury. Linear, nondepressed skull fractures usually require no specific intervention. Fractures that cross the course of the middle meningeal artery of the temporal bone or that cross the course of the dural sinuses (superior sagittal, transverse) may cause epidural hematomas. Vertical occipital fractures are associated with contrecoup injuries of the frontal lobes. Frontal bone fractures involving the sinuses may cause an intracranial infection.

56.   Choose the true statement about posttraumatic seizures:

a. Depressed skull fractures associated with an intracranial hematoma have no increased incidence of posttraumatic seizures.

b. Only 15% of these seizures occur within 1 year of injury.

c. Posttraumatic seizures do not require anticonvulsant therapy.

d. Posttraumatic seizures are the first seizures occurring after 1 week from the initial trauma.

e. Posttraumatic seizures occur in more than 10% of patients with head injuries.

The answer is d. An outpatient who presents with delayed posttraumatic seizures should receive a loading dose of phenytoin and should continue on a maintenance dose until a 2-year, seizure-free interval has passed. Posttraumatic seizures are the first seizures occurring after 1 week from the initial trauma. Approximately 85% of these seizures occur within 1 year of injury. Consider a CT or MRI study to exclude intracerebral pathology for the patient with his/her first posttraumatic seizures. There is an incidence of 2–6% of patients with head injuries.

57.   Which of the following patient–fracture pairings is most likely?

a. 5-year-old boy who fell on an outstretched arm → linear, nonimpacted, nondisplaced ulna fracture.

b. 20-year-old man fell 10 ft and landed on feet on concrete with both legs extended → Y-shaped intercondylar femur fracture.

c. 18-year-old football player tackled while turning to run → linear fracture of tibia.

d. 23-year-old mechanic struck in leg by car bumper → oblique tibial fracture with a butterfly fragment.

e. 2-year-old girl with fall down carpeted steps → multiple rib fractures.

The answer is b. The mechanism of injury should correlate with the skeletal pathology. Fractures are caused by direct or indirect forces. The nightstick fracture of the ulna is an example of a direct blow causing a linear fracture. A fall on an outstretched arm would be unlikely to cause a simple nonimpacted linear fracture. Penetrating trauma or crush injuries are other obvious types of direct fractures (e.g., the femoral intercondylar fracture). Many fractures are caused by indirect forces. Axial loading forces will result in T- or Y-shaped fractures (the femoral intercondylar fracture). Rotational forces cause spiral fractures. Rotational and axial forces result in oblique fractures. Angulation with axial forces produces butterfly fractures.

58.   A 65-year-old man was extricated from an automobile after a high-speed motor-vehicle crash. He is making respiratory efforts as evidenced by abdominal wall motion. His eyes are open. His palpable blood pressure is 70 mm Hg. Despite 20 cc/kg of crystalloid infusion, the patient remains hypotensive. Bilateral breath sounds are markedly diminished. The next step in the management of this patient would be to:

a. Perform needle thoracostomy.

b. Orotracheally intubate.

c. Perform pericardiocentesis.

d. Perform cricothyrotomy.

e. None of the above.

The answer is b. Bilaterally diminished or absent breath sounds may indicate a bilateral tension pneumothorax. Absent breath sounds may mean an obstructed upper airway. Respiratory effort is not synonymous with effective ventilation. The presence or absence of airway sounds may be difficult to appreciate in a noisy ED. A simple method to assess airway patency is to have the patient speak. Upper airway obstruction, partial or complete, may be caused by an aspirated foreign body, direct laryngeal injury, and occlusion of the airway by the tongue. This patient has an abnormal pattern of respirations. Management of his airway would include cervical immobilization, chin lift, removal of foreign bodies (dentures, etc.), placement of a nasopharyngeal airway, BVM ventilation, and possible orotracheal intubation. Bilateral needle thoracostomies should correct the ventilatory impairment secondary to the tension pneumothoraces. Oropharyngeal airways are placed in unconscious patients.

59. **Epidural hematomas:**

a. Have a higher mortality rate than acute subdural hematomas.

b. Usually involve a frontal or occipital bone fracture.

c. Usually involve a middle meningeal artery bleed.

d. Show up as a crescent-moon shape on CT scan.

e. Present with contralateral fixed and dilated pupil.

The answer is c. Epidural hematomas (EDH) may occur as the result of an arterial or venous injury. EDH has a mortality rate of 0–20%. The most common cause of an EDH is middle meningeal artery injury. The classic scenario is a closed head injury, an altered level of consciousness, a lucid interval, then rapid neurologic deterioration with ipsilateral pupillary dilatation, and contralateral hemiparesis. Since the underlying brain injury is not severe, the prognosis is excellent with prompt diagnosis and early surgical intervention. Patients with cerebral atrophy are more susceptible to subdural hematomas (SDH). SDH has a mortality rate of 30–60%. On CT scan, an EDH has a lenticular (football-shaped) appearance, in contrast to the crescent-shape lesion of a SDH.

60. **Neurologic evaluation of a trauma patient reveals eye opening only to pain, no verbal response, and decorticate rigidity. The Glasgow Coma Score is:**

a. 5.

b. 6.

c. 7.

d. 8.

e. 9.

The answer is b. This patient would receive the following Glasgow Coma Score: eye opening to pain, 2 points; no verbal response, 1 point; abnormal flexion, 3 points. Total score, 6.

61. **Choose the correct pairing of mechanism and injury:**

a. Neck hyperflexion → bilateral fracture through the pedicles of C2.

b. Axial load compression → unilateral facet dislocation.

c. Hyperflexion → bilateral facet dislocation.

d. Hyperextension → anterior subluxation.

e. Severe rotation → burst fracture of atlas.

The answer is c. Cervical spine injuries are classified by mechanism and stability of the injury. Flexion or hyperflexion causes anterior subluxation, bilateral facet dislocation, simple wedge fractures, clay-shoveler's fracture, and the flexion teardrop fracture. Flexion/rotation forces cause unilateral facet dislocations. Vertical forces (axial loading) cause vertebral body burst fractures (C1 = Jefferson fracture). Extension and hyperextension injuries cause hangman's fracture of C2, extension teardrop fractures, and fracture of the posterior arch of C1. Odontoid fractures result from a combination of applied forces. Pillar fractures are caused by extension/rotational forces.

62.   **A 70-year-old woman fell while getting out of her bathtub and struck her chin against the tub. Her arms are much weaker than her legs and she notes mild sensory deficits of the lower extremities. Radiographs show a C4 extension teardrop fracture. These findings are most consistent with:**

   a. Anterior cord syndrome.

   b. Brown-Séquard syndrome.

   c. Transverse cord syndrome.

   d. Central cord syndrome.

   e. Incomplete spinal shock.

   The answer is d. The central cord syndrome is characterized by weakness greater in the upper extremities (hands > proximal muscles) than the lower extremities. This syndrome typically occurs in older patients with hyperextension injuries of the cervical spine. The anterior cord syndrome is characterized by motor paralysis and loss of pain and temperature sensation distal to the lesion. Posterior column function is spared (vibration, proprioception, and light touch). Hemisection of the cord causes the Brown-Séquard syndrome. There is ipsilateral paralysis and loss of vibration and proprioception, and contralateral loss of pain and temperature sensation.

63.   **Listed in order, the radiographic findings most *specific* and most *common* for traumatic rupture of the aorta are:**

   a. Apical capping → downward displacement of the left mainstem bronchus.

   b. Mediastinal widening → displacement of the right paraspinous interspace.

   c. Deviation of the esophagus (NG tube) to the right → first rib fracture.

   d. Deviation of the esophagus (NG tube) to the right → mediastinal widening.

   e. Blurring of the aortic knob → left pleural effusion.

   The answer is d. Widening of the superior mediastinum (>8 cm) is the most common sign of radiographic finding of a traumatic aortic rupture (TAR). The most accurate radiographic sign of a TAR is deviation of the esophagus more than 1–2 cm to the right of the T4 spinous process. The second most accurate sign of a TAR is obscuration of the aortic knob or descending aorta. Other CXR signs include: a left apical cap, displacement of the left mainstem bronchus >40 degrees below horizontal, widening of the paravertebral stripe, and obliteration of the aortopulmonary window. Whether fractures of the first and second ribs are associated with a significantly increased incidence of TAR is controversial. An initial normal CXR does not rule out TAR. Characteristic changes may develop over several hours. Up to 66% of patients older than 65 years with TAR may not show mediastinal widening. An aortogram may be ordered based upon clinical suspicion and/or mechanism of injury.

64.   **The clinical finding most consistent with a displaced fracture of the femoral neck is:**

   a. Normal anatomic position, but shortened.

   b. Externally rotated, abducted, and shortened.

   c. Externally rotated, adducted, and shortened.

   d. Internally rotated, abducted, and shortened.

   e. Internally rotated, adducted, and shortened.

   The answer is b. Patients with a displaced femoral neck fracture complain of severe pain, limited range of motion, and the inability to ambulate. Displaced fracture of the femoral neck results in limited range of motion with inability to ambulate and severe pain. The patient will present with a shortened, abducted, and externally rotated leg.

65.   **Choose the true statement regarding ankle injuries:**

a. Injury to the talotibial ligament often coexists with injury to the anterior talofibular ligament.

b. The most commonly injured ankle ligament is the deltoid ligament.

c. The position responsible for the majority of ankle injuries is internal rotation, inversion, and plantar flexion.

d. The talofibular ligaments stabilize the ankle mortise.

e. Disruption of the anterior tibiofibular ligament causes anterior talar subluxation.

The answer is c. More than 90% of ankle sprains involve the anterior and posterior talofibular, and the calcaneofibular ligaments. A positive anterior drawer sign indicates rupture of at least the anterior talofibular ligament. The deltoid (medial) ligament is rarely injured alone. Injury to the deltoid ligament is usually accompanied by an avulsion fracture of the fibula, a tear of the anterior or posterior tibiofibular ligaments, or a separation of the tibiofibular syndesmosis. Disruption of the anterior talofibular ligament causes anterior talar subluxation. The tibiofibular ligaments stabilize the ankle mortise.

66.   **An unrestrained automobile driver involved in rapid deceleration injury presents with shortening, internal rotation, and adduction of his right leg. He probably has:**

a. Anterior dislocation of the hip.

b. Posterior dislocation of the hip.

c. Intertrochanteric fracture of the hip.

d. Subtrochanteric fracture of the hip.

e. Femoral neck fracture.

The answer is b. Posterior hip dislocations are more common (80–90%) than anterior hip dislocations (10–20%). The mechanism of action is an axial force applied to a flexed knee. Posterior dislocations are associated with acetabular fractures and sciatic nerve injury. The leg is shortened, internally rotated, and adducted. Anterior hip dislocations present as an externally rotated and abducted lower extremity. Early reduction minimizes the risk of avascular necrosis of the femoral head.

67.   **A 33-year-old man was shot in the chest. The entrance wound is 2 cm medial to the right nipple, and the exit wound just medial to the right scapula. The patient is awake and alert. He has significant hemoptysis and complains of dyspnea. You put a chest tube in the right hemithorax and immediately get 800 mL of blood, but there is a large air leak. The patient suddenly develops a left hemiparesis and pulseless electrical activity. Your next step in the management of this patient would be:**

a. Intubation, low right thoracotomy, and clamping of the pulmonary hilum.

b. Intubation, CPR, and intravenous epinephrine.

c. Intubation, left thoracotomy, cross-clamp ascending aorta, and open-chest cardiac massage after needle aspiration of the left ventricle.

d. Intubation, left thoracotomy, cross-clamp ascending aorta, and open-chest cardiac massage after needle aspiration of the left ventricle and emergency right temporal burr holes.

e. Intubation, low right thoracotomy and clamping of the pulmonary hilum, left thoracotomy, and needle aspiration of the left ventricle and ascending aorta.

The answer is e. Systemic air embolism may develop in patients with penetrating thorax trauma and hemoptysis. Risk factors include high ventilatory pressures, significant hemoptysis, and large air leaks in the setting of penetrating trauma. There is a high mortality and morbidity from this event. Treatment includes lowering the patient's head, thoracotomy with clamping of the injured area, and aspiration of air from the heart and ascending aorta. Open cardiac massage with clamping of the ascending aorta may be helpful. If available, initiate cardiopulmonary bypass.

68. **Traumatic pneumomediastinum:**

   a. Is associated with a crunching sound over the precordium in 50% of cases.

   b. Is invariably associated with a pneumothorax.

   c. Is nearly always associated with a discernible injury to the airway or digestive tract.

   d. Produces severe disability.

   e. Is frequently confused with traumatic esophageal rupture.

   The answer is a. Hamman sign is a crunching sound heard over the heart during systole. Traumatic pneumomediastinum should be suspected from subcutaneous air of the neck. Consider an injury to the pharynx, larynx, trachea, bronchi, or esophagus. Traumatic pneumomediastinum is usually asymptomatic.

69. **Choose the correct statement about patellar injuries:**

   a. Widely separated fracture fragments do not imply an injury to the knee joint.

   b. You should reduce a patellar dislocation by flexing the knee and extending the hip, then sliding the patella into place.

   c. Patellar fractures are associated with acetabular and femoral neck fractures and anterior dislocations of the hip in motor vehicle collisions.

   d. The patella and knee do not need to be x-rayed after patellar reduction.

   e. Nondisplaced patellar fractures may be treated with a cylinder cast.

   The answer is e. The patella most commonly dislocates over the lateral condyle. Reduction is performed by hyperextending the knee, flexing the hip, then sliding the patella into place. Patellar fractures occur from direct trauma or quadriceps muscle contraction (avulsion type). In motor vehicle collisions, patellar fracture is a sign of significant force transmitted through the femur. Patellar fractures are associated with posterior hip dislocations and acetabular injuries. Widely comminuted patellar fractures are associated with knee joint injury.

70. **A possible complication of penetrating trauma to the anterior triangle of the neck is:**

   a. Fat embolism.

   b. Stroke.

   c. Subclavian vessel injury.

   d. Thoracic spine injury.

   e. Ischemic necrosis of the hand.

   The answer is b. The sternocleidomastoid muscle (SCM) divides the neck into anterior and posterior triangles. The anterior triangle contains the carotid artery, internal jugular vein, vagus nerve, and the airway. The posterior triangle boundaries are the SCM, trapezius, and clavicle. The posterior triangle is divided into "carefree and careful zones" by the spinal accessory nerve. The subclavian vessels lie at the base of the posterior triangle; not within the anterior triangle. Air embolism results from venous injury. Arteriovenous fistulas are a possible complication. All neck injuries should be evaluated for cervical spine injuries. Cerebrovascular infarcts are due to carotid artery dissection, intimal flap formation, or embolic injury. Any wound that violates the platysma requires surgical consultation and possible operative intervention.

71. **The injury significantly associated with traumatic diaphragm rupture is:**

    a. Pelvic fractures.

    b. Right-sided blunt thoracic trauma.

    c. Left-sided blunt thoracic trauma.

    d. Stab wounds to the second intercostal space of the anterior thorax.

    e. Comminuted fracture of the T12 vertebral body.

    The answer is a. Penetrating trauma between the fourth intercostal space and the umbilicus can cause diaphragmatic injury. There is an association between penetrating abdominal trauma and a pneumothorax. Blunt trauma most commonly involves rupture of the left hemidiaphragm. Radiographic abnormalities include elevation of the hemidiaphragm, effusions, and bowel gas or a NG tube in the hemithorax. The incidence of a ruptured diaphragm due to blunt trauma is 5%. The incidence doubles if there is fracture of the pelvis. Splenic and hepatic injuries are associated with traumatic diaphragmatic rupture. With penetrating trauma, the diagnosis is often made at laparotomy or thoracotomy. Other techniques for this diagnosis include peritoneal lavage fluid exiting a chest tube, UGI series revealing abdominal viscera in the thorax, or CT scan with contrast.

72. **A 66-year-old woman was the unrestrained driver of an automobile, which struck a large tree at high speed. She is disoriented and has dysphonia. Her blood pressure is normal, but her heart rate is 110/min. She has considerable sternal and interscapular pain. Physical examination is significant for a II/VI systolic murmur over the left precordium. Her cervical spine series, chest, and pelvic radiographs are all normal. Your next step is:**

    a. An aortogram.

    b. An echocardiogram.

    c. Transfer to the CCU for monitoring, serial cardiac enzymes, and repeat EKG.

    d. Indirect laryngoscopy.

    e. CT scan of the head and chest.

    The answer is a. The differential diagnosis based on mechanism of injury includes, but is not limited to, myocardial contusion, traumatic rupture of the aorta, valvular injury, and hemopericardium. The highest priority is to exclude traumatic aortic rupture (TAR). Physical findings of TAR include hoarseness, upper extremity hypertension, superior vena cava syndrome, paraplegia, systolic murmur over the back, and pulse deficits. The most common site of TAR in patients who arrive in the ED alive is between the left subclavian artery and the ligamentum arteriosum. The second most common sites are the origin of the innominate artery or left subclavian artery. Contrast-enhanced CT scanning is primarily used as a screening tool. Transesophageal echocardiography appears to be more sensitive than aortography for diagnosing TAR. Aortography is still considered the gold standard.

73. **Spontaneous eye opening:**

    a. Implies awareness.

    b. Is graded as a 5 on the appropriate section of the Glasgow Coma Scale.

    c. Is scored lower than eye opening to verbal command in the Glasgow Coma Scale.

    d. Is not reproducible and should not be used to judge the patient's level of consciousness.

    e. Suggests that the reticular activating center is functioning.

    The answer is e. Spontaneous eye opening suggests that the reticular activating system is functioning, but does not imply awareness. The Glasgow Coma Scale awards 4 points for spontaneous eye opening and 3 points for opening eyes to verbal command. The Glasgow Coma Scale provides a quantitative assessment of the patient's level of consciousness based on the best responses of the following: eye opening, best motor response, and best verbal response.

74.   Regarding examination of an injured knee:

a. The Lachman test is the most sensitive test for diagnosing a posterior cruciate injury.

b. Medial instability in full extension (straight medial instability) indicates that at least the posterior cruciate and medial collateral ligaments are torn.

c. Rotary instability exists if lateral or medial stress testing is positive in both full extension and with 20–30 degrees of flexion.

d. The PCL must be torn if rotary instability testing is positive.

e. Neurovascular injuries are not associated with injury to the PCL.

The answer is b. The knee should be placed in 30 degrees of flexion to determine varus (lateral collateral ligament) and valgus (medial collateral ligament) instability. If the knee demonstrates instability, then stress testing should be performed with the knee in full extension. Medial instability in full extension indicates a severe injury to the cruciate and medial ligament and the posterior capsule. Lateral instability in full extension indicates a severe injury to the posterolateral joint, the lateral collateral and cruciate ligaments, and possibly the peroneal nerve. An effusion may limit the reliability of the anterior draw maneuver. The posterior draw sign tests for injury to the posterior cruciate ligament. In summary: joint instability in extension = joint instability in flexion = severe ligamentous injury. The converse is not true.

75.   Choose the true statement regarding hand and wrist injuries:

a. Anatomic snuffbox tenderness with negative radiographs rules out a fracture.

b. A Barton fracture is an extra-articular fracture of the distal ulna with possible carpal displacement.

c. A Smith fracture is a dorsal angulated fracture of the distal radius.

d. Rotatory alignment is within normal limits if the flexed metacarpophalangeal (MCP) joints result in the fingertips pointing to the radial styloid.

e. The ability to flex or extend a digit excludes significant tendon laceration.

The answer is d. Navicular fractures may have negative x-rays. Avascular necrosis of the proximal portion of the bone is the major complication of this injury. Posttraumatic tenderness of the anatomic snuffbox should be treated as a fractured scaphoid; thumb spica splint and orthopedic referral are indicated. Important considerations of wrist radiographs are bony displacement, angulation, and intra-articular involvement. Tendon injuries of the hands may be difficult to diagnose. Partial tendon lacerations should be suspected when there is pain against resistance, motor weakness, or a tendon sheath laceration. When evaluating for an injury to the flexor digitorum superficialis tendon, the fingers not being tested should be held in extension to block the action of the profundus tendon. A Barton fracture is an intra-articular fracture of the dorsal or volar rim of the distal radius with possible carpal displacement. A Smith fracture is a volar angulated fracture of the distal radius.

76.   The amount of hematuria that reliably corresponds to significant genitourinary trauma is:

a. A positive urine dipstick test for blood.

b. A spun "urinocrit" greater than 2%.

c. More than 50 RBCs per high-power field.

d. Gross hematuria.

e. None of the above.

The answer is e. Gross hematuria following blunt trauma is an indication for immediate radiologic evaluation of the genitourinary tract. However, the degree of hematuria cannot be used as an index of the severity of injury. Dipstick urine testing may be falsely positive secondary to myoglobinuria.

77. **Choose the true statement about fractures of the humerus:**

    a. Closed fractures of the humeral shaft are frequently associated with medial nerve injury.

    b. Acute radial neuropathy is a poor sign for recovery.

    c. Finger extension following fractures of the humeral shaft does not exclude radial nerve neuropraxia.

    d. Displaced supracondylar humeral fractures associated with a diminished radial pulse can tolerate delayed reduction.

    e. Compartment syndrome is not a complication of a displaced supracondylar fracture.

    The answer is c. Humeral fractures are frequently accompanied by radial or axillary nerve injuries. Document the patient's neurovascular status prior to manipulation. Radial nerve motor deficits are manifested by a wrist drop. The prognosis is good for recovery of full radial nerve function if paralysis occurred immediately following the humeral fracture. Displaced supracondylar fractures are an orthopedic emergency. Acute complications of a supracondylar fracture include nerve injuries (radial, median, ulnar), vascular injuries (diminished radial pulse commonly due to transient vasospasm), and compartment syndrome/Volkmann ischemic contracture. Supracondylar fractures are more common in children.

78. **Choose the true statement regarding pressure injection injuries of the hand:**

    a. The high pressures cause large entrance sites.

    b. The injuries are well localized to the entrance.

    c. These injuries rarely require surgical exploration.

    d. Initial treatment includes elevation, prophylactic antibiotics, and tetanus immunization.

    e. Unless associated with a degloving injury, pressure injection injuries are usually benign.

    The answer is d. A pressure injection injury of the hand appears innocent. The entrance site is usually small but there is dissemination of contaminating materials (grease or paint) via the tendon sheaths and spaces of the hands. Preliminary care includes antibiotic prophylaxis, tetanus immunization, and hand elevation. Definitive treatment requires a hand surgeon.

79. **The most significant immediate complication associated with pelvic fracture is:**

    a. Hemorrhage.

    b. Rectal or vaginal lacerations.

    c. Sciatic nerve injury.

    d. Infection.

    e. Myositis ossificans.

    The answer is a. Hemorrhage is a major cause of death in pelvic fractures. Two to six liters of blood may accumulate within the retroperitoneum. Hemorrhage from the major branches of the internal iliac, the superior gluteal, and the internal pudendal arteries may require surgical ligation or angiographic embolization. The use of MAST garments (or PASG) remains controversial.

80.   Proper principles of orthopedics require you to:

    a. Accept moderate rotational and angular deformity in pediatric fractures, as there will be excellent remodeling as the child grows.

    b. Univalve a cast if a patient complains of underlying paresthesias.

    c. Use antihistamines to relieve pruritus under a cast.

    d. Snugly smooth the plaster of a cylindrical cast to ensure that it is form-fitting.

    e. None of the above.

The answer is e. Splinting fractures prevents injury and reduces pain. Although minimal angulation deformities are acceptable in children, rotational deformities are not. Children usually require the immobilization of joints above and below the fracture. If the ED physician elects to apply a circumferential cast, plaster should be rolled on over adequate padding using only the large flat surfaces of the hand to mold, since fingers may cause pressure points to form. Inserting objects under casts to relieve itching should be strongly discouraged. Patients should return for a cast check within 24 hours or sooner if any of the "six Ps" (pain, pallor, pulselessness, paralysis, paresthesias, and poikilothermia) occur. Any patient presenting with these signs should have the cast bivalved.

81.   Choose the correct statement about scalp injuries:

    a. The scalp consists of six separate layers of tissue.

    b. The third layer of the scalp must be closed by cutaneous or subcutaneous sutures.

    c. Scalp hematomas cannot cause hypotension in any age group.

    d. No significant cosmetic deformities can result from improper closure of scalp lacerations.

    e. Brain or epidural abscesses following scalp lacerations are usually due to occult skull fractures.

The answer is b. The scalp is composed of five layers and can be remembered by the mnemonic SCALP (Skin, Connective tissue, Aponeurosis [galea], Loose connective tissue, Periosteum). The galea has connections to the muscles of the scalp. Improper closure will result in cosmetic deformities. Most scalp hematomas have minimal significance. An infected scalp hematoma may cause an intracranial infection even in the absence of a skull fracture. A soft tissue infection may seed the intracranial vessels via the penetrating skull veins. Scalp hematomas in infants may sequester a significant quantity of blood to cause hypovolemic shock. Pressure dressings applied to hematomas can reduce their size.

82.   A patient with a right-sided epidural hematoma and uncal herniation will have:

    a. Decorticate posturing.

    b. Ipsilateral dilated pupil.

    c. Hyperventilation.

    d. Ipsilateral hemiparesis.

    e. Pinpoint pupils.

The answer is b. Increased intracranial pressure may cause uncal herniation and brainstem compression. Uncal herniation causes cranial nerve III compression and causes an ipsilateral pupillary dilatation. Compression of the ipsilateral cerebral peduncle causes a contralateral hemiparesis since the motor tract fibers cross below this level. However, the contralateral cerebral peduncle can be compressed against the edge of the tentorium and may cause paralysis ipsilateral to the dilated pupil. This "false" localizing sign should not dissuade one from the diagnosis. Temporizing measures include intubation/hyperventilation and the administration of mannitol and corticosteroids. Definitive treatment includes neurosurgical consultation and decompression. Decerebrate (extensor) posturing is associated with uncal herniation.

83.   **Choose the correct statement:**

a. Osmotic agents like mannitol cause an increase in intracranial pressure.

b. Epidural hematomas in children younger than 2 years (i.e., with open sutures or fontanelles) do not cause hypotension secondary to blood loss.

c. Initial management of the unconscious hypotensive patient should include vasopressors.

d. Intubation/hyperventilation is the initial treatment of choice for a patient presenting with a closed head injury and a GCS <10.

e. Intubation/hyperventilation is the initial treatment of choice for a child presenting with a closed head injury, decreased consciousness, and an ipsilateral dilated pupil.

The answer is e. Vasopressors are used to treat neurogenic shock only when all other etiologies of hypotension have been excluded. Hemorrhagic shock is the most common etiology for hypotension in the trauma patient. Maintenance IV fluids are usually sufficient to correct the modest decline in systolic blood pressure that is often seen in neurogenic shock. Patients with head injury and evidence of unilateral or bilateral uncal herniation or lateralizing motor deficits should be intubated and hyperventilated immediately while preparations are made for emergency CT scanning and surgery. Intravenous mannitol or glycerol should be used in patients with severe head injury and elevated intracranial pressure (ICP). Problems associated with mannitol or glycerol include a transient rise in the ICP as fluid is drawn into the vascular space. Intracranial hematomas may expand as the brain swelling subsides. Finally, hypotension may result if these agents are used in patients with hypovolemia. These drugs generally should not be used until the patient (1) is being adequately ventilated, (2) has adequate circulating blood volume, and (3) has had preparations for CT scan and/or surgery made. Patients with clear evidence of uncal herniation or rapidly deteriorating neurologic status will require emergency surgical intervention. Other measures to reduce intracranial pressure include elevating the head of the bed and the administration of sedatives and neuromuscular relaxants.

84.   **Operative intervention for neurotrauma is indicated in a patient suffering from:**

a. Significant mass effect from contusion or hemorrhage, resulting in a 5-mm shift of intracranial structures.

b. Penetrating head injury with necrotic foreign body tracks.

c. Significantly depressed skull fractures.

d. Foreign body removal if compromising neurologic function.

e. Any of the above.

The answer is e. Indications for operative treatment in patients with neurotrauma are indicated for all of the above situations and, additionally, in the instance of extra-axial collections.

85.   A 3-year-old girl has a 4-cm wide, deep stellate thigh laceration sustained when she fell into a septic tank overflow pool 2 hours ago. Potential infection is minimized by:

a. High-pressure saline irrigation, excisional debridement, and primary closure with peri- and postoperative antibiotics.

b. High-pressure saline irrigation, abrasive debridement, and delayed primary closure with peri- and postoperative antibiotics.

c. High-pressure saline irrigation, excisional debridement in the operating room, and open wound management with delayed primary closure on day 4.

d. Low-pressure irrigation with 10% povidone–iodine solution, abrasive sponge debridement, and primary closure with peri- and postoperative antibiotics.

e. Low-pressure saline irrigation, abrasive sponge debridement, and open wound management to promote drainage of the inevitable infection.

The answer is c. Bacteria often remain on wound surfaces grossly contaminated by pus or feces. Delayed primary closure should be used if there is a high probability for infection. The wound is packed open with sterile fine mesh gauze. Primary closure occurs on day 4. Low-pressure irrigation fails to remove fine dirt particles and bacteria. High-pressure irrigation may traumatize tissue and should be used for heavily contaminated wounds. Heavily contaminated wounds with extensive devitalized soft tissue require operative debridement. Antibiotic therapy is justified for open wound management.

86.   A patient with a C8 cervical radiculopathy will have difficulty with:

a. Arm abduction.

b. Elbow extension.

c. Elbow flexion.

d. Hand grasp.

e. Wrist extension.

The answer is d.

C6: Decreased forearm flexion and hand extension, decreased shoulder adduction, weak biceps reflex.

C7: Weak triceps and finger extension; weak triceps reflex.

C8: Weak hypothenar and hand flexors; weak elbow extension.

87.   Which of the following is correct concerning pediatric head trauma?

a. Sutures provide pliability to the pediatric skull that protects not only the skull, but also the brain parenchyma from injury.

b. The pediatric brain is well myelinated.

c. Seizures that occur later (longer than 20 minutes after the insult) portend the greater possibility of both internal injury and the development of seizures at a later date.

d. Impact seizures are associated with intracranial parenchymal injury.

e. Subdural hematomas in children are almost always associated with the presence of overlying fractures.

The answer is e. The sutures in the child's skull are both protective and detrimental regarding head injury in these patients. The cranium is more pliable and resistant to skull fractures, but forces are generated internally that can damage the brain parenchyma without fracturing the skull. The pediatric brain is less myelinated, predisposing it to shearing forces and further injury. A brief seizure that occurs immediately after the insult (with rapid return of normal level of consciousness) is commonly called an impact seizure and is unassociated with intracranial parenchymal injury. However, seizures that occur longer than 20 minutes after the insult indicate greater possibility of both internal injury and the development of seizures at a later date.

88. **Which of the following is true of clinicians regarding forensics:**

    a. Clinicians should describe gunshot wounds as entrance or exit wounds.
    b. The ED physician should make an educated speculation regarding the caliber of the bullet.
    c. Wounds should be described according to standard anatomic position with the arms to the side and palms up.
    d. The term "powder burn" should be used to describe the carbonaceous material associated with close-range wounds.
    e. The physician must record the manner of a gunshot wound victim's death in the medical record as homicide, suicide, or accidental.

The answer is c. Documentation of gunshot wounds should include the location, size, shape, and characteristics of the wound. Clinicians should not describe wounds as entrance or exit, but should document a detailed description of the appearance and location of a wound without speculating on an interpretation or the caliber of the bullet. Exit wounds are not always larger than the entrance wound. The term soot rather than powder burns, should be used to describe the carbonaceous material associated with close-range wounds. Powder burns are literally the burns associated with the coincidental ignition of clothing by the flaming black powder used in muzzleloaders, antique weapons, and blank cartridges. This does not occur with the smokeless powder used in modern commercial ammunition. Powder burns, therefore, is an obsolete and potentially misleading expression. It is unnecessary to write in the medical record, the manner of a gunshot victim's death. The determination of whether a death is accidental, suicidal, or homicidal is the responsibility of the coroner or medical examiner and only after a detailed investigation of the scene and circumstances of the incident.

CHAPTER 19 Pediatric Emergencies

Raemma Paredes Luck, MD, MBA

1. **A 3-year-old boy was bitten on his right hand yesterday by the family's pet cat. He now presents to the ED with redness, swelling, and tenderness of his dorsal right hand. His mother tells you that he developed a severe rash once when given penicillin. The most appropriate antibiotic for this bite would be:**

   a. Ciprofloxacin.

   b. Azithromycin.

   c. Trimethoprim-sulfamethoxazole and clindamycin.

   d. Amoxicillin/clavulanic acid.

   e. Cephalexin.

   The answer is c. Dogs and cats are responsible for 90% of all animal bites. Approximately 3–18% of all dog bites and 28–80% of all cat bites get infected. Cat bites produce puncture wounds, which cause inoculation of bacteria deep into the tissues. Infection is often noted within 24–72 hours of the bite. *Pasteurella* species is the most common organism isolated in dog bites (50%) and cat bites (75%). It is highly sensitive to penicillin. However, because other aerobic and anaerobic organisms such as *Staphylococcus, Streptococcus, Bacteroides* and *Fusobacterium* are present, amoxicillin/clavulanate is recommended. Ciprofloxacin should be avoided in patients younger than 18 years, as it is associated with long-term damage to developing cartilage. Azithromycin does not have adequate coverage for *Pasteurella*. A first-generation cephalosporin may cover *Staphylococcus*, but is inadequate for *Pasteurella*. Trimethoprim-sulfamethoxazole has adequate coverage for *Pasteurella, Staphylococcus,* and *Eikenella*, but not for anaerobic infections. Hence, in patients allergic to penicillin, the addition of clindamycin to trimethoprim-sulfamethoxazole would cover anaerobic infections as well.

2.   **A 5-year-old boy fell from the monkey bars and landed on his outstretched left hand. In the ED, you note moderate swelling of his left elbow with inability to extend his arm. The elbow radiograph is shown in Figure 19-1. Choose the true statement:**

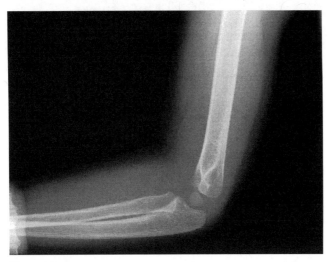

Figure 19–1

a. The most common mechanism for this injury is a fall on the outstretched hand with hyperextension of the elbow.

b. An elevated anterior fat pad is pathognomonic for fracture.

c. All elbow fractures require immediate orthopedic consultation.

d. The distal humeral fragment is usually displaced anteriorly.

e. Neurovascular complications are uncommon.

The answer is a. Supracondylar fractures comprise approximately 50% of all elbow fractures in the pediatric age group. The most common mechanism is a fall on the outstretched hand (FOOSH) with hyperextension of the elbow. Posterior displacement or angulation of the distal humerus usually occurs. The radiograph often reveals elevation of both anterior and posterior fat pads with the anterior humeral line transecting through the anterior edge of the capitellum rather than the middle third. Significant neurovascular deficits, deformities, and limitation of motion can arise if the fracture is missed or management is suboptimal. Nondisplaced or minimally displaced fractures (type 1) can be managed with a long-arm posterior splint with the forearm in pronation or neutral position and the elbow at 90 degrees. Close orthopedic follow-up is needed. Otherwise, immediate orthopedic referral is required for all other types of supracondylar fractures.

3. **You are examining a 12-month-old boy who woke up early this morning with a sudden onset of noisy breathing and a barking cough. He has stridor on inspiration and tachypnea, as well as suprasternal and subcostal retractions. Optimal management for this patient is to give him:**

   a. An intramuscular dose of ceftriaxone.

   b. Intravenous fluids and admit him to the hospital.

   c. A beta-agonist medication by nebulization.

   d. Nebulized racemic epinephrine and oral dexamethasone.

   e. Saline mist therapy.

   The answer is d. Croup or laryngotracheobronchitis, is the most common cause of upper airway obstruction in infants and children and is usually seen during the fall and winter months. Parainfluenza virus types 1 and 2 cause the majority of cases. Although stridor, barking cough, and respiratory distress are the most prominent symptoms, lower respiratory tract symptoms such as wheezing and rhonchi can also be noted. You have to consider the possibility of bacterial tracheitis, epiglottitis, or foreign body aspiration in any patient presenting with severe distress, toxicity, or a course not consistent with viral croup. The management of croup is supportive. Mild croup can be treated with oral dexamethasone at a dose of 0.15–0.6 mg/kg. Patients with moderate to severe croup may also be given nebulized racemic epinephrine in addition to dexamethasone. Antibiotics are not indicated for viral croup. Mist therapy and albuterol treatments are not definitive therapies. Most patients can be sent home after a period of observation in the ED. Indications for admission are dehydration, stridor at rest, moderate to severe respiratory distress, and presence of comorbid conditions.

4. **A 2-year-old girl was prescribed high-dose amoxicillin (80 mg/kg/d) for acute otitis media (AOM) by her pediatrician. She comes to the ED crying in pain and with persistent fever but no ear drainage. Knowing the epidemiology of persistent otitis media, the best management is to change the antibiotic to:**

   a. Azithromycin.

   b. Erythromycin.

   c. Trimethoprim-sulfamethoxazole.

   d. Amoxicillin/clavulanate.

   e. Ciprofloxacin eardrops.

   The answer is d. The most common bacterial causes of AOM are *Streptococcus pneumoniae* (25–40%), *Hemophilus influenzae* (35–50%), and *Moraxella catarrhalis* (5–10%). With the incorporation of the pneumococcal conjugate vaccine in the routine immunization schedule for infants at 2, 4, and 6 months of age, the incidence of otitis media secondary to *S. pneumoniae* has decreased. Meanwhile, the incidence of nontypeable *H. influenzae* has increased in recent years. Both these bacteria have developed resistance to the oral antibiotics commonly used to treat AOM. The ability of *S. pneumoniae* to alter its penicillin-binding proteins decreases the ability of beta-lactam antibiotics, such as amoxicillin, to bind to the bacteria's cell wall. *H. influenzae* and *M. catarrhalis* produce beta-lactamases, which are enzymes that cleave the beta-lactam ring of beta-lactam antibiotics. Hence, in a child who does not respond to the first-line drug, amoxicillin, you should suspect beta-lactamase producing bacteria as the etiology of the otitis. Azithromycin, trimethoprim-sulfamethoxazole, and erythromycin are not effective against these beta-lactamase producing bacteria. Antibiotic eardrops are not indicated in otitis media without perforation or tympanostomy tubes. Amoxicillin/clavulanate, a beta-lactamase inhibitor, is the best treatment option and is recommended by the American Academy of Pediatrics in severe cases of otitis. And as always, administration of an oral analgesic medication to relieve the ear pain is a must!

5.   **A mother carries her 18-month-old son to the ED because he has refused to walk on his right leg since he woke up this morning. She says that he is always running around the house, but denies any history of a fall or fever. Physical examination shows minimal swelling of his right leg but no point tenderness. His hip and knee examination is normal. His radiograph is shown in Figure 19-2. Choose the true statement:**

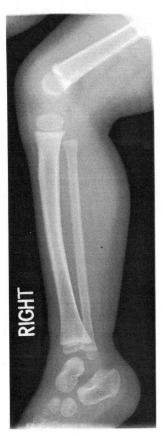

Figure 19–2

a. This injury is commonly seen in infants younger than 9 months.

b. Child abuse should be considered in all toddlers with this finding.

c. The child has a large knee effusion and probably has a septic joint.

d. A history of a fall or trauma is always obtained.

e. Management consists of a splint and pain management.

The answer is e. Spiral fractures of the distal tibia, or so-called "toddler fractures," are often caused by seemingly trivial falls or by a twisting motion of the leg on a planted foot. A history of a fall or injury may not always be obtained, and the subtle or absent physical findings only add to the diagnostic dilemma. If a toddler's fracture is suspected but the radiographs are normal, you can repeat the plain films after 10 days to see new bone formation or periosteal reaction around the fracture edges. Management of a todder's fracture consists of immobilization of the tibia with a posterior splint to provide pain relief and to promote healing. The presence of spiral fractures in the tibia, fibula, or femur in a nonambulating child is highly suggestive of nonaccidental trauma, and a skeletal survey is indicated in children younger than 2 years who cannot verbalize the cause of the injury or in those with fractures highly specific for nonaccidental trauma or suspicious circumstances surrounding the injury.

6. A football coach brings a 13-year-old boy for evaluation of right knee pain. He slipped and fell today and since then has been limping slightly. On physical examination, both his knees and thighs are normal. There is a slight limitation on internal rotation on his right hip but there is no hip pain or tenderness. His radiograph is shown in Figure 19-3. This condition:

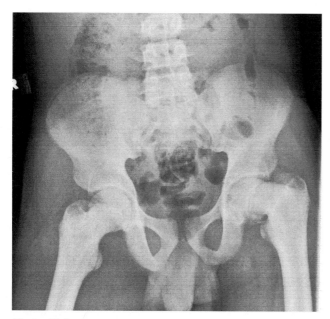

Figure 19–3

a. Is more common in females after 15 years of age.

b. Is more common in obese Hispanic adolescents.

c. Usually affects both hip joints concurrently.

d. Is commonly seen in obese African American boys between 8 and 15 years of age.

e. Is treated with intra-articular steroids and crutches with minimal weight bearing.

The answer is d. Slipped capital femoral epiphysis (SCFE) is a condition in which the femoral epiphysis is displaced from the metaphysis through the open growth plate. It affects males more commonly than females (4:1 ratio), one hip more than both hips (10–40% of SCFE have bilateral slips), African American adolescents, and those who are obese. Most patients present with vague chronic hip or knee pain, but some present acutely after minor trauma. The hip is often in external rotation with limited range of motion or pain on internal rotation, flexion, and abduction. Plain films should include anterior–posterior as well as frog-leg views of the entire pelvis. SCFE is classified as stable if the child can ambulate and unstable if he cannot. Management includes no weight bearing to prevent further slippage of the femoral head and an urgent orthopedic consult for prompt internal fixation.

7.   **A 15-month-old boy is brought by his parents for evaluation of right knee swelling, fever, and refusal to walk. On physical examination, you find redness, swelling, and limited range of motion of the right knee. Plain films show widening of the joint space with soft tissue swelling. Choose the statement that best describes the etiology and antibiotics needed to treat this infection:**

   a. *Kingella kingae*, intravenous cefuroxime.

   b. *Streptococcus pneumoniae*, intravenous ceftriaxone.

   c. *Staphyloccocus aureus*, intravenous vancomycin.

   d. Group A *Streptococcus*, intravenous ampicillin/sulbactam.

   e. *Escherichia coli*, intravenous ampicillin and gentamicin.

   The answer is c. Septic arthritis is an infection of the joint space primarily from a hematogenous spread of bacteria. The majority of cases (70%) occur in children younger than 4 years with a peak age of 6–24 months. Most cases (75%) involve the lower extremities, with the knee and hip joints the most commonly affected. Monoarticular involvement is the rule in 90% of cases. *S. aureus* is the most common organism implicated followed by *S. pneumoniae*. In neonates, Group B *Streptococcus* is an important cause while *Neisseria gonorrhoeae* gains importance during adolescence. Evaluation of the synovial fluid is necessary for diagnosis and should be done before initiating antibiotic therapy. Blood cultures are positive in 20–50% of cases. Management includes immediate admission, parenteral antibiotics with staphylococcal coverage such as vancomycin, and surgical intervention.

8.   **You are seeing a 5-month-old infant who has been irritable with fever of 24 hours. Mom states that the infant refuses her formula, has not been active, and cries whenever she is moved. On physical examination, you note a bulging anterior fontanel. Laboratory results show a WBC of $30 \times 10^3/\mu$L (30×10^9/L) with 20% immature forms. Evaluation of the cerebrospinal fluid shows a glucose level of 15 mg/dL, protein concentration of 130 mg/dL, WBC of 500/μL, and a Gram stain positive for Gram-positive diplococci. Appropriate antibiotic management for this patient should include:**

   a. Vancomycin and cefotaxime.

   b. Cefazolin and clindamycin.

   c. Ampicillin/sulbactam and gentamicin.

   d. Ceftazidime and gentamicin.

   e. Clarithromycin and ceftriaxone.

   The answer is a. This infant has bacterial meningitis. The most common bacterial causes in infants between 0 and 3 months of age are group B *Streptococcus*, *E coli*, *Listeria*, *Enterococcus* and other Gram-negative enteric bacilli. In patients from 3 months to 21 years, *N. meningitidis* and *S. pneumoniae* predominate. In the first month of life, the treatment is amipicillin with gentamicin or a third-generation cephalosporin. After the first month of life, treatment is vancomycin and a third-generation parenteral cephalosporin such as cefotaxime or ceftriaxone until the organism is identified. Third-generation cephalosporins are active against gram-negative enteric bacteria, *H. influenzae*, *M. catarrhalis*, *S. pneumoniae*, *Neisseria meningitidis*, and group A streptococci, all of which are serious causes of meningitis in infants and children. Ceftazidime has excellent activity against *Pseudomonas aeruginosa* but is less active with *S. pneumonia*, Group A *Streptococcus*, and *Staphylococcus aureus*. Oral antibiotics are not indicated for bacterial meningitis.

9. **You are evaluating a 5-year-old child for ataxia of 3-days duration. This morning, her mother noted some right facial asymmetry. The patient has been afebrile with no symptoms other than the difficulty walking. Physical examination shows weak knee reflexes and no ankle reflexes. In order to make the proper diagnosis, you should now perform:**

    a. Electroencephalography.

    b. CT scan of the head.

    c. MRI of the spine.

    d. Lumbar puncture.

    e. Urine toxicology screen.

    The answer is d. The presence of ataxia, nerve palsies, and areflexia is highly suggestive of Guillain-Barré syndrome. Most authorities believe that the demyelination of the motor and sensory nerves is due to autoimmune mechanisms. Motor complaints such as weakness and cranial nerve deficits are common presenting symptoms. Sensory abnormalities such paresthesias and pain or numbness are also commonly seen. The sensory and motor symptoms are usually ascending and symmetric with depression on the deep tendon reflexes early on. Lumbar puncture shows a characteristic elevated protein level with normal glucose and less than 10 WBC/mm^3 (albuminocytologic dissociation). EEG, CT scan of the head, MRI of the brain or spine, and urine toxicology screen will not give the diagnosis.

10. **You are evaluating a 3-week-old infant with vomiting for the past 3 hours. The mother states that he has been doing well with his cow's milk based formula until 3 hours ago. The vomitus was described as undigested milk mixed with green material. The diagnostic workup of choice for this infant is:**

    a. Emergent abdominal ultrasound.

    b. Emergent barium enema.

    c. Emergency upper GI series.

    d. CBC and lipase levels.

    e. Change his diet to a protein hydrolysate formula.

    The answer is c. Bilious vomiting in the neonatal period always necessitates an emergent evaluation since 20% of these infants will require surgical intervention. Conditions that present with bilious vomiting in this age group are malrotation with or without a midgut volvulus, annular pancreas, duodenal and jejunal atresia, mecomium ileus, and Hirschsprung disease. Malrotation with midgut volvulus is the most life threatening of these causes and is a surgical emergency. Approximately 50% of cases present in the first month of life. Barium enema is not as reliable as an upper GI series in diagnosing malrotation. It is most useful in evaluating distal bowel obstruction such as Hirschsprung disease. Abdominal ultrasound is useful in diagnosing pyloric stenosis. A CBC and lipase levels are not helpful in making the definitive diagnosis. Changing the formula in an infant who is vomiting bile is not indicated.

11. **An 18-year-old boy comes to your ED for a maculopapular rash on his palms and soles, pain and tenderness on his right knee, and swollen fingers. He denies urethral discharge but felt warm yesterday. You suspect disseminated gonococcal infection (DGI). The best treatment option for this boy is to:**

  a. Give oral cefixime and 1 g azithromycin.
  b. Prescribe doxycycline 100 mg twice daily for 14 days.
  c. Give a single dose of intramuscular ceftriaxone 250 mg.
  d. Admit for intravenous ceftriaxone therapy for 7 days.
  e. Give oral ciprofloxacin twice daily for 7 days.

  The answer is d. Patients with DGI often have fever and chills, accompanied by painful large joints in 50% of cases, tenosynovitis in more than 60% of cases, and subtle skin lesions in 75% of cases. The lesions may be papular or macular, occasionally pustular, with purpuric or hemorrhagic centers. Most patients with DGI have no genitourinary, pharyngeal, or anorectal symptoms. Hospitalization is indicated in all patients with signs and symptoms suggestive of DGI. The drug of choice is ceftriaxone, 1 g intravenously, given daily for 7 days. Other parenteral third-generation cephalosporin such as cefotaxime or ceftizoxime may also be used. Alternatively, parenteral therapy may be continued for 24–48 hours after clinical improvement is noted and then switched to oral therapy. Thereafter, oral cefixime (400 mg twice a day) or levofloxacin (500 mg once a day) may be used to complete 1 week of therapy.

12. **An 18-month-old girl has had several episodes of nonbilious vomiting that started an hour before her ED visit. The patient's mother denies any rhinorrhea, fever, cough, or a history of a fall, although she notes that the girl has been crying more than usual. The girl is noted to be lethargic, pale, and weak on arrival. After intravenous fluids, she continued to vomit. An abdominal radiograph is suggestive of intussusception. You know that:**

  a. Intussusception is the most common cause of intestinal obstruction in infants between 6 and 36 months of age.
  b. A normal abdominal radiograph rules out intussusception.
  c. The classic triad of colicky abdominal pain, palpable abdominal mass, and currant jelly stools is seen more than 90% of the time.
  d. Contrast enema is the preferred method of diagnosis and treatment in patients with intussusception without signs of perforation or peritonitis.
  e. The lack of stools mixed with blood and mucous ("currant jelly" stools) virtually rules out this condition.

  The answer is a. Intussusception is the most common cause of intestinal obstruction in infants between 6 and 36 months of age. It results from the invagination or telescoping of a portion of the proximal intestines into an area just distal to it. The classic triad of colicky abdominal pain, palpable abdominal mass, and currant jelly stools is seen in only 15% of the time. Some patients present with lethargy or an encephalopathic picture due to the release of endorphins from the ischemic bowels into the bloodstream. Several radiographic findings, such as the crescent sign and the target sign, if present, make the diagnosis more likely. Up to 25% of cases have normal abdominal radiographs. Ultrasound is used most often to make the diagnosis. Air enema, rather than contrast enema, is the preferred method of diagnosis and treatment in patients with intussusception without signs of perforation or peritonitis. Approximately 10% will have recurrence of the intussusception within 24–48 hours after reduction.

13. **You are treating an irritable 10-month-old child with supraventricular tachycardia (SVT). The best treatment option to stop the dysrhythmia in this child is:**

    a. Vagal stimulation alone.

    b. Adenosine as rapid intravenous push.

    c. Oral digoxin.

    d. Intravenous verapamil.

    e. Cardioversion at 4 J/kg.

    The answer is b. SVT is the most common dysrhythmia in the pediatric population. Infants or children usually present with a history of poor feeding, rapid breathing, and irritability or pallor. The origin of the arrhythmia is above the bundle of His and most often uses an accessory pathway to complete the circuit. An electrical impulse travels down the AV node and activates the ventricle but goes back up the accessory pathway to depolarize the atrium again. This is seen on EKG as a narrow complex tachycardia at rates of 230–300/min. Adenosine is the safest and fastest acting antiarrhythmic agent that blocks the AV node and breaks the circuit. Verapamil, a calcium channel blocker, is contraindicated in infants younger than 1 year because it can cause hypotension and cardiovascular collapse. Vagal stimulation via carotid massage is not recommended in young children. In a patient who is symptomatic, oral digoxin is not the drug of choice as it takes sometime to work. Its use may also enhance conduction in the accessory pathway especially in patients with WPW. Cardioversion is used for unstable patients at 0.5–1.0 J/kg, not 4 J/kg. New onset SVT should be hospitalized for further evaluation and management.

14. **A 3-year-old boy choked on a disc battery. X-ray shows that the battery is in his stomach. Appropriate management involves:**

    a. Parental reassurance and home observation.

    b. Ipecac to induce expulsion of the battery.

    c. Cathartics to speed transit through the gastrointestinal tract.

    d. Admission to the hospital for observation.

    e. Laparotomy if the battery is still in the small bowel at 48 hours.

    The answer is a. There are three varieties of disc batteries: silver oxide, manganese dioxide, and mercuric oxide. Disc batteries that have passed the esophagus into the stomach need not be retrieved in the asymptomatic patient. The vast majority will pass into the GI tract without complications. Obviously, in the rare patient who develops symptoms suggestive of obstruction or other GI injury, endoscopic or operative retrieval is indicated. Ipecac and cathartics have no place in the management of button battery ingestion. Admission to the hospital is not necessary in the asymptomatic child.

15.   **A 6-month-old girl has scabies. The most effective medication to use is:**

   a. Crotamiton (Eurax).

   b. Topical diphenhydramine (Benadryl).

   c. Lindane (Kwell).

   d. Permethrin (Elimite).

   e. Topical hydrocortisone.

   The answer is d. Permethrin 5% cream (Elimite) is the recommended treatment for scabies in infants and small children. Permethrin 5% cream is applied from the head to the toes and left for 8–12 hours or overnight once and may be repeated in 2 weeks. It is more effective than crotamiton (Eurax) in eliminating the mite, in reducing secondary bacterial infection, and in reducing pruritus. Because of its potential for neurotoxicity, lindane is contraindicated in preterm infants and patients with seizure disorders, pregnant women, and nursing mothers. Patients who do not respond to permethrin may respond to lindane. Postscabietic nodules and pruritus may persist for months, even after successful treatment. Topical diphenhydramine is absorbed through open skin lesions and can cause anticholinergic toxicity, so should be avoided. Topical steroids may ameliorate pruritus but does not cure scabies. All members of the family and close household contacts should be treated as well.

16.   **A 4-week-old girl presents with fever, cough, and increased work of breathing. Vital signs: rectal temperature 38.3°C (100.9°F); respiratory rate, 60/min; heart rate, 160/min. You hear coarse breath sounds and rhonchi. The abdomen is soft and the remainder of the examination is unremarkable. The WBC count is 18,000/mm^3 and chest radiograph shows a dense air-space consolidation of the right lower lobe. The most common bacterial cause of pneumonia in this neonatal period is:**

   a. Group B *Streptococcus.*

   b. *Streptococcus pneumoniae.*

   c. *Staphylococcus aureus.*

   d. *Haemophilus influenzae.*

   e. *Mycoplasma pneumoniae.*

   The answer is a. Bacterial causes of pneumonia in the neonatal age group are group B streptococci, *Listeria monocytogenes, E. coli,* and other gram-negative bacilli. *Chlamydia trachomatis* and *Ureaplasma urealyticum* are important causes in infants younger than 16 weeks. Beyond the neonatal period, *S. pneumoniae* is the predominant bacterial pathogen in all age groups, although its incidence has been decreasing since the introduction of the heptavalent pneumococcal conjugate vaccine. *H. influenzae* has become a less common cause of pneumonia especially after the introduction of the HIB vaccine. *S. aureus, M. pneumoniae,* and *Chlamydia pneumoniae* are less frequent causes after *S. pneumoniae.* Viral causes of pneumonia in the neonate include Herpes simplex virus, CMV, and rubella. RSV and parainfluenza are the most common viral causes of pneumonia from 1 to 24 months of age. From 6 months to 5 years of age, influenza, Epstein-Barr virus (EBV), and adenovirus predominate.

17.   **Choose the most accurate statement regarding the diagnosis of pediatric urinary tract infections:**

   a. A properly collected bag specimen is recommended for infants and non–toilet-trained children.

   b. The combination of positive nitrite and leukocyte esterase markers on urine dipstick is both sensitive and specific for UTI.

   c. Fever in a child with UTI is suggestive of cystitis.

   d. A negative urine dipstick rules out a UTI.

   e. A urine culture with greater than 10^4 CFU/mL is considered positive for a midstream specimen.

The answer is b. Urine culture is considered the gold standard in the diagnosis of pediatric UTI. Criteria for a definite urinary tract infection depend on the technique used to obtain the urine culture. A positive culture is defined as: 10^2 CFU/mL of a single urinary pathogen obtained by suprapubic bladder aspiration, 10^4 CFU/mL of a single pathogen obtained by urethral catheterization, and 10^5 CFU/mL of a single pathogen from a midstream clean-catch specimen. Bag specimens are not recommended for infants and non–toilet-trained children because of their high degree of contamination. A urine dipstick or urinalysis may be negative in up to 50% of patients with UTI. Positive nitrite and leukocyte esterase on urine dipstick have the highest combined sensitivity and specificity for infection. A positive Gram stain of the urine has a sensitivity of 93%. A child or infant with fever and systemic signs and symptoms of UTI should be presumed to have pyelonephritis. Cystitis is associated with more local symptoms such as dysuria or suprapubic tenderness.

18. **You diagnose a 1-year-old well-appearing febrile female infant with UTI. The best management option is to:**

    a. Admit all infants with presumed pyelonephritis for parenteral therapy.
    b. Give one dose of ceftriaxone and send home on oral antibiotics.
    c. Send home on 10 days of oral antibiotics with close follow-up.
    d. Get an urgent ultrasound of the bladder and a voiding cystourethrogram (VCUG) prior to sending home.
    e. Give intravenous hydration, obtain blood cultures, and start parenteral antibiotics.

    The answer is c. Antibiotic therapy is indicated in all infants and children with presumed UTI based on clinical signs and results of urinalysis. Pending cultures, antibiotic therapy is based on the most common etiologic organisms. *E. coli* is the predominant bacteria isolated followed by *Enterobacter* and *Klebsiella* and less commonly by gram-positive organisms such as *Enterococcus* and *Staphylococcus*. Group B streptococci are isolated primarily during the neonatal period and pregnancy. *P. aeruginosa* is seen more often in patients who are immunocompromised and in those with anatomic abnormalities or indwelling catheters. Indications for parenteral antibiotics and admission are systemic toxicity, inability to tolerate fluids and medications, age younger than 3 months, failure to respond to oral antibiotics, anatomic obstruction to urine flow, and a urine culture with known organism resistant to oral antibiotics. Otherwise, well-appearing infants and children with UTI, even if febrile, can be sent home on oral antibiotics for 10–14 days with close follow-up. An urgent ultrasound of the bladder and a VCUG are not indicated during the emergency department visit. It should be done in male infants with their first UTI and female infants with recurrent UTI after the infection has been treated.

19. **An 18-month-old child has several mouth lesions that look like small cold sores on his cheeks and gums. He has fever, vomiting, a foul-smelling breath, and refuses to eat or drink. You know that:**

    a. This condition is caused by a coxsackievirus.
    b. The lesions last approximately 3 days.
    c. Dehydration is a frequent complication.
    d. The condition is caused by herpes simplex 2.
    e. Fever usually lasts for lass then 24 hours.

    The answer is c. The child has gingivostomatitis caused by primary herpes simplex 1 virus. Children younger than 5 years are most commonly affected, and the mouth is the most common site of involvement. The lesions start as vesicles then erode to become ulcers noted on the lips, gums, tongue, and palate. The high fever usually lasts for 3–5 days. The condition lasts approximately 10–14 days with dehydration a common complication because of the child's refusal to eat. Pain control usually with oral agents such as acetaminophen with codeine or ibuprofen and topical anesthetic such as "miracle mouthwash" is important in the management.

20.   A 12-year-old boy presents with what appears to be a first episode of shingles on the left T4 dermatome. You know that:

a. In children, it occurs almost exclusively in the immunocompromised patient.

b. It occurs exclusively in patients who had the varicella vaccine.

c. Lesions last approximately 4–5 weeks preceded by pain along the dermatomal distribution by 1 week.

d. Antiviral medications are not effective.

e. Postherpetic neuralgia only occurs in immunocompromised hosts.

The answer is c. Herpes zoster is due to a reactivation of the varicella-zoster virus residing in the dorsal root ganglia. It is seen most exclusively in patients who had primary chickenpox infections. Most reactivations are seen in healthy individuals. Pain along the distribution of 1–3 sensory dermatomes usually precedes the lesions by approximately a week. Lesions last approximately 4–5 weeks. Postherpetic neuralgia may last for months and usually is not responsive to standard analgesics. Antiviral medications such as valacyclovir and famciclovir are recommended in adults and immunocompromised patients. However, insufficient data exist on the use of these drugs in infants and children.

21.   A 9-day-old baby presents to the emergency department with purulent conjunctivitis. Topical erythromycin prophylaxis was given in the nursery. The most likely cause of this neonate's conjunctivitis is:

a. Syphilis.

b. *Neisseria gonorrhoeae.*

c. Group B *Streptococcus.*

d. Herpes simplex virus.

e. *Chlamydia trachomatis.*

The answer is e. Neonatal conjunctivitis (ophthalmia neonatorum) occurs within the first month of life. Previously, the most common cause was chemical irritation from application of silver nitrate eyedrops as antimicrobial prophylaxis at birth, which is usually seen 1–2 days after birth. Presently, most hospitals use erythromycin ointment as the standard prophylaxis and as a result, the incidence of chemical conjunctivitis has gone down. However, erythromycin ointment does not prevent all gonococcal and other bacterial ocular infections and is not effective against *C. trachomatis.* Although *N. gonorrhoeae* is no longer a major cause of neonatal conjunctivitis in the United States, it should be presumed in infants who have purulent conjunctivitis until proven otherwise. Corneal perforation is a known complication. You should do a Gram stain of the eye discharge looking for Gram–negative diplococci, as well as gonococcal and chlamydial cultures or nucleic acid amplication (PCR) tests. Gonococcal conjunctivitis is commonly seen between 3 and 5 days after birth. By the end of first week of life and throughout the first month of life, *C. trachomatis* becomes the most frequent cause of conjunctivitis. Other important but less common bacterial causes are *Haemophilus influenzae* and *Streptococcus pneumoniae.*

22.   A 3-month-old boy is brought to the ED by his 16-year-old mother after the infant reportedly stopped breathing and became dusky. The mother reports that she quickly "blew into his mouth" and some formula came out of his nose. Thereafter, he started breathing again and his appearance turned pink and healthy. Your examination is remarkable only for generalized hypotonia. Your most appropriate action is to:

a. Discuss postprandial regurgitation with the mother and discharge the baby with instructions to keep the head elevated after feeding.

b. Start the infant on theophylline 6 mg/kg per day and arrange follow-up with a pediatrician the following day.

c. Admit the infant to the hospital for further evaluation.

d. Arrange for a home apnea monitor and schedule an outpatient workup with a pediatrician.

e. Reassure the mother that this is a normal event and discharge to infant home.

The answer is c. According to the National Institute of Health, an *apparent life-threatening event* or ALTE is "an episode that is frightening to the observer and is characterized by some combination of apnea (central or occasionally obstructive), color change (usually cyanotic or pallid but occasionally erythematous or plethoric), marked change in muscle tone (usually limpness), choking, or gagging." The infant who presents with a history of ALTE may have a normal physical examination and may act normal at the time of the evaluation. The causes of an ALTE are varied and include seizures, gastroesophageal reflux, anemia, arrhythmia, trauma, ingestion, metabolic derangements, hypoglycemia, congenital heart disease, and infection. These infants, especially those requiring vigorous stimulation or mouth-to-mouth resuscitation, may be at increased risk of subsequent death and therefore require hospitalization for observation and further evaluation. Basic evaluation in the emergency department should include a CBC, electrolytes, urinalysis, EKG, chest radiograph, and cultures from blood and urine. Further evaluation should be left to the inpatient physician or primary care physician depending on the patient's history, physical examination, and hospital course.

23. **Choose the true statement about simple febrile seizure:**

   a. A family history of simple febrile seizures is uncommon.

   b. They occur in patients between 6 months and 5 years of age

   c. Focal postictal neurologic deficits are frequently present.

   d. Recurrence after the first episode is rare.

   e. They are not associated with an increased risk of epilepsy.

The answer is b. Simple febrile seizures are seizures occurring in neurologically and developmentally normal patients between 6 months and 5 years of age. These seizures are generalized, last less than 15 minutes, occur once in a 24-hour period, and are seen in febrile pediatric patients without evidence of intracranial infection or other cause. They are believed to occur during a rapid rise in temperature, although approximately half of the children have documented fevers of less than 39°C (102.2°F). Overall, febrile seizures affect approximately 5% of all children. Simple febrile seizures become complex febrile seizures when multiple seizures occur during the same illness, seizure events are prolonged, or there is a focal component to the seizure. Focal postictal neurologic deficits, however, are typically absent. A family history of febrile seizures is common (25–40% of patients). Recurrence occurs in 30–40% of children and is more likely when the first febrile seizure occurs before 1 year of age. Children with simple febrile seizures have an approximately 2–3% chance of developing epilepsy, compared with a 1% rate of epilepsy in the general population.

24. **Choose the true statement about radial head subluxation (nursemaid elbow):**

   a. It is commonly seen in infants younger than 1 year.

   b. The usual mechanism of injury is a history of a pull by the arm or a fall.

   c. Physical examination is positive for mild swelling and tenderness around the elbow.

   d. Radiographs are recommended for proper diagnosis.

   e. The method of choice for reduction is the flexion and pronation technique.

The answer is b. Nursemaid's elbow is the most common upper extremity injury in patients between 6 months and 5 years of age seen in the pediatric emergency department. The peak age is between 2 and 3 years of age. Patients present with a history of either a pull of the arm, a twisting of the arm or in a third of cases, a history of a fall on the arm. It is believed to be due to the entrapment of the annular ligament in the radiohumeral joint. The patient refuses to use the arm and cries when it is moved. The arm is held near the body, in pronation with the elbows slightly flexed. There is no swelling, redness, or deformity but pain on range of motion of the elbow. Nursemaid's elbow is a clinical diagnosis. Radiographs are necessary only if multiple attempts of reduction fail or there is significant swelling and tenderness around the elbow. The method of choice presently is the hyperpronation technique where the elbow and wrist of the affected arm are stabilized and the arm is hyperpronated. It is more successful than the flexion–supination maneuver.

25.   A 7-year-old girl has palpable purpura and petechiae on her legs and buttocks and is complaining of abdominal pain. You know that:

a. The most common presentation also includes arthralgias and microscopic hematuria.

b. This is a hypersensitivity vasculitis with immune complex deposition affecting the blood vessels, especially the veins, exclusively of the lower extremities.

c. An indolent form of meningococcemia may mimic this condition.

d. The condition lasts for approximately 2 weeks.

e. All patients with this condition should be hospitalized for further management.

The answer is a. Henoch-Schönlein purpura is a systemic vasculitis usually seen in children between the ages of 4 and 11 years. There is immune complex deposition of immunoglobulin A in the arterioles and capillaries anywhere in the body. Patients usually have abdominal complaints in 70% of cases. The classic presentation is that of a child with abdominal pain, arthralgias, microscopic hematuria, and the characteristic palpable purpuric and petechial rash in the lower extremities and buttocks. A child with meningococcemia may present similarly, although with more toxicity and abruptness of symptoms. Criteria for admission include severe abdominal pain, severe arthralgias, uncertain diagnosis, or inability to exclude meningococcemia, and intractable vomiting. Steroids are reserved for patients with severe abdominal pain, hematuria, and disabling arthralgias. The course remits and relapses over a course of several weeks to months.

26.   You suspect rotavirus in a 1-year-old listless infant with moderate dehydration. You know:

a. Rotavirus infections are responsible for approximately 90% of all diarrheal illness in infancy.

b. Rotavirus infections are self-limited and cause little morbidity and mortality.

c. Rotavirus infections can present with high fevers, copious diarrhea, and vomiting.

d. Rotavirus vaccine will prevent most of the infections.

e. Most patients with rotavirus require hospitalization for moderate to severe dehydration.

The answer is c. Rotaviruses are the most common cause of severe gastroenteritis in children younger than 5 years, accounting for one-third of all children with diarrhea. It peaks during the winter and spring seasons. The child usually presents with copious diarrhea, high fever, and vomiting that lasts up to 8 days. Almost all children are infected by the time they reached their third birthday. The virus is a major source of morbidity with a large percentage of patients requiring hospitalization for dehydration. Enzyme immunoassay techniques that are highly sensitive and specific for stool rotavirus antigens are available in most hospital laboratories. In February 2006, oral pentavalent rotavirus vaccine (Rotarix, RotaTeq) was approved for use among US infants. A previous product, Rotashield, was removed from the market due to a high association with intussusception. The recommendation calls for routine vaccination of infants at 2, 4, and 6 months of age for a total of three doses.

27.   A true statement about the differences between a child and adult airway is:

a. The soft tissues of the oropharynx are relatively small compared to the oral cavity.

b. The cylindrical larynx has a more posterior or caudal location in the neck.

c. The large occiput causes passive flexion of the cervical spine in the supine position.

d. The infant's trachea is long relative to its thorax but shorter than the adult trachea.

e. The large occiput enables the child to preserve neutral spine alignment throughout the torso.

The correct answer is c. The smaller the child the greater is his occiput relative to his midface. This causes passive flexion of the cervical spine in the supine position. To prevent this, the child's midface must be kept parallel to the spine board in the "sniffing position." Placement of a layer of padding in the entire torso may also be necessary to preserve neutral spine alignment. The soft tissues of the oropharynx are large compared to the oral cavity. Compared to the adult larynx, the child's larynx is funnel-shaped, is located more cephalad, and the vocal cords are located in a more anterior angle. Thus, these differences make it more difficult to visualize the larynx and vocal cords during intubation.

28. **The newest guidelines from the American Heart Association regarding pediatric advanced life support (PALS) states that:**

    a. Use of either cuffed or uncuffed endotracheal tubes in patients younger than 8 years is acceptable.

    b. Exhaled CO_2 monitoring is recommended only during intubation.

    c. Routine use of high-dose epinephrine is still recommended.

    d. Biphasic shocks with an automated external defibrillator (AED) are still not recommended for infants younger than 1 year.

    e. Unlike in adults, you should do three shocks prior to chest compressions when performing CPR.

    The answer is a. There were many new recommendations from the 2005 International Consensus on Cardiopulmonary Resuscitation (CPR) and Emergency Cardiovascular Care (ECC) Science with Treatment Recommendations. The new motto is: "Push hard, push fast, minimize interruptions; allow full chest recoil, and don't hyperventilate." Another recommendation is that providers can now use both cuffed and uncuffed endotracheal tubes in children younger than 8 years. Another recommendation is that AEDs can now be used in both infants and children. High-dose epinephrine is no longer recommended and may be harmful. In all settings, whether a patient is being intubated or transported, confirmation of endotracheal tube placement by detection of exhaled CO_2 should be performed using a colorimetric detector or capnography. When performing defibrillation, the first shock is followed by five cycles or 2 minutes of CPR rather than the previous recommendation of three shocks followed by CPR.

29. **You need to give approximately 1.5 times the maintenance intravenous fluids to a 15-kg child who has received saline boluses for moderate dehydration. The correct rate is:**

    a. 75 mL/h.

    b. 100 mL/h.

    c. 60 mL/h.

    d. 10 mL/kg/h.

    e. 4 mL/kg/h for the first 20 kg.

    The answer is a. To calculate maintenance fluids, the Holliday-Segar formula is 4 mL/kg/h for the first 10 kg, 2 mL/kg/h between 11 and 20 kg, and 1 mL/kg/h after 20 kg. For this child, he would need 50 mL/h as maintenance rate and 1.5× would be 75 mL/h.

30.   Choose the accurate statement regarding bronchiolitis:

a. Typically occurs in children between 2 and 5 years of age.

b. Commonly associated with tachypnea, wheezing, and rales.

c. Diagnosis is confirmed with sputum culture.

d. Steroids are often used to prevent recurrence.

e. Aerosolized ribavirin is indicated in all cases.

The answer is b. Bronchiolitis is the most common lower respiratory track infection in infancy. The pathophysiology consists of acute inflammation, edema, increased mucus production, and bronchospasm. The condition starts as rhinitis followed by tachypnea, wheezing, cough, crackles, use of accessory muscles, and/or nasal flaring a few days later. Respiratory syncytial virus (RSV) is the cause in 50–70% of cases, with the highest incidence occurring between December and March. Almost all infants will have an RSV infection by the time they reach 2 years of age, although infection does not grant permanent or long-term immunity. Reinfections are common throughout life. Other viruses causing bronchiolitis are human metapneumovirus, influenza, adenovirus, and parainfluenza. The American Academy of Pediatrics does not recommend routine chest radiographs or laboratory testing on patients with mild to moderate bronchiolitis. Treatment is primarily supportive. Racemic epinephrine, nebulized beta-agonist may be helpful in certain cases but should not be routinely used. Steroids have not been shown to be beneficial.

31.   A previously healthy 4-year-old girl presents with hypoventilation and hypoxemia secondary to pneumonia. You decide to intubate her with a:

a. 4 mm internal diameter (ID) cuffed endotracheal tube.

b. 4 mm ID uncuffed endotracheal tube.

c. 5 mm ID uncuffed endotracheal tube.

d. 5 mm ID cuffed endotracheal tube.

e. 5.5 mm ID uncuffed endotracheal tube.

The answer is c. In general, uncuffed tubes are used in children younger than 8 years because the subglottic trachea, surrounded by the cricoid cartilage, is the narrowest part of the pediatric airway. In children older than 1 year, the following formula is used to determine an appropriate tube size: Tube size (mm ID) = (age in years + 16)/4. If using a cuffed tube, the formula is: (age in years/4) + 3.

32.   A mother tells you that her 2-month-old infant rolled over and fell from the bed and started crying. You find a swollen and tender right thigh. An infant can start to roll over at:

a. 1 month.

b. 2 months.

c. 4 months.

d. 6 months.

e. 9 months.

The answer is c. One of the red flags of abuse is injury that is inconsistent with normal developmental milestones. Hence, the emergency physician needs to have a basic knowledge of developmental pediatrics so as to appropriately evaluate child abuse. For example, a 1-month-old infant can raise her head from prone position and has a tight grasp. In this vignette, a 2-month-old infant does not have the ability to roll over yet and so the injury is suspicious for abuse. At 2 months, she should be able to hold her head in midline position, lift her chest off the table, coo, and recognize her parent. At 4 months, she should be able to roll over, shift her weight, laugh, orient to voice, and look around. At 6 months, she should be able to sit unsupported, put her feet in her mouth and babble. At 9 months, she should be able to crawl, pull to stand, and cruise.

33. **A 9-month-old infant with a ventriculoperitoneal (VP) shunt placed 9 weeks ago presents with a temperature of 102°F and vomiting. You know that:**

   a. VP shunt infections are due to Gram-negative organisms.

   b. VP shunt infections most often occur in the first 4 months after placement.

   c. All patients with VP shunts presenting with fever need to be tapped.

   d. Lethargy and decreased spontaneity are not specific symptoms of shunt infections.

   e. CT scans need to be ordered in all patients with VP shunts presenting to the ED.

   The answer is b. Patients with VP shunts are usually evaluated in the ED for shunt malfunction or shunt infections. The majority of shunt infections are due to coagulase-negative staphylococci and occur in the first 3–4 months after placement. After this time, other causes or sources of fever need to be considered. The most sensitive symptoms for shunt infection are lethargy and decreased spontaneity. Nonspecific symptoms include irritability, anorexia, vomiting, and abdominal pain. Not all patients with shunts and fever need to be tapped unless the shunt was changed within the past 4 months. CT scans are needed only if you are ruling out shunt malfunction; it should not be ordered routinely in every patient with a shunt who presents to the ED.

34. **An 11-month-old child had a generalized seizure of 30 minutes duration. His temperature is 103.5°F, heart rate 140/min, respiratory rate 32/min, and a normal BP. He is now sleeping but arousable with a normal physical and neurologic examination. The father states he had febrile seizures when he was younger. The parents are now concerned if he will develop epilepsy. A well-documented risk factor for epilepsy in a child with febrile seizures is:**

   a. Family history of febrile seizures.

   b. Fever >103°F.

   c. Age younger than 1 year.

   d. Complex febrile seizure.

   e. Previous febrile seizure.

   The answer is b. The American Academy of Pediatrics developed a practice parameter on the long-term treatment of a child with simple febrile seizures in 1999. As defined in this parameter, the child who has a febrile seizure lasting more than 15 minutes, as in the vignette, has a complex febrile seizure. Other features are (1) focal seizures or (2) recurrence within 24 hours. Complex febrile seizure increases the risk of developing epilepsy in the future. Other well-known risk factors are the presence of developmental or neurologic abnormalities at the time of the seizure, family history of epilepsy, >3 febrile seizures in the past, and less than 1 hour duration between onset of fever and seizure. The risk factors for recurrent febrile seizures are family history of febrile seizures, onset of febrile seizure at age less than 1 year, and low degree of fever at the time of seizure.

35. **A 6-year-old immigrant from Afghanistan complains of a severe sore throat and foul breath. His neck is swollen and voice hoarse. Examination reveals fever, tachypnea, anterior cervical adenopathy, and whitish-gray adherent pharyngeal exudates. You notice tachycardia with frequent ectopic beats when you listen to his heart. WBC is 12,000/mm³ with a left shift. Chest radiograph demonstrates cardiomegaly. The patient has no previous history of medical problems. You suspect diphtheria and know that:**

    a. Spread occurs hematogenously.

    b. Morbidity results primarily from localized infection in the pharynx.

    c. Steroids should be administered in all cases.

    d. Debridement of pharyngeal exudates is essential for resolution.

    e. Definitive treatment includes parenteral antibiotics and antitoxin.

    The answer is e. Diphtheria is a rare but serious cause of pharyngitis. Morbidity is secondary to both local infection and systemic toxicity. *Corynebacterium diphtheriae*, which is spread by contact with nasopharyngeal secretions, invades the pharynx and causes progressive tissue necrosis and pseudomembrane formation. If severe, airway obstruction can occur. Elaborated toxin causes myocarditis, nephritis, hepatitis, and neuritis with both bulbar and peripheral paralysis. Patients typically present with acute onset of fever, sore throat, and a hoarse or muffled voice. Physical examination reveals an exudative pharyngitis with a white to gray, closely adherent pseudomembrane, marked cervical adenopathy ("bull neck"), and fetid breath ("dirty mouse smell"). Definitive treatment includes parenteral antibiotics (penicillin or erythromycin) and equine serum diphtheria antitoxin. No data supports the use of steroids. The most serious complications include airway obstruction, congestive heart failure, conduction disturbances, and muscle paralysis. All patients should be hospitalized for isolation and airway monitoring. Close contacts of the patient should be located and treated.

36. **Conjunctivitis is commonly associated with:**

    a. Hand-foot-and-mouth disease.

    b. Fifth disease.

    c. Rubeola (measles).

    d. Mononucleosis.

    e. Reye's syndrome.

    The answer is c. Viruses are the most frequent cause of conjunctivitis and adenovirus is the most frequent virus implicated. Other diseases may present with conjunctivitis as part of their clinical syndrome. These include Kawasaki disease, measles (rubeola), and seasonal allergies. Measles, caused by a paramyxovirus, begins with a prodrome of gradually increasing fevers and URI symptoms (cough, coryza, conjunctivitis). The prodrome is followed 2–4 days later with the appearance of a maculopapular rash that appears first on the head and spreads inferiorly to the trunk and extremities (including the palms and soles). Koplik spots, white papules on an erythematous base, on the buccal mucosa are pathognomonic.

37. **Which of the following findings is suggestive of child abuse?**

    a. Retinal hemorrhages in an 8-month-old.

    b. Spiral midshaft tibia fracture in a 15-month-old.

    c. Currant jelly stools in an 8-month-old.

    d. Anterior shin bruises in an 18-month-old.

    e. All of the above.

The answer is a. Two-thirds of all victims of child abuse are younger than 3 years and one-third of these are younger than 6 months. Noting unusual injuries or injuries out of proportion to the alleged trauma, and a consideration of the child's developmental age are important to avoid missing abuse cases and also to prevent unjustified accusations. Infants younger than 6 months are incapable of ingesting poisons or drugs. Retinal hemorrhages, lens dislocations, and retinal detachment may occur in children subjected to shaking or head trauma (shaken baby syndrome). The "double bubble" sign of duodenal hematoma formation would be distinctly unusual in a child of this age in the absence of trauma. Burns of the posterior thighs, buttocks, and genitalia are seen as the result of inappropriate discipline during toilet training. Common fractures associated with child abuse include spiral fractures, metaphyseal chip or "corner" fractures, rib fractures, and complex skull fractures. Toddlers learning to walk may display bruises on predictable body surfaces, but bruise marks over multiple areas or over areas that are not typically injured accidentally (ear pinnae, buttocks, mouth) should be noted.

38. **A 4-year-old boy is brought to the ED with bilious vomiting. On examination, his abdomen is distended and tympanitic, with mild nonspecific tenderness and no peritoneal signs. The remainder of the examination is unremarkable. Chest radiograph is normal. Abdominal radiographs show multiple dilated air-filled loops of small bowel with air-fluid levels, but no free air. Your next appropriate study would be:**

    a. Barium upper GI series with small bowel follow-through.

    b. Diatrizoate upper GI series with small bowel follow-through.

    c. CT scan of the abdomen with contrast.

    d. Diatrizoate enema.

    e. Barium enema.

    The answer is e. This patient has signs of complete distal mechanical small bowel obstruction with no evidence of perforation. Hernias would be the most common cause in this age group, but none was identified on physical examination. The next step is to perform a barium enema, which will identify the site of obstruction if it involves the large bowel (appendicitis with obstruction, intussusception) and may identify malrotations of the gut associated with obstruction. A diatrizoate enema is a suboptimal study and unnecessary as there is no perforation. A barium upper GI study may be indicated, although in most cases it will not change the management. Diatrizoate is used as an alternative to barium sulfate for medical imaging of the gastrointestinal tract in patients who are allergic to barium, or in cases where the barium might leak into the abdominal cavity. It is also used to kill tapeworms. A diatrizoate upper GI is contraindicated, since if the patient vomits and aspirates, even small amounts of diatrizoate cause fulminant and often fatal pulmonary edema.

39. **In treating a patient with suspected with Reye's syndrome, your initial management should include:**

    a. Aspirin for fever control.

    b. Intravenous fluids at 1.5 times maintenance.

    c. Broad-spectrum antibiotics.

    d. Pentobarbital coma.

    e. Admission to an ICU setting.

    The answer is e. All patients with suspected Reye's syndrome require admission to the ICU. The management of these patients is based upon the severity and stage of their illness. In clinical stages I and II (noncomatose patients), treatment includes intravenous D10W to help counter their severe liver dysfunction, nasogastric neomycin and/or lactulose to reduce ammonia production, and other means of supportive care. Intravenous fluids should be given initially at or below maintenance to avoid cerebral edema. In stages III to V (comatose patients), the primary goal is aggressive control of intracranial pressure. Measures to manage increased intracranial pressure include hyperventilation, intravenous furosemide, intravenous mannitol, and in refractory cases pentobarbital coma. Even with the above measures the overall mortality still remains 15% and approaches 95% in stage V.

40.   **Concerning infantile spasms:**

   a. They occur during sleep and involve twisting of the mouth.

   b. They are rarely associated with an underlying CNS disorder.

   c. EEG is almost always normal.

   d. Prognosis is generally excellent.

   e. They are commonly associated with developmental regression.

   The answer is e. Infantile spasms present during the first year of life and consist of rapid flexor or extensor spasms of the head and trunk. These spasms may occur as a single event or in clusters of 5–20 at a time. Onset typically occurs between 3 and 9 months of age and frequently is accompanied by developmental regression. Approximately two-thirds of children with infantile spasms have an underlying CNS disorder such as a congenital brain malformation or tuberous sclerosis. EEG is almost always abnormal with a characteristic pattern called hypsarrthymia (extremely high voltage slow waves) present in 50% of the cases. Although early treatment with ACTH or prednisone may optimize outcome, the prognosis is still generally poor. Only half of these children will attain remission of seizures and 90–95% will become mentally retarded.

41.   **A 2-week-old full-term infant is brought to the ED with a history of difficulty breathing during feeding. Examination reveals a noncyanotic, tachypneic infant. The heart rate is 140/min, and you can easily hear a widely radiating systolic murmur. Chest radiography shows cardiomegaly and pulmonary congestion. The child most likely has:**

   a. Patent ductus arteriosus.

   b. Hypoplastic left ventricle.

   c. Coarctation of the aorta.

   d. Transposition of the great vessels.

   e. Ventricular septal defect.

   The answer is c. The first step in evaluating heart disease in the infant is to establish whether it is cyanotic or acyanotic. In the infant with heart failure, the diagnosis is aided by knowledge of the time course. Immediately after birth, congestive heart failure (CHF) is most often caused by noncardiac diseases such as hypoxia, hypoglycemia, hypocalcemia, acidosis, and sepsis. Patent ductus arteriosus is the most common cause of CHF in premature infants, but hypoplastic left ventricle is the most common cause of CHF in the term infant's first week. Coarctation commonly presents as acute CHF in the second week. Transposition of the great vessels usually occurs in the first 3 days with cyanosis and failure. CHF due to a ventricular septal defect usually presents approximately 1 month after birth. After 3 months, CHF is most likely due to acquired diseases like myocarditis, anemia, and rheumatic fever.

42.   **A 5-week-old infant is brought to the ED for the evaluation of a new cough. The mother states that aside from some nasal congestion and eye redness over the last couple of days, he has been well since birth. On examination, the child is afebrile but quite tachypneic. Pulse oximetry reveals a saturation of 93%. On chest radiograph you note bilateral interstitial infiltrates. The organism most likely producing this constellation of symptoms is:**

   a. Group B *Streptococcus.*

   b. *Staphylococcus aureus.*

   c. *Haemophilus influenzae.*

   d. *Chlamydia trachomatis.*

   e. *Mycoplasma pneumoniae.*

The answer is d. Chlamydia pneumonia ("afebrile pneumonia of infancy") occurs in infants 2–16 weeks after birth. *C. trachomatis* is acquired as the infant passes through the vaginal canal during delivery. Infants typically present with the gradual onset of a "staccato" cough. Fever is generally absent. Associated findings include nasal congestion and bilateral conjunctivitis. Eosinophilia is often noted on the laboratory workup. Diffuse interstitial infiltrates on CXR are most common. If *C. trachomatis* is suspected, erythromycin should be added to the treatment regimen.

43.   **Choose the most accurate statement regarding the diagnosis and management of meningitis in infants and children:**

a. A bulging fontanelle is an early sign of meningitis.
b. Head CT should be obtained on a routine basis prior to LP.
c. Empiric antibiotics should never be delayed in suspected cases of meningitis.
d. In an infant with lethargy and irritability when being handled, a normal spinal tap is grounds for discharge.
e. A positive Gram stain in the absence of other CSF abnormalities can reasonably be judged to be a skin contaminant.

The answer is c. Meningitis generally occurs as a complication of primary bacteremia. Signs and symptoms are age dependent. Infants may present with fever, poor feeding, lethargy, and irritability when being handled. A bulging fontanelle is specific for increased intracranial pressure, but it is a late sign in meningitis. Older children present with more typical symptoms of meningitis including headache, photophobia, and neck rigidity. Head CT need not be obtained on a routine basis prior to LP. CT should be performed emergently if there is evidence of increased ICP, trauma, or focal lesions. CSF findings suggestive of bacterial meningitis include increased WBCs with a preponderance of PMNs, increased protein, and decreased glucose. A negative tap, however, does not exclude the diagnosis. A child with a history highly suggestive of meningitis with a negative tap should be admitted for close observation and repeat lumbar puncture. Of note, a positive CSF Gram stain may predate other CSF changes. In patients with suspected meningitis, administration of antibiotics should never be delayed. Antibiotic selection is based on likely organisms, which in turn is based on age.

44.   **A 6-month-old boy presents with a 2-week history of cough and a 3-day history of fever. The mother says the child seemed to have a cold, and then got better, but for the last 3 days has developed progressive fever. Physical examination is significant for a respiratory rate of 40/min, temperature of 39°C (102.2°F), and heart rate of 150/min. The left chest is dull to percussion and breath sounds are decreased at the left base. Chest radiograph shows consolidation of the left lower lobe with an effusion and small pneumothorax. Partial consolidation of the upper lobe with several thin-walled cystic areas is also visible. You must choose an antibiotic that will treat:**

a. *Mycobacterium tuberculosis.*
b. *Streptococcus pneumoniae.*
c. Group B *Streptococcus.*
d. *Staphylococcus aureus.*
e. *Escherichia coli.*

The answer is d. *S. aureus* is an uncommon cause of pneumonia, but is particularly likely to occur following viral infections such as influenza. Effusions (empyema), pneumothorax, and, in children, pneumatoceles are nearly pathognomonic of staphylococcal pneumonia. Patients should be admitted to the hospital for parenteral IV antistaphylococcal antibiotics and tube thoracostomy drainage of associated empyema.

45. Which of the following statements regarding pediatric chest radiographs is most accurate:

a. The thymus is present from birth to 5 years.

b. A cardiothoracic ratio greater than 0.4 in infants indicates cardiomegaly.

c. The thymus is differentiated from cardiomegaly by its scalloped border.

d. Decreased pulmonary vasculature is seen with pulmonary hypertension or left to right shunting.

e. Increased pulmonary vasculature is seen in congenital heart disease with right to left shunting.

The answer is c. Cardiomegaly is defined in infants as a cardiothoracic ratio greater than 0.55 on the PA view. On the lateral view, cardiomegaly appears as posterior mediastinal enlargement. The thymus, which is present from birth to approximately 2 years, appears retrosternally on the lateral view. Through contact with the rib margins, the thymus takes on a characteristic scalloped appearance. This helps to differentiate the thymus from cardiomegaly. A right heart border "sail" appearance is due to the thymus bordering the cardiac silhouette, which results in a squared off superior right heart border. It should not be confused with an infiltrate. Increased pulmonary vasculature is seen with pulmonary hypertension or left to right shunting. Cyanotic lesions with right to left shunting, such as tetralogy of Fallot and tricuspid atresia, are characterized by a decrease in pulmonary vasculature.

46. Choose the correct statement regarding acute otitis media (AOM):

a. The most reliable examination finding is loss of bony landmarks.

b. Drug-resistant *Streptococcus pneumoniae* is more frequent in children attending daycare.

c. Decongestants and antihistamines are helpful adjuncts in treating AOM.

d. ENT referral for possible tympanostomy tubes is indicated in all cases of AOM.

e. Failure to improve after initiation of antibiotic therapy is common.

The answer is b. Acute otitis media commonly affects infants and young children because of the relative immaturity of their upper respiratory tracts. The peak age of incidence is 6–18 months. The most virulent pathogen is *S. pneumoniae*, which accounts for approximately 40% of the cases. *Haemophilus influenzae* (nontypeable) and *Moraxella catarrhalis* account for another 40–50% of the cases but have a high rate of spontaneous resolution. The most reliable examination finding is decreased mobility of the tympanic membrane on pneumatic otoscopy. Other findings include a red, dull, or bulging tympanic membrane and loss of bony landmarks. Although the need for antibiotics is controversial (80% of cases of AOM resolve spontaneously without antibiotics), most authorities still recommend the routine use of antibiotics. Because of its cost, efficacy, and safety profile, amoxicillin is still considered first-line therapy. The use of high-dose amoxicillin (80–90 mg/kg/d) is now recommended in patients at high risk for drug-resistant *S. pneumoniae* (younger than 2 years, daycare, recent antibiotics). Alternatives include amoxicillin-clavulanate, cefuroxine, trimethoprim-sulfamethoxazole (if penicillin allergic). There is no indication for antihistamines, decongestants, steroids, or tympanostomy tubes with an episode of AOM. Most children will be afebrile and asymptomatic within 2–3 days after initiation of antibiotic therapy.

47. A 5-year-old boy presents with honey-colored crusting lesions around his nose consistent with impetigo. Which of the following is most accurate regarding this skin infection?

a. Routine coverage for *Staphylococcus aureus* is not necessary.

b. Topical mupirocin should always be combined with an oral antibiotic.

c. Vigorous scrubbing of the lesions with warm saline hastens resolution.

d. Poststreptococcal glomerulonephritis is a possible complication.

e. Rheumatic fever is a known sequela of this infection.

The answer is d. Appropriate treatment of impetigo requires antibiotic coverage of *Streptococcus* and *Staphylococcus* species. A first-generation cephalosporin, erythromycin, or topical mupirocin alone can be used as appropriate therapy. Vigorous scrubbing has not been shown to be of any benefit in the healing process, although good hand washing and personal hygiene will limit the spread of infection to others. Complications of impetigo include cellulitis, regional lymphadenitis, and acute poststreptococcal glomerulonephritis. The incidence of poststreptococcal glomerulonephritis is less than 1%. Unfortunately, antibiotic therapy does not prevent this complication. Rheumatic fever is not a known sequela of impetigo.

48. **A 7-year-old child requires a closed reduction of a wrist fracture. Of the agents listed, the single best choice for sedation and analgesia is:**

    a. Morphine.

    b. Meperidine.

    c. Fentanyl.

    d. Midazolam.

    e. Chloral hydrate.

    The answer is c. Fentanyl is indicated for brief, painful procedures lasting 30–45 minutes. Morphine and meperidine are indicated for procedures lasting one hour or longer. Midazolam and chloral hydrate are sedatives without analgesic properties. In clinical practice, the combination of an opiate such as fentanyl with a benzodiazepine such as midazolam is particularly effective for sedation and analgesia. Because these agents have respiratory depressant effects, skilled personnel and equipment for airway management need to be immediately available when using these agents.

49. **The most appropriate choice of management for a child with Kawasaki disease is:**

    a. Admission for IV gamma-globulin and high-dose aspirin therapy.

    b. Admission for antibiotics and steroids.

    c. Discharge on high-dose aspirin therapy and follow up in 2–3 days.

    d. Discharge on high-dose aspirin therapy and a second-generation cephalosporin.

    e. Discharge on high-dose steroids.

    The answer is a. Kawasaki disease, the most frequent cause of acquired pediatric cardiac disease, is an acute multisystem vasculitis of small and medium sized arteries. It occurs primarily in infants and children, with a peak incidence between 1 and 2 years of age. Diagnosis is based on the presence of fever for 5 or more days in association with four of the following five conditions: bilateral conjunctivitis, cervical lymphadenopathy, polymorphous rash, mucous membrane changes, and extremity findings. Erythrocyte sedimentation rate (ESR) and C-reactive protein (CRP) are often markedly elevated. The clinical course is divided into three phases. The acute phase (days 1–11) is characterized by fever and myocarditis. The subacute phase (days 11–20) is characterized by resolution of the fever, rash, and adenopathy as well as the development of thrombocytosis and periungal desquamation. Risk for developing coronary artery thrombosis and sudden death is the greatest at this time. The convalescent phase (days 21–60) begins when the clinical findings have resolved and continues until the ESR is normal. All patients should be admitted for IV gamma-globulin and high-dose aspirin therapy. Neither steroids nor antibiotics are indicated. Steroids may actually be detrimental.

50.   **You deliver a child at 36-weeks gestation and intestines are protruding from a defect in the abdominal wall. On inspection, you note that the intestines lack a peritoneal covering:**

a. A gastroschisis is a defect in the umbilical ring that allows the intestines to protrude out of the abdominal cavity in a sac.

b. An omphalocele is a defect in the abdominal wall that allows the evisceration of abdominal structures without a sac being present.

c. Gastroschisis and omphalocele are invariably fatal within hours.

d. You are twice as likely to encounter gastroschisis as you are to see omphalocele.

e. Emergency department treatment for gastroschisis involves gastric decompression; this same treatment is contraindicated in omphalocele.

The answer is d. Gastroschisis is a defect in the abdominal wall that allows the antenatal evisceration of abdominal structures without a sac being present. Omphalocele is a defect in the umbilical ring that allows the intestines to protrude out of the abdominal cavity in a sac. Gastroschisis occurs twice as frequently as omphalocele. ED treatment involved gastric decompression and placing an occlusive plastic covering to prevent heat and water loss.

51.   **A 3-month-old girl is irritable, feeds poorly, and breaks into a profuse sweat whenever she takes the nipple. She is tachypneic and pale. You determine that her heart rate is 280/min. Chest x-ray shows a large heart with alveolar infiltrates. You know that:**

a. Jugular venous distension and peripheral edema are commonly found in infants with this condition.

b. Volume replacement is the most essential treatment.

c. Heart rate is the least malleable of the cardiovascular parameters.

d. Cardioversion with 0.01 J/kg is indicated for profound shock.

e. Digoxin and diuretics are the mainstay of treatment. Stable patients may be treated with vagal maneuvers.

The answer is e. The most common cause of congestive heart failure (CHF) in children is congenital heart disease, which often masquerades as other problems such as pneumonia or sepsis. The predominant symptoms of congenital heart disease include poor feeding, excessive diaphoresis, irritability or lethargy with feeding, weak cry and, in severe cases, grunting and nasal flaring. Tachypnea is a cardinal sign. Since feeding is the infant's primary form of exertion, dyspnea and sweating during feeding can often be elicited in the history. Peripheral edema, jugular venous distention, and rales are unusual and late signs in infants. Heart rate is the most malleable of the cardiac physiologic parameters. The most common pediatric dysrhythmia is paroxysmal supraventricular tachycardia. Initial management of unstable patients with narrow complex tachycardia consists of immediate synchronized cardioversion at 0.5 J/kg with increases in power output to 2 J/kg as needed. In the stable patient, vagal maneuvers are the intervention of choice. If vagal maneuvers are not successful in the stable patient, IV adenosine (0.1 mg/kg, maximum first dose 6 mg) followed by a higher dose (0.2 mg/kg, maximum 12 mg) can be used.

52.   **A 2-year-old child mistook a bottle of her uncle's "cancer vitamins" for candy. She is comatose, hypotensive, and bradycardic, but her skin is pink. Antidotal therapy includes:**

a. Sodium nitrite to induce methemoglobinemia.

b. Methylene blue to induce methemoglobinemia.

c. Sodium thiosulfate to produce cyanomethemoglobin.

d. Sodium nitrite to bind cyanide.

e. Amyl nitrite to induce a methemoglobinemia of 50%.

The answer is a. Amygdalin is a cyanogenic glycoside that is found in particularly high concentrations in apricot pits and bitter almonds. It is the principal constituent of laetrile, a compound popular for nontraditional cancer therapies in the late 1970s (still available through the Internet). The clinical signs and symptoms of cyanide poisoning mimic those of hypoxia, with one exception: unless respiratory arrest has occurred, patients are not cyanotic. The pediatric antidote doses are 0.33 mL/kg of 10% sodium nitrite and 1.65 mL/kg of 25% sodium thiosulfate. Methemoglobin (MetHb) formation is the goal of the sodium nitrite: cyanide has a high affinity for MetHb and readily leaves cytochrome oxidase to form cyanomethemoglobin.

53. **The component of the medical evaluation considered most important in identifying sexual abuse in the prepubertal child is:**
    a. Greeting.
    b. History containing the child's disclosure.
    c. Physical examination.
    d. Laboratory cultures for sexually transmitted diseases.
    e. Photographs of the child.

    The answer is b. In incidents of child sexual abuse, the interview with the child typically is the most valuable component of the medical evaluation. Elicited history frequently is the only diagnostic information that is discovered. Additionally, if performed in a sensitive and knowledgeable manner, the history-taking process can be a first step in the healing process for the child who has been sexually traumatized. Regardless of the history provided, the members of the interdisciplinary team need to demonstrate an open, nonjudgmental, and caring attitude toward the child, which clearly demonstrates their willingness to advocate for the child as the evaluation unfolds. All of the listed characteristics, however, can contribute to the diagnosis of sexual abuse.

CHAPTER 20 Medical Imaging

Thomas G. Costantino, MD

1. A 60-year-old woman with a history of high blood pressure presents with left flank pain that started suddenly and has been present for 6 hours. Her heart rate is 120/min, and her blood pressure is 180/120 mm Hg. Ultrasound of the mid abdomen in the sagittal plane is shown in Figure 20-1. Your next step should be:

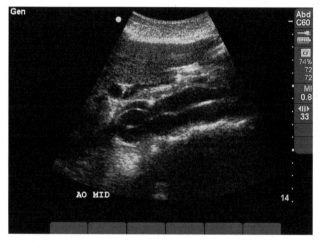

Figure 20–1

a. Consult vascular surgery immediately, as the patient has an abdominal aortic aneurysm (AAA).

b. Start intravenous antihypertensive medication with a goal of mean arterial pressure (MAP) of 90 mm Hg and prepare for further imaging to determine type of aortic dissection (AD).

c. Ask the patient if she is serving as a surrogate mother, as the image clearly shows a developing fetus.

d. Give intravenous analgesia since the patient has kidney stones.

e. Reassure the patient that there is nothing wrong.

The answer is b. While the aorta has a normal diameter of <3 cm, it does show a linear density in the lumen consistent with an intimal flap. The presence of an undulating intimal flap is pathognomonic for aortic dissection. Transthoracic echocardiography has a reported sensitivity of 80% for diagnosing aortic dissection, while transesophageal echocardiography brings that closer to 90%. Transabdominal ultrasound can only detect dissection that extends from the thoracic into the abdominal aorta. Contrast-enhanced multidetector chest CT is becoming accepted as test of choice to diagnose and classify aortic dissection, with a sensitivity reported to be 93% (Khandheria et al., 1989:17–24; Marx et al., 2006:1328).

2.   **A 65-year-old man complains of a sudden onset of back pain while he was drying dishes. His blood pressure is 70/50 mm Hg, with a heart rate of 133/min. Ultrasound images of the right upper quadrant in longitudinal plane and of the mid abdomen in transverse plane are shown in Figure 20-2A and B. What should you do next?**

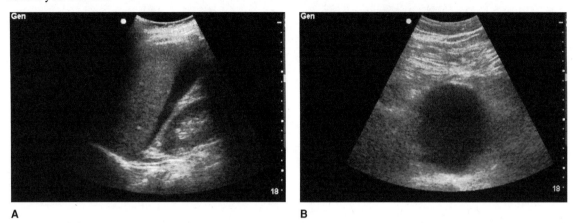

A   B

Figure 20–2

a.   The patient has free intraperitoneal fluid but a normal aorta. This is probably ascites. Treat with colloid fluid and arrange or perform paracentesis.

b.   The patient has an aortic dissection. You should immediately move the probe to the heart looking for pericardial tamponade.

c.   There is a clot in the inferior vena cava. Order intravenous tPA for suspected saddle pulmonary embolism.

d.   The large abdominal aortic aneurysm and free intraperitoneal fluid in this patient suggest ruptured abdominal aortic aneurysm (AAA). The patient should immediately go to the operating room for repair by vascular surgery.

e.   The gall bladder is distended with a thickened wall and pericholecystic fluid. Start intravenous antibiotics and arrange for surgical consultation.

The answer is d: Emergency physicians have been shown to diagnose AAA with a sensitivity of nearly 100%. In the setting of an unstable patient, bedside ultrasound is the best modality to diagnose ruptured AAA. These images show a 10-cm AAA with free fluid in Morrison's pouch, representing intraperitoneal rupture. Only approximately 35% of ruptured AAAs bleed in the peritoneum. CT angiography is 100% sensitive and provides anatomic detail as well as detects small ruptures, so is the test of choice in more stable patients. With overall mortality of 80–90% once ruptured, and at least 50% for those who make it to the operating room, emergent operative repair is the procedure of choice (Tayal et al., 2003:867–871; Marx et al., 2006:1339).

3. A 21-year-old woman complains of vaginal bleeding for 2 days. Her last menstrual period was 4 weeks ago, but lighter than normal. Her vital signs are within normal limits. Quantitative serum beta-hCG is 17,000. Her blood type is O positive. Transvaginal ultrasound images are shown in Figure 20-3A and B. Your next step should be:

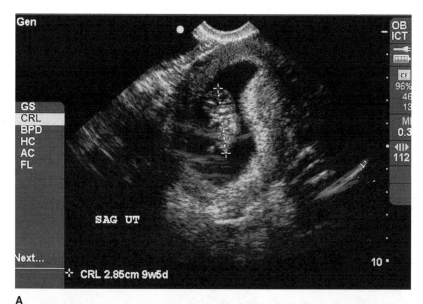

A

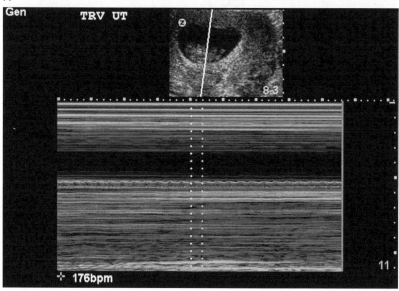

B

Figure 20–3

a. Consult obstetrics for emergent laparoscopy for ruptured ectopic pregnancy.
b. Give intramuscular methotrexate to treat for nonruptured tubal pregnancy.
c. Arrange follow-up in 2 or 3 days for repeat quantitative beta-hCG if symptoms persist.
d. Tell her she had a miscarriage.
e. Tell her she can expect twins.

The answer is c. Approximately 25% of women with a clinically recognized pregnancy experience some vaginal bleeding, with nearly half of those resulting in miscarriage. However, if a normal heart rate can be identified with ultrasound, more than 85% will reach term. In addition, ultrasound identification of intrauterine pregnancy (IUP) makes the risk of concurrent ectopic pregnancy less than 1 in 4000. A yolk sac can be seen with a beta-hCG of approximately 1700, and is the earliest ultrasound marker of an IUP. Fetal heart motion is usually seen with beat-hCG levels of around 17,000. When a heartbeat is identified, M-mode ultrasound is used to measure fetal heart rate as demonstrated in Figure 20-3B (Houry and Abbott, 2006:2741).

4.   **Another 21-year-old woman complains of vaginal bleeding for 2 days. Her last menstrual period was 4 weeks ago, but lighter than normal. Her vital signs are within normal limits. Quantitative serum beta-hCG is 17,000. Her blood type is O positive. Transvaginal ultrasound images are shown in Figure 20-4A and B. Your next step should be:**

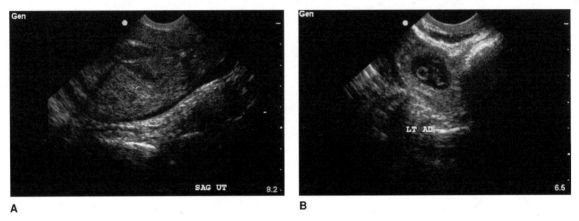

Figure 20–4

a. Consult obstetrics for emergent laparoscopy for ruptured ectopic pregnancy.

b. Give intramuscular methotrexate to treat for nonruptured tubal pregnancy.

c. Arrange follow-up in 2 or 3 days for repeat quantitative beta-hCG if symptoms persist.

d. Tell her she had a miscarriage.

e. Tell her she can expect twins.

The answer is a. Ultrasound is the primary diagnostic method to detect ectopic pregnancy and should be done on every symptomatic first trimester patient without a known intrauterine pregnancy (IUP). Although ectopic pregnancy will be present in approximately 10% of symptomatic first trimester ER patients, ultrasound will only be definitely diagnostic in approximately one-third of these on the initial visit. Figure 20-4A shows a uterus with a thick endometrial stripe but no IUP. Also noted is a black stripe posterior to the uterus in the pouch of Douglas, which represents free peritoneal fluid (blood). Figure 20-4B shows a gestational sac with a fetal pole and yolk sac in the left adnexa. This is a definite ectopic pregnancy. The presence of free fluid suggesting rupture and an hCG level >15,000 are relative contraindications for methotrexate; this would require operative removal (Marx et al., 2006: 2743–2746).

5. A third 21-year-old woman complains of vaginal bleeding for 2 days. Her last menstrual period was 4 weeks ago, but lighter than normal. Her vital signs are within normal limits. Quantitative serum beta-hCG is 317,000. Her blood type is O positive. Transvaginal ultrasound images are shown in Figure 20-5. Your next step should be:

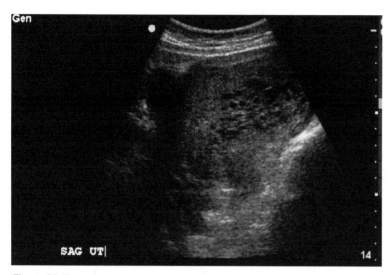

Figure 20–5

a. Consult obstetrics for molar pregnancy.

b. Give methotrexate.

c. Arrange for follow-up in 2–3 days for repeat hCG if symptoms persist.

d. Tell her she had a miscarriage.

e. Tell her she can expect triplets.

The answer is a. This image demonstrates one of the classic ultrasonographic appearances of a molar pregnancy. Often described as a cluster of grapes, it is an echogenic intrauterine mass with multiple small hypoechoic vesicles. Alternately a more echogenic appearance is referred to as a "snowstorm." Ultrasound is only 17% sensitive for partial moles and 58% sensitive for complete moles in the first trimester, so this condition is more frequently diagnosed in the second trimester. Prompt surgical removal is the preferred treatment and usually leads to favorable outcome. Approximately 80% of gestational trophoblastic disease is benign molar pregnancy, with 12% being invasive mole, and 8% choriocarcinoma. It is often diagnosed on ultrasound with symptomatic vaginal bleeding and a markedly elevated serum hCG level of >100,000 mIU/mL (Marx et al., 2006:2747).

6.   A 40-year-old woman was involved in a motor vehicle crash. She has normal vital signs and only mild abdominal pain. You perform an ultrasound to evaluate for hemoperitoneum. While sweeping the right upper quadrant, you obtain the image shown in Figure 20-6, which demonstrates:

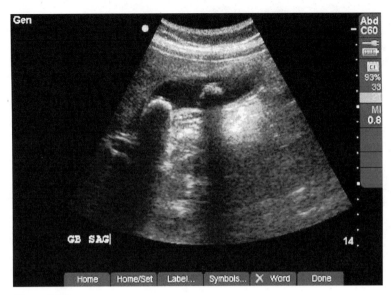

Figure 20–6

a. Sludge in the gallbladder.

b. A normal gallbladder.

c. Cholelithiasis.

d. Liver laceration.

e. Ruptured diaphragm.

The answer is c. Cholelithiasis occurs in 20% of women older than 40 years in the United States. Approximately 80% of these will remain asymptomatic, while 20% develop biliary colic and one-quarter of these (5% overall) develop acute cholecystitis. Gallstones are echogenic on ultrasound and cast a posterior acoustic shadow. In an asymptomatic patient, where gallstones are incidentally found, no treatment is recommended. In patients with more than one episode of biliary colic, laparoscopic cholecystectomy is the recommended treatment (Marx et al., 2006:1420).

7. **A 40-year-old woman complains of epigastric pain, vomiting, and fever for 12 hours. Symptoms occurred 2 hours after she ate popcorn at a movie. You suspect acute cholecystitis and perform a right upper quadrant ultrasound, shown in Figure 20-7, which shows:**

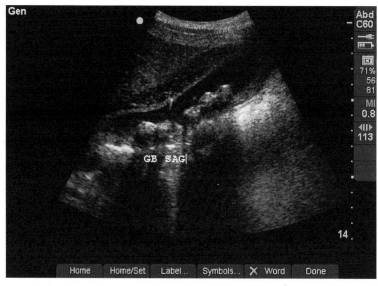

Figure 20–7

a. Multiple gallstones with a thickened gallbladder wall and pericholecystic fluid confirming acute cholecystitis.

b. Gallstones but no other abnormalities, suggesting biliary colic.

c. A normal gallbladder, suggesting a nonbiliary cause of her symptoms.

d. A loop of duodenum, keep looking for the gallbladder.

e. A rare hepatic ectopic pregnancy.

The answer is a. The image shows multiple echogenic areas casting dark shadows within an anechoic lumen. This is consistent with a gallbladder with multiple gallstones. Although not measured in this image, the gallbladder wall appears thickened and measured 1.5 cm on ultrasound and pathology. The findings of gallstones and a thick gallbladder wall (>3 mm) have a 95% positive predictive value for acute cholecystitis. A positive sonographic Murphy sign and pericholecystic fluid are other markers of acute cholecystitis. Admission to the hospital for analgesia and antibiotics is the initial treatment with early surgical intervention for most patients (Marx et al., 2006:1422).

8.   A 28-year-old woman complains of sharp right flank pain radiating to her right lower abdomen for 2 days. The pain is intermittent, with colicky episodes lasting several minutes. Her vital signs are normal and her pregnancy test is negative. Her urinalysis shows microscopic blood. She has right costovertebral tenderness to percussion. You perform an emergency ultrasound of her right kidney (see Figure 20-8). Based on this image and her clinical features, your next step should be:

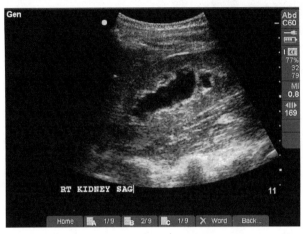

Figure 20–8

a. Admit her for intravenous antibiotics.

b. Call the surgeon to take her for exploratory laparotomy for intraperitoneal hemorrhage.

c. Congratulate her on her new pregnancy.

d. Achieve pain control, ensure she can tolerate oral intake, and discharge her for follow-up with a urologist.

e. Talk with your urologist about emergent ureteral stent placement.

The answer is d. This ultrasound image shows moderate hydronephrosis. Although it has poor sensitivity in detecting ureteral stones, ultrasound is approximately 90% sensitive for detecting hydronephrosis and in the proper clinical setting is a good imaging choice for renal colic. However not all patients with renal colic require imaging. CT scan is the test of choice if the diagnosis is in doubt. Inpatient care is required for patients with urinary tract infections and those with intractable vomiting or pain. Most others can be discharged with urologic follow-up within 2 weeks and proper analgesia, even if their stone size suggests low likelihood of spontaneous passage (Marx et al., 2006:1590–1592).

9.   A 22-year-old man was the driver of a motorcycle that collided with a tractor-trailer. He arrives unconscious with a heart rate of 144/min and a blood pressure of 80/55 mm Hg. You perform rapid sequence intubation and initialize resuscitation by ATLS protocol. You then perform a FAST (focused assessment by sonography in trauma) examination, shown in Figure 20-9. Your next step should be:

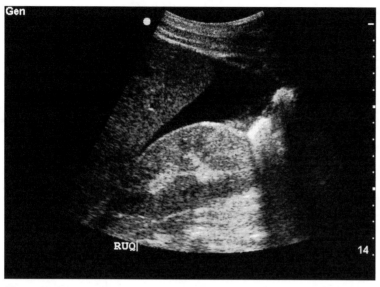

Figure 20–9

a. Arrange for the patient to immediately go to the operating room for an exploratory laparotomy for intraperitoneal hemorrhage.

b. Arrange for the patient to undergo emergent surgery for traumatic aortic rupture.

c. Perform a bedside thoracotomy to relieve pericardial tamponade.

d. Insert bilateral large bore thoracostomy tubes for hemothorax.

e. Perform diagnostic peritoneal lavage prior to making any further decision.

The answer is a. This image shows free intraperitoneal fluid in Morrison's pouch, the potential space between the liver and right kidney. This is the single most sensitive part of the FAST examination. Overall, FAST has a sensitivity of approximately 90% for hemoperitoneum. FAST has largely replaced DPL as a screening tool for intraperitoneal hemorrhage in trauma evaluations. Although ultrasound has also been shown to have high sensitivity for pericardial effusion and hemothorax and those are part of the FAST examination, this image does not show those. In the trauma patient with a positive fast and signs of hemorrhagic shock (low BP, elevated HR), immediate exploratory laparotomy is the procedure of choice (Marx et al., 2006:312).

10.   **A 30-year-old man was in a motor vehicle crash and now complains of difficulty breathing and left chest pain. Vital signs are: heart rate 120/min, BP 120/90 mm Hg, respiratory rate 32/min, and pulse oximetry 96%. His portable chest x-ray is interpreted as unremarkable. During the FAST, you obtain the image shown in Figure 20-10. Your next step should be:**

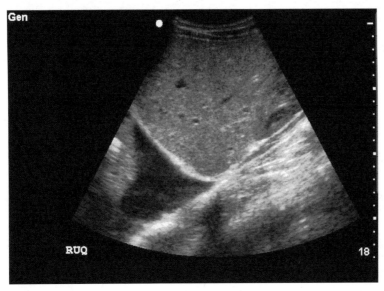

Figure 20–10

a.   Arrange for him to go immediately to the operating room for an exploratory laparotomy for intraperitoneal hemorrhage.

b.   Perform bedside thoracotomy for pericardial tamponade.

c.   Insert a large bore tube in the left chest to treat massive hemothorax.

d.   Insert a rectal tube to decompress the large bowel.

e.   Perform diagnostic peritoneal lavage before making any further decision.

The answer is c. Ultrasound has been shown to be more than 90% sensitive for hemothorax from blunt trauma, comparable to chest radiography. Hemothorax is identified by seeing an anechoic (black) area above the diaphragm in the right or left upper quadrant view of the FAST examination and by seeing the posterior thoracic wall. Normally this area would have similar echogenicity to the liver or spleen due to an artifact and the posterior thoracic wall would not be seen. In blunt chest trauma leading to hemothorax, placement of a large bore chest tube is the procedure of choice (Ma and Mateer, 2003:78).

11. A 55-year-old man complains of shortness of breath. He is drenched in sweat. Vital signs: oral temperature 98.7°F; heart rate 130/min; blood pressure 85/70 mm Hg. His EKG shows only sinus tachycardia. You begin resuscitation with intravenous normal saline solution. You consider other causes for shock and perform an ultrasound of his heart and aorta, with one view shown in Figure 20-11. You diagnose:

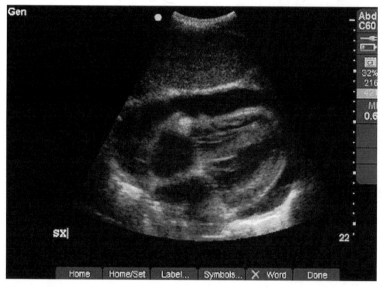

Figure 20–11

a. Pericardial tamponade and prepare for emergency pericardiocentesis.

b. Pulmonary embolism and prepare to give tPA.

c. Acute MI and alert the catheterization laboratory.

d. Tension pneumothorax and reach for a needle to perform emergent decompression.

e. Atrial myxoma and prepare to write a case report.

The answer is a. This is a subxyphoid view of the heart showing a large pericardial effusion. The right ventricle is relatively collapsed during this diastolic view (as evidenced by the noncollapsed left ventricle). True cardiac tamponade is defined as a pericardial effusion causing circulatory collapse, as manifested by this patient's hypotension and tachycardia. Although cardiac tamponade is a rare cause of unexplained hypotension presenting to the ED (approximately 1%), it is immediately reversible and should be diagnosed as rapidly as possible (Tayal et al., 2003:92–93).

12.   **A 38-year-old previously healthy man complains of a left thigh rash for 2 days. His leg is erythematous and warm to the touch. The lesion is approximately 5 cm in diameter but not fluctuant. You perform an ultrasound of the area, shown in Figure 20-12. Which of the following is your next step?**

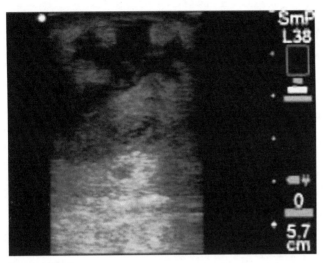

Figure 20–12

    a. Perform an incision and drainage to evacuate the pus, then pack the wound for continued drainage.

    b. Give intravenous vancomycin and admit for further treatment of MRSA cellulitis.

    c. Draw a line around the erythematous area, start oral antibiotics, and have the patient return for a wound check in 24 hours.

    d. Start intravenous heparin for a deep venous thrombosis and arrange admission.

    e. Start subcutaneous low molecular weight heparin and arrange for appropriate outpatient follow-up.

The answer is a. Subcutaneous abscesses usually have a hypoechoic appearance on ultrasound with some hyperechoic debris that may be seen moving within the abscess on real-time sonography. There is also some thickening of the surrounding subcutaneous tissue. Cellulitis often has thickening of the subcutaneous tissue with "cobblestoning" of lucent irregular lines in the subcutaneous fat but no discreet collection. Simple incision and drainage is still the treatment of choice for most subcutaneous abscesses (Dewitz and Frazee, 2003:363–364).

13.   A 42-year-old man has been short of breath for 2 days. You find a swollen right leg, which the patient had noted initially about 2 weeks ago. You perform bedside ultrasound of the right leg, and see the image shown in Figure 20-13 just below the right inguinal crease in the transverse position. When you apply downward pressure on the probe, appearance of the image does not change. What is your next step?

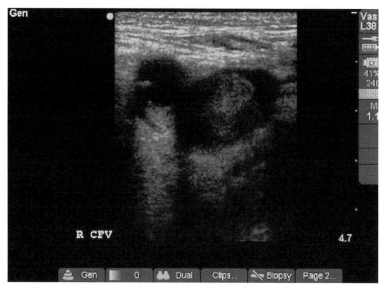

Figure 20–13

a. You should arrange for formal studies, as without color flow or Doppler you cannot interpret this image.

b. Although the image is normal, pulmonary embolism is a concern and further imaging of the chest is warranted.

c. Start intravenous antibiotics and search for signs of infection as this image shows a large inguinal lymph node.

d. Start intravenous heparin for right common femoral vein deep venous thrombosis. With the patient's dyspnea, pulmonary embolism is also a concern and further imaging to confirm this is warranted.

e. Arrange for orthopedic follow-up so the patient can get definitive diagnosis and treatment for his soft-tissue tumor.

The answer is d. This image shows an echogenic collection in the right common femoral vein. The lack of compression confirms the diagnosis of DVT. Vein compression alone is sufficient to diagnose or exclude DVT in most studies with Doppler flow relegated to a secondary role. Lower extremity DVT is the most common source for pulmonary embolism and a patient with a DVT with symptoms suggesting a PE should have further imaging (chest CT, ventilation–perfusion scan, or pulmonary angiography) to diagnose this (Blaivas, 2003:335–347).

14. **A 70-year-old man is diagnosed with pneumonia, but is otherwise stable. He is being admitted to the hospital, but the nurse tells you she and two other nurses have been unable to establish an intravenous line for antibiotic administration. Your next step should be:**

a. Start an intravenous line in the common femoral vein.

b. Use standard landmarks to insert an intravenous line in the internal jugular vein or subclavian vein.

c. Use real-time ultrasound guidance to insert an intravenous line in the jugular vein or subclavian vein.

d. Perform a proximal saphenous vein cutdown.

e. Insert an intraosseous line in the proximal tibia.

The answer is c. In a 2001 report titled "Making Healthcare Safer," the Agency for Healthcare Research and Quality listed real-time ultrasound guidance of all central venous catheters as one of 11 patient safety practices that should be widely implemented to reduce medical error. Ultrasound guidance has been shown to increase success, and decrease complications, time, and the number of percutaneous punctures from central venous access. When available, ultrasound guidance should be routinely used (Roberts and Hedges, 2003:434; www.ahrq.gov/Clinic/ptsafety/summary.htm).

15. A 7-month-old boy fell and hit his head. He had a brief loss of consciousness followed by two episodes of vomiting prior to arrival. You notice a 3-cm scalp hematoma, but he is otherwise uninjured. Vital Signs are within normal limits. A slice from his noncontrast head CT is shown in Figure 20-14. Shortly after he returns from radiology, he becomes obtunded with a Glasgow Coma Scale score of 7 and you decide to intubate the patient. In performing rapid sequence intubation, the most appropriate choice of medications for this patient is:

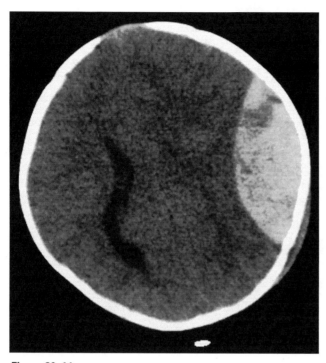

Figure 20–14

a. Etomidate (0.3 mg/kg IV) and succinylcholine (2 mg/kg IV).

b. Ketamine (2 mg/kg IV) and vecuronium (0.2 mg/kg IV).

c. Ketamine (2 mg/kg IV) and succinylcholine (2 mg/kg IV).

d. Lidocaine (1.5 mg/kg IV), thiopental (3 mg/kg IV), and vecuronium (0.2 mg/kg IV).

e. Etomidate (0.3 mg/kg IV), succinylcholine (2 mg/kg IV), and fentanyl (3 μg/kg IV).

The answer is d. This patient has a traumatic epidural hematoma on his noncontrast head CT. Care should be taken to avoid using RSI agents such as ketamine that may increase intracranial pressure in head-injured patients in order to reduce the risk of herniation. Giving succinylcholine without pretreating with a nondepolarizing agent also risks increasing ICP. Pretreatment with agents known to reduce intracranial pressure such as lidocaine or fentanyl is ideal. Given the lack of systemic injury, thiopental is an acceptable alternative to etomidate, although both agents are known decrease intracranial pressure (Danzl and Vissers, 2003:108–119).

16. **A 75-year-old man fell 1 week ago at home. He has had a mild headache since then, but is otherwise well. One hour ago, he fell again with a brief loss of consciousness but now has a GCS of 15. On examination, he has a left occipital hematoma. You are at a small rural hospital and obtain the CT image shown in Figure 20-15. What does the CT reveal?**

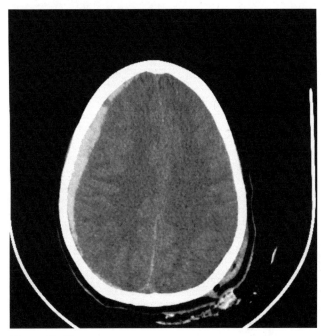

Figure 20–15

a. This shows a subacute subdural hematoma. The patient can be admitted to his primary care physician's service and be seen by social services for placement owing to frequent falls.

b. This shows an acute subdural hematoma. The patient should be transferred to the nearest facility with a neurosurgeon, as he may need emergent operative drainage.

c. The patient only has an extracranial hematoma and can be discharged with an icepack.

d. There is no time for transfer. You must perform an emergent burr hole on the right as the patient has an expanding epidural hematoma.

e. This shows a chronic subdural hematoma and the patient can be followed as an outpatient.

The answer is b. This image shows an acute right frontal-parietal subdural hematoma. The patient also has a left occipital extracranial hematoma. This represents the classic coup and contrecoup injury pattern seen in many head injuries. Acute blood (immediate up to 3 days) is hyperdense on CT scan with Hounsfield units (HU) between 50 and 90. Subacute subdurals (3 days to 2 weeks) is isodense on CT scan with between 20 and 50 HU. Chronic subdurals (greater than 2 weeks) are hypodense on CT scans, approximately 5–10 HU. A mixture of densities suggests a mixture of subdural types. Subdural hematomas are more common in elderly patients with only 20% surviving to hospital discharge. All acute subdural hematomas should be evaluated by a neurosurgeon (Marx et al., 2006:346, 373).

17.   **A 50-year-old woman is brought from home after being found unresponsive. She is obtunded with rectal temperature 99.5°F, heart rate 110/min, blood pressure 170/100 mm Hg. Following rapid sequence intubation, you obtain the CT shown in Figure 20-16. Your next step should be:**

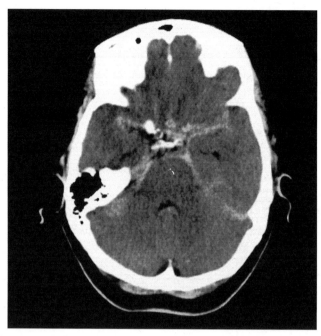

Figure 20–16

   a. Perform an emergent burrhole.
   b. Give intravenous tPA and consult neurology.
   c. Give nimodipine, acetaminophen, and consult neurosurgery.
   d. Admit to the ICU with supportive care, as the head CT is normal.
   e. Give intravenous antibiotics and steroids.

The answer is c. Figure 20-16 shows a subarachnoid hemorrhage (SAH) with blood in the suprasellar cistern. Eighty percent of SAH occurs from ruptured saccular aneurysms from the circle of Willis. CT scan is the test of choice for SAH with a sensitivity of nearly 100% in the first 12 hours but dropping to 90% by 24 hours. Lumbar puncture has a sensitivity of 100% and should be considered in patients with a suggestive clinical picture and negative CT scan. Her obtunded state on arrival puts her at a Hunt and Hess scale grade 5 SAH, which has the poorest prognosis. Patients with grade 3 or higher are at risk for hypercapnia, which can lead to increased intracranial pressure, and so should be intubated. Nimodipine 60 mg orally should be given to lessen the occurance of spasm and ischemic stroke. Analgesia can be used to decrease pain and resultant catecholamine surges. Antipyretics are also used for hyperthermia. The role of surgery versus coiling is controversial and should be done in consultation with neurosurgery (Marx et al., 2006:1635–1636).

18.   A 29-year-old man complains of vague abdominal pain for 2 days with vomiting, diarrhea and anorexia. Vital signs: oral temperature 99.1°F, heart rate 85/min, blood pressure 114/68 mm Hg. He has bilateral lower abdominal tenderness with peritoneal signs. He recounts two previous, similar episodes in the past 5 years that spontaneously resolved. A slice of his abdominal CT is shown in Figure 20-17. Your next step should be:

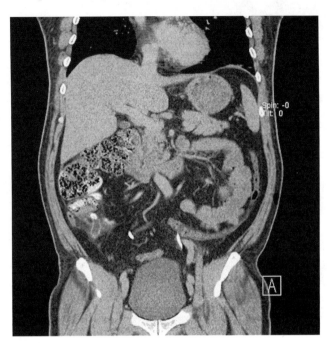

Figure 20–17

a. Consult surgery for acute appendicitis.

b. Consult surgery for pneumoperitoneum.

c. Consult gastroenterology for suspected Crohn's disease.

d. Consult surgery for spontaneous splenic rupture.

e. Admit for pancreatitis.

The answer is a. This coronal CT reconstruction of the abdomen shows an appendicolith with distal appendiceal thickening and periappendiceal stranding in the right lower quadrant. The appendix is a hollow, closed end tube arising from the posterior medial surface of the cecum. It is usually about 10 cm long. The majority of cases of acute appendicitis are caused by an acute obstruction of the lumen by an appendicolith. Abdominal CT has been shown to increase the accuracy of the diagnosis of appendicitis with a sensitivity of 87–100% and specificity of 89–98%. The presence of an appendicolith with appendiceal thickening (>6 mm) and pericecal stranding are used to diagnose appendicitis on CT. Rectal contrast works best but oral contrast with a 90-minute delay is also effective. Although controversy exists about the routine use of CT scanning, for patients with a moderate suspicion and other likely diagnoses, CT is recommended. Surgical removal is the treatment of choice (Marx et al., 2006:1451–1457).

19. A 28-year-old woman complains of sharp right chest pain, worse when she breathes, since smoking marijuana earlier that day. Vital signs: oral temperature 98.9°F, heart rate 90/min, blood pressure 110/55 mm Hg, pulse oximetry 99% on room air. Her physical examination is unremarkable. Her chest x-ray is shown in Figure 20-18. Your next step should be:

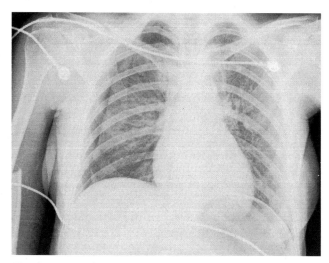

Figure 20–18

a. Order a stat echocardiogram.

b. Insert a nasogastric tube, insufflate with 200 mL of air, and repeat the chest x-ray.

c. Place on 100% oxygen and observe for 6 hours. Patient may be discharged home if the repeat chest x-ray is ok with follow-up within 24 hours.

d. Arrange for emergent chest CT with contrast to rule-out aortic dissection.

e. Give appropriate analgesia and discharge home—this is a negative study.

The answer is c. This chest x-ray shows a small (25%) pneumothorax on the right. The size of the pneumothorax can be determined by measuring the intrapleural distance in 3 spots. The average distance in millimeters is approximately the average percent of pneumothorax. For small spontaneous pneumothorax, symptoms often resolve within 24 hours and the physical examination in unreliable. Upright chest x-ray is the classic test of choice to diagnose pneumothorax with expiratory films adding little value. Management of small primary spontaneous pneumothorax is controversial with observation, simple aspiration, and classic tube thoracostomy all being appropriate interventions. The risk of recurrence is approximately 33% (Marx et al., 2006:1143–1148).

20.   **A 58-year-old man has a long history of dyspepsia for which he frequently takes over the counter antacids. For the past 2 days his epigastric pain is worse and is constant. Vital signs: oral temperature 99.0°F, heart rate 110/min, blood pressure 158/90 mm Hg. His abdomen is rigid and you note decreased bowel sounds. The x-ray showed in Figure 20-19 was obtained. Your next step would be to:**

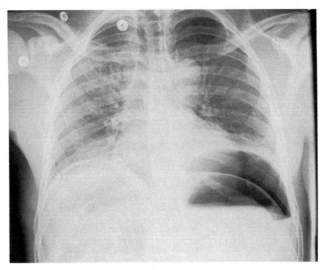

Figure 20–19

a. Perform an immediate paracentesis.

b. Consult surgery for perforated hollow viscus.

c. Give oral contrast and take to CT scan for further evaluation.

d. Start a proton pump inhibitor and refer to a gastroenterologist.

e. Begin high-dose somatostatin therapy and consult gastroenterology.

The answer is b: This upright chest x-ray shows free air under the diaphragms, consistent with perforated peptic ulcer. PUD is common in the United States but only 7% experience perforation. Ninety-five percent of these patients will require emergent operative intervention. The upright chest x-ray is approximately 70% sensitive for detecting perforation from peptic ulcer disease. Although, instillation of 500 mL of air, or lateral decubitus films may help improve the sensitivity, CT abdomen (either no contrast or with oral contrast) is the next best test if perforation is suspected and the initial x-ray is negative (Sabiston, 852–857).

CHAPTER 21

Administrative Emergency Medicine, Emergency Medical Services, and Ethics

Richard Martin, MD, FAAEM, Liza D. Lê, MD, and Scott H. Plantz, MD, FAAEM

1. **For a hospital to maximize the value of its emergency department, it must realize that the ED serves as:**

   a. The window through which the community sees and judges the hospital.

   b. Only a minor source of admissions to the hospital.

   c. An area of low risk.

   d. The place from which to screen away people unable to pay for inpatient care.

   e. An area that can generate very large profits.

   The answer is a. The emergency department is the window through which the community sees the hospital, and for many serves as the front door of the hospital. The majority of hospital beds are filled by patients admitted through the ED. But the ED is also an area of instability in which there is the potential for major adverse events. The hospital has a moral obligation to provide access to the community for emergencies, and a legal mandate to provide care to all who seek it.

2. **Emergency department throughput is most effected by:**

   a. Internal departmental operations.

   b. Radiology turnaround times.

   c. Laboratory turnaround times.

   d. Waiting times for admitted patients.

   e. Consultant availability.

   The answer is d. The time from triage to disposition of the ED patient is affected by the overall functioning of the entire hospital, and cannot be solved by modifying ED operational issues in isolation. The largest single impact on ED throughput is the bed space occupied by patients awaiting admission. Prolonged ED waiting times can have major legal repercussions, by delaying treatment of critically ill patients.

3. **Emergency physician billing is based on levels of care, as defined by the Centers for Medicare and Medicaid Services (CMS), previously known as the Health Care Financing Administration (HCFA), with level I being the briefest patient encounter, and level VI being intensive care of the critically ill patient:**
   a. Most admitted patients should be at least level V.
   b. The average reimbursement difference between level IV and V is $40.
   c. With sufficient documentation, an ankle sprain can be a level V.
   d. The "decision-making" section of the chart, including differential, must be filled out for a level V.
   e. For a level V, medical, social, and family history must all be documented.

   The answer is a. Most admitted patients will receive a full evaluation in the ED, and thus can be appropriately documented as level V. A substantial number, but not the majority, will have prolonged monitoring and/or critical care procedures, to be level VI. Level V requires documentation of two out of three of medical, social, and family histories. For level V, medical decision-making must be addressed, with differential diagnoses and plan of management. Simple problems, such as an ankle sprain, will not rise above level III, no matter how extensive the documentation.

4. **Cost containment measures in the ED can be approached in a systemic fashion, recognizing that:**
   a. CT scans are both expensive to perform and result in high charges to the patient.
   b. The Joint Commission (formerly The Joint Commission on the Accreditation of Healthcare Organizations, or JCAHO), requires documentation of cost-containment efforts.
   c. The number of tests ordered will have a major impact on reimbursement for most hospitalized patients.
   d. Obtaining pulse oximetry on each patient will not lead to significant increase in charges.
   e. Use of oral rather than parenteral medications will have a significant impact on cost containment.

   The answer is e. JCAHO does not require that cost-containment issues be addressed. CT scans are expensive in terms of billing, but the marginal cost of obtaining a CT scan is minimal. Oral rather than parenteral medications are less costly to provide, in terms of the actual cost of the medication and in the additional nursing time required for the parenteral form. Pulse oximetry is a valuable fifth vital sign, but increases charges significantly.

5. **Emergency department management of pneumonia is the focus of certain quality indicators in ED performance measurement:**
   a. The quality indicators for pneumonia—blood culture and timely administration of antibiotics—are derived from expert consensus panels and are generally accepted as appropriate by the EM community.
   b. The Joint Commission requires all patients with pneumonia to receive antibiotics within 6 hours of arrival.
   c. Compliance with indicators can have an adverse effect on nonmandated processes.
   d. Results of blood cultures direct a change in therapy only approximately 10% of the time.
   e. Indicators for pneumonia do not restrict physician judgment in selecting specific antibiotic therapy.

   The answer is c. Focus on pneumonia necessarily draws resources from other clinical problems. Not all patients with pneumonia are required to receive antibiotics within 6 hours, as long as it is documented that the clinical presentation was atypical and not suggestive of pneumonia. The results of blood cultures rarely influence individual patient management. Most patients with pneumonia should have antibiotics chosen in concordance with the combined American Thoracic Society/Infectious Disease Society consensus guidelines. The indicators that have been chosen are not universally accepted as valid and are the subject of ongoing controversy within the ED community.

6. **Committee meetings direct much hospital policy and performance. Such meetings:**

   a. Generally have clear criteria and objectives.

   b. May cost the hospital as much as $1200 per meeting.

   c. Are most effective when specific plans for follow-up are made.

   d. Are not productive without a disciplined agenda.

   e. Are not of importance to the busy clinician.

   The answer is c. Meetings are of most value when there is specific responsibility for follow-up of each decision, with delineated responsibility for implementation. Meetings are quite expensive, in terms of the salaried time of the participants, but are often ineffective, due to lack of planning and purpose. However, because unexpected issues arise, it is not always most productive to follow a rigid agenda. Clinicians who choose not to participate in meetings should then expect to have to follow policies that were constructed without their input.

7. **Emergency Medical Treatment and Active Labor Act (EMTALA) laws are applicable to every patient arriving at the ED. To remain EMTALA-compliant, it should be understood that:**

   a. A tertiary hospital cannot refuse a patient in transfer.

   b. ED-to-ED transfers are EMTALA violations.

   c. It is not a violation to transfer an unstable patient.

   d. EMTALA fines are covered by malpractice insurance.

   e. Referrals from the ED to a specialist's office are potential EMTALA violations.

   The answer is e. A tertiary care center must accept patients for whom it is has the specialty resources to care for, but is not required to accept patients for whom it can provide no additional benefit. ED-to-ED transfers are permissible, when the patient is going to a higher level of care and appropriate measures have been taken to stabilize the patient. While some patients must be transferred in an unstable state, it is a violation if all measures that could be taken to stabilize have not been performed. EMTALA fines are not covered by professional liability policies. Under strict interpretation of EMTALA, it is required that the specialist come to the ED to see the patient.

8. **Physician profiling consists of establishing data on the practice patterns of every hospital-based physician. Physician profiling:**

   a. Can directly assess quality of care.

   b. Is voluntary and not required by The Joint Commission.

   c. Is not protected from legal discovery.

   d. Commonly incorporates throughput statistics from the ED.

   e. Can use adverse events to reliably detect outliers.

   The answer is d. Physician profiling is expected by the Joint Commission. Profiling can only indirectly assess quality of care. Because adverse events per physician represent a small number of patients compared to the total number of patients seen, outliers may not always be detected. Physician profiles are confidential and not part of the legal discovery process. Efficiency of patient care—throughput—is commonly part of the profile.

9. **Utilization refers to the appropriate use of hospital resources:**

    a. When a physician forms a clinical judgment that a patient requires hospitalization, the third-party payer can deny the length of stay but not the whole hospitalization.

    b. Utilization is not antithetical to quality assurance.

    c. The use of hospitalists has been demonstrated to improve utilization.

    d. The hospital Utilization Committee can mandate certain clinical practices.

    e. The Joint Commission mandates the use of Utilization Committees.

    The answer is c. Studies have confirmed that hospitalists improve utilization, including shortening hospital stays. There is an inherent conflict between quality assurance and utilization. Utilization takes a backseat to quality assurance, and the utilization committee cannot mandate clinical practices. However, reimbursement from third-party payers may be denied if hospitalization decisions do not conform to standard utilization guidelines.

10. **Patient safety is a major initiative of regulatory agencies. It is important to understand that:**

    a. The majority of errors in patient care can be traced to personnel issues.

    b. Most safety procedures are focused on physicians rather than nurses.

    c. Medication errors are the most commonly identified safety issues.

    d. Hospitals generally do not have specified procedures for patient restraint and prevention of falls.

    e. The purpose of root cause analysis is to determine who is responsible for a particular error.

    The answer is c. Medication errors continue to be common, but increasing attention to such errors is having a significant impact. The focus of safety initiatives is to prevent errors that occur in the functioning of the system, rather than to focus on individual mistakes.

11. **A 60-year-old man is treated in the ED in the morning for a wrist fracture sustained in a fall. That evening, he is admitted to another hospital with an acute MI. The possible cognitive error might have been:**

    a. Premature closure.

    b. Unpacking principle.

    c. Diagnosis momentum.

    d. Anchoring.

    e. Any of the above.

    The answer is e. The atmosphere of the emergency department predisposes emergency practitioners to error. More than 30 cognitive dispositions to respond (CDRs) have been described in the medical literature. Any of them listed here may have been responsible for the missed diagnosis. Premature closure to the decision-making process means accepting a diagnosis before it has been fully verified; the consequences of this bias are reflected in the maxim, "When the diagnosis is made, the thinking stops." Unpacking principle is the failure to elicit all relevant information (unpacking) in establishing a differential diagnosis and can result in missing other significant possibilities. Once diagnostic labels are attached to patients, they tend to become stickier and stickier (diagnosis momentum); what might have started as a possibility gathers increasing momentum until it becomes definite, and all other possibilities are excluded. Anchoring is the tendency to perceptually lock onto salient features in the patient's initial presentation too early in the diagnostic process, and then failing to adjust this initial impression in the light of later information.

12.   The most important requirement of performance improvement is:

a. Complete and accurate documentation.

b. Selection of the most important indicators.

c. Identification of problem issues.

d. Documentation of practice change.

e. Compliance with quality-of-care standards.

The answer is d. All of the above are aspects of Performance Improvement, but a PI program is not acceptable unless it can document changes and quantifiable improvement.

13.   An example of quality assurance/performance improvement is:

a. X-ray callbacks.

b. Assessing throughput.

c. Utilization studies.

d. Staff training in patient communication.

e. Continuing medical education.

The answer is b. ED throughput is considered an important component of QA/PI in the ED, as it has huge impact on patient care. Callbacks of x-ray discrepancies are, in and of itself, risk management. Utilization studies and staff training and education may lead to QA/PI but are not part of the basic process.

14.   When there is interdepartmental conflict, it is most important to:

a. Access the hospital policy/procedure manual.

b. Perform literature review to identify evidence-based practice.

c. Interview all participants.

d. Not discuss anything until you have consulted the hospital lawyers.

e. Listen to the other side.

The answer is e. Conflict itself is unavoidable, and contains within itself the potential for both positive and negative effects. Conflict resolvers try to find ways to make conflicts as constructive as possible for everyone involved. While conflict resolution may vary from culture to culture, people in the United States generally seek a "win-win" situation. Frequently the simple process of venting one's feeling leads away from the impasse to a solution. The appropriate starting point in any conflict resolution is to listen to the other side's point of view and work from there.

15. **At the scene of an accident, the skills a first responder can perform include:**

    a. Spinal immobilization.
    b. Needle decompression of a tension pneumothorax.
    c. Manual defibrillation.
    d. Establishing an intravenous line.
    e. Using adjunctive airway devices.

    The answer is a. The first responder is a nontransport provider, a BLS or ALS police officer or firefighter, the first person who quickly responds to the scene of an emergency to provide initial care. He does the initial event and patient assessment, as well as limited lifesaving interventions that include CPR, AED use, basic airway management, spinal immobilization, and control of bleeding. EMT-intermediate can establish intravenous access, manually defibrillate, use adjunctive airway devices, and administer limited medications. EMT-paramedic is the most advanced prehospital provider. He can interpret cardiac rhythms and perform invasive lifesaving procedures that include needle thoracostomy.

16. **An absolute contraindication to the prehospital use of the military antishock trouser (MAST) garment is:**

    a. Pregnancy.
    b. Pulmonary edema.
    c. Thoracic injuries.
    d. Abdominal content evisceration.
    e. Impaled objects.

    The answer is b. MAST garment is a device that surrounds the legs and lower abdomen. When inflated, it applies external pressure to the enclosed body parts. Its use has fallen out of favor because there is little evidence that shows that it improves patient survival in hemorrhagic shock secondary to trauma, and may actually be harmful to patients with penetrating thoracic trauma with short transport times. Relative contraindications for MAST include: pregnancy, impaled objects, evisceration of abdominal contents, and thoracic/diaphragmatic injuries. Pulmonary edema remains an absolute contraindication.

17. **In a discussion with your local ambulance company the question comes up about helmet removal in the field. You tell your ambulance crew that they should:**

    a. Leave motorcycle helmets on in the field.
    b. Remove football helmets in the field.
    c. Remove football shoulder pads in the field.
    d. Remove motorcycle helmets in the field.
    e. Leave football helmet facemasks on in the field.

    The answer is d. The facemask of football helmets should be removed as soon as possible after an accident, before transportation, regardless of the patient's respiratory status. A properly fitted football helmet with shoulder pads maintains the head in neutral spinal alignment and must stay on during transport. Motorcycle helmets should be removed in the field after an accident because they are not fitted and do not fit securely on the head. Since motorcycle helmets are worn without shoulder pads, they do not maintain the neutral spine position when patients lie supine on the ground.

18. **The goal of disaster triage to:**

    a. First assess the nonambulatory patients.

    b. First assess the "walking wounded."

    c. Give priority to the most salvageable patients with the most urgent conditions.

    d. Give priority to the most critically ill patients to ensure that they receive rapid care.

    e. Provide an initial needs assessment.

    The answer is c. Give priority to the most salvageable patients with the most urgent conditions. In everyday hospital triage, priority is given to the most salvageable patients with the most urgent conditions. The goal of disaster triage is different—to maximize the benefit to an entire population of patients, which may require letting some patients die with only comfort care.

19. **START stands for Simple Triage and Rapid Assessment, which primarily involves assessment of:**

    a. Respirations.

    b. Temperature.

    c. Oxygen saturation.

    d. Blood pressure.

    e. Hemorrhage.

    The answer is a. START involves a quick assessment of respiration, perfusion, and mental status. Victims who can ambulate are asked to move away from the immediate area. These victims are classified as the "walking wounded." Rescuers triage patients quickly by checking respiratory rate, pulse, and mental status (e.g., ability to follow commands).

20. **Proper decontamination involves:**

    a. Spraying off particulate matter that remains on the skin with water.

    b. Intubating critically ill patients before gross decontamination.

    c. Irrigating ocular exposures after the whole-body decontamination.

    d. Removing clothing quickly.

    e. Leaving wounds that were irrigated and debrided open during showering.

    The answer is d. Decontamination decreases the victim's absorbed dose as well as secondary contamination of health care providers. It is thought that 80% of the decontamination process is accomplished with removal of the contaminated clothes. Particular matter should be brushed away before showering, because some chemicals may create an exothermic reaction with water. Critically ill contaminated patients should have a patent airway, immobilized cervical spine, oxygen, assisted ventilation, and pressure on arterial bleeding before the decontamination process. Intubation and intravenous line insertion should be delayed until completion of gross decontamination. Ocular exposures take precedence in the decontamination process and should be irrigated prehospital. Wounds are the next decontamination priority after ocular exposures. They are irrigated, debrided, and covered with a water-occlusive dressing to prevent recontamination during showering.

21. **A level III disaster requires assistance from:**

a. Red Cross only.

b. Nongovernment organization (NGO) local resources only.

c. Regional mutual aid.

d. State and federal aid.

e. International aid.

The answer is d. State and federal aid disasters are divided into three levels. Level I disaster only requires local resources. Level II disaster requires regional mutual aid. Level III disaster requires state and federal aid.

22. **You should consider using helicopter EMS when:**

a. Weather conditions are too poor for ground transport.

b. The patient requests it.

c. Stable patients who do not require time critical treatment but with good insurance coverage.

d. Transferring facilities request it to "get the patient out of here as quickly as possible."

e. Prehospital personnel report an entrapped trauma patient with extrication time greater than 20 minutes.

The answer is e. Entrapped trauma patients and patients with extrication time greater than 20 minutes both prompt consideration for helicopter air transport. None of the other answers is appropriate.

23. **Off-line, or indirect, medical control, involves:**

a. Logistics.

b. Protocol development.

c. Operations.

d. Planning.

e. Incident command.

The answer is b. Protocols are preestablished guidelines that outline the standard of care for most illnesses or injuries encountered by prehospital providers. Standing orders for predefined patient conditions allows providers to perform specific procedures or administer limited medications before communication with hospital personnel. These actions are performed under the medical license of a medical director.

24. **Of the American Heart Association's four-steps for the "Chain of Survival," the link with the least benefit to survival is:**

a. Early access to emergency medical system.

b. Early cardiopulmonary resuscitation (CPR).

c. Early defibrillation.

d. Early basic life support.

e. Early advanced cardiac life support.

The answer is e. American Heart Association's four-step "Chain of Survival" concept has been promoted as a means of optimizing community responses. Better survival has been associated with the first three links in the chain: (1) early access to emergency medical care, (2) early CPR, and (3) early defibrillation. Early advanced cardiac life support, the fourth link, is often considered of benefit in that it provides advanced airway management (endotracheal intubation) and intravenous drug therapy.

25. **Children are more vulnerable to weapons of mass destruction than adults because they have:**
    a. A slower respiratory rate.
    b. Thinner skin.
    c. Smaller surface area-to-volume ratio.
    d. Larger fluid reserves.
    e. Slower metabolic rates.

    The answer is b. Children are more susceptible to weapons of mass destruction than adults because they breathe at a faster rate, which increases their relative exposure to aerosolized agents. Some chemicals, like sarin, are heavier than air. Thus they accumulate at the level of air density where children are more likely to inhale them. Because children have thinner skin, it makes them more vulnerable to agents that act on or through their skin. Children have smaller fluid reserves and higher metabolic rates. This makes them prone to dehydration from vomiting and diarrhea, leading to an increase toxicity exposure.

26. **A 17-year-old Navy plebe sprained his ankle skateboarding and wants to leave the emergency department to seek treatment at the Naval Academy Medical Clinic. You do a medical screening examination and find the patient has capacity to make decisions, but are worried because he is underage. You should:**
    a. Allow the patient to refuse treatment.
    b. Contact the patient's parents and obtain consent for discharge.
    c. Have the patient sign out Against Medical Advice (AMA).
    d. Obtain the commanding officer's consent.
    e. Complete transfer paperwork and arrange transport to the clinic.

    The answer is a. Military personnel younger than 18 years are considered emancipated minors. As long as the patient is alert, understands the risks and benefits, and there is no eminent life threat, he may refuse treatment.

27. **A 14-year-old runaway thinks he got a sexually transmitted disease while working as a prostitute to support himself. You should:**
    a. Hold the patient until his parents can be contacted in order to obtain consent to treat.
    b. Treat the patient for STDs and discharge.
    c. Consult the hospital attorney.
    d. Contact the police.
    e. Consult Child Protective Services.

    The answer is e. Although it appears the child is an emancipated minor, there is a strong possibility the child may be suffering from abuse or neglect. Consulting Child Protective Services and also treat the STD would be most appropriate.

28.   **An 86-year-old man with advanced Alzheimer disease is found confused in his home by the next-door neighbor. The air conditioning has been off all day due to a power outage. The neighbor says that the patient's son is the legal guardian and has been caring for him. He does not know how to contact the son. Can you treat this patient?**

   a. No, the son must give consent before you begin treatment.

   b. No, only the patient can give consent if the son is not available.

   c. Yes, the neighbor can give consent since this is an emergency situation.

   d. Yes, but only if you get the police involved.

   e. Yes, implied consent applies because the patient may be having a heatstroke.

   The answer is e. The patient should be treated based on implied consent because a potential emergency exists. If there is any reason to believe the son has not been checking on the patient frequently the incident should be reported to Adult Protective Services.

29.   **The police bring in a 16-year-old adolescent male driver of an automobile that had a low-speed collision with a tree. The patient says he is diabetic and he says he feels like he is going to pass out. Finger-stick glucose is 40 mg/dL. You give him a glass of orange juice and a sandwich and he now feels fine. The police officer requests that you obtain a blood sample. The patient refuses the test. Should you carry out the request?**

   a. No, the patient can refuse the test as long as he is not under arrest.

   b. No, the patient's parents must give consent.

   c. No, the patient is an emancipated minor and may refuse further tests and treatment.

   d. Yes, the patient may not refuse a reasonable police request.

   e. Yes, if you don't draw the blood the police may charge you with obstructing justice.

   The correct answer is d. In most states a driver may not refuse a blood sample and the request should be honored as long as obtaining the evidence does not endanger the patient or delay his care. Even though the patient is a minor, and he cannot legally sign out on his own accord, and the parents should be contacted, their consent is not necessary to obtain the blood for alcohol and drug testing.

30.   **The police bring a 44-year-old woman to the emergency department. She was found walking down the middle of the street naked at 2 AM. The police ask you to sedate the patient and hold her until morning. The patient is calm, says she feels fine, has a bad problem of walking in her sleep and she wants to go home to "take her sleeping pill and go to bed." She admits to a history of depression, but says she is neither suicidal nor homicidal, and she does not appear delusional. Her vital signs are normal and her blood glucose is 114 mg/dL. She refuses further treatment. Can you restrain her physically or chemically and treat without her consent?**

   a. Yes, the patient has no right to refuse treatment.

   b. No, the patient is not confused and she doesn't have a life-threatening emergency so she can refuse treatment.

   c. Yes, the patient has a history of being impaired so you can treat her.

   d. Yes, the patient has an acute psychiatric emergency so you can treat her.

   e. Yes, the police requested treatment so it is legal to treat her.

   The answer is b. This is a tough call. Although the patient might have a mental illness, her public display of nudity does not pose a threat to herself or others and she now appears able to care for herself. As no emergency currently exists, you should not treat if she refuses treatment.

31. **The 1966 National Highway Safety Act authorized the United States Department of Transportation to fund:**
    a. New highway construction and repair of existing unsafe highways and bridges.
    b. Increased law enforcement personnel to patrol the nation's highways.
    c. Ambulances, communications, and training programs for prehospital services.
    d. New hospital construction and expansion of existing services to treat accident victims.
    e. Publicly funded prehospital helicopters rescue services.

    The answer is c. The publication of a National Academy of Sciences "white paper" in 1966 led to the passage of the Highway Safety Act, which provided funds for prehospital emergency services. Seven years later, Public Law 93-154 was legislated by Congress to further improve emergency medical services (EMS) on a nationwide scale. Funds were provided for 15 different areas, including manpower and training, lay participation, disaster services, and independent review of emergency services. Implementation and development of services were delegated to the state and local level.

32. **Choose the correct statement about a prehospital disaster plan and its contents:**
    a. The Incident Commander is, by default, the senior physician on the scene.
    b. Most patients presenting to an emergency department in a disaster have injuries that require advanced trauma services.
    c. Physician training for mass casualty situations is a requirement for medical staff privileges.
    d. The Joint Commission (JCAHO) only reviews a hospital's external disaster plan; internal disasters are not considered reviewable by a national organization.
    e. As the hospital disaster response is activated, the more seriously injured patients brought in later often receive delayed treatment.

    The answer is e. Physicians should understand that they are not in charge at the scene of a prehospital incident; the Incident Commander may guide a physician to where his/her skills are most needed. In general, physicians should remain at the hospital while victims are brought to them. The Joint Commission requires that member hospitals have a written and rehearsed plan for the timely care of casualties arising from both external and internal disasters. Most casualties are transported to a hospital over a relatively short period of time. Most patients presenting to an emergency department in a disaster have minor injuries and do not require advanced trauma services.

33. **Choose the correct statement regarding prehospital caregivers:**

    a. As standards for prehospital care evolve, the participation of noncertified lay people (i.e., the general public) in providing care will diminish.

    b. In most systems, first responders have extensive medical training.

    c. Multitiered systems, providing either BLS or ALS, are the wave of the future.

    d. An EMT-P (paramedic) is trained to manage airways, interpret cardiac rhythms, administer selected drug therapy in the field, and perform some invasive procedures.

    e. Since early defibrillation does not influence survival rates, most prehospital providers are not trained in the use of defibrillators.

The answer is d. Public participation in prehospital emergency care cannot be overlooked. Advanced first-aid courses and lifeguard training by the Red Cross and basic CPR courses sanctioned by the American Heart Association are provided because the difference between life and death may depend on the skills of the first person to reach the scene. The public must also be assured of having a voice in the administration and review of an EMS system. Since different communities provide different levels of training for their EMT personnel, it is important that the emergency physician be acquainted with the local services. Single-tiered ALS response teams are proving to be cost-effective, and fewer multi-tiered systems are in existence today. As studies continue to define what prehospital services are effective, these standards will undoubtedly change. Early defibrillation has been shown in numerous studies to increase survival.

34. **Authorities have announced that the strongest hurricane of the century will strike an area within the next 48 hours. The most difficult part of the mass evacuation response will be:**

    a. Getting people to leave the area.

    b. Notifying the public with accurate information about the disaster.

    c. Long delays caused by heavily congested traffic from the concurrent withdrawal of thousands of people.

    d. Evacuating hospitals, nursing homes, jails, and mental institutions.

    e. Finding temporary shelter for the evacuees during the hurricane.

The answer is d. The Disaster Research Center cites results of an EPA study that show that once people decide to go, they do so in an orderly fashion using their cars. The major problem that occurs later is the premature return of people to their homes, often before authorities have announced it safe to do so.

35. **EMTs report by radio that they are attempting to treat a man whose wife states that he has tried to commit suicide by swallowing more than 60 antidepressant tablets and consuming a large amount of alcohol. The man is awake and combative. He refuses to go to the hospital and is threatening to sue anybody who touches him. You should instruct the paramedics to:**

    a. Have the patient sign a release-of-responsibility form stating he refuses, and have his wife witness and acknowledge his refusal to accept treatment and the possibility he might die.

    b. Wait to see if the patient becomes unresponsive from the drug ingestion and then transport him to the hospital.

    c. Forcibly subdue the patient and bring him to the emergency department.

    d. Have the patient swallow a bottle of ipecac, document his refusal for treatment, and assure his wife she can call back if he changes his mind or becomes more ill.

    e. Contact the police for assistance in transporting the patient to the hospital.

The answer is e. Patients suspected of having a head injury, intoxicated by drugs or alcohol, or mentally ill or retarded must be assumed to be mentally incompetent, and transportation to the hospital for evaluation of a potential medical problem is mandatory. While the standards and protocols for dealing with this issue should be addressed by individual EMS systems, the best choice in this instance would be to contact the police for assistance. An "against medical advice" release-of-responsibility waiver is meaningless in the circumstance of a mentally incompetent patient, since by definition he cannot understand the consequences of his action. Nontreatment of incompetent patients is a frequent cause of malpractice suits.

36. **Choose the correct statement about minimizing risk in the emergency department:**

    a. There is no reason to acknowledge information in the registrar's form or nurse's note, since their liability is covered by the hospital and not your responsibility.

    b. Writing clear, concise, and complete admission orders as a courtesy to the admitting physician can expedite transfer of a patient to an intensive care bed.

    c. Discuss findings, treatment, and expected outcomes with the patient and family and document having done so.

    d. It is reasonable for the triage nurse to tell patients in the waiting room about prolonged delays and to encourage them to follow-up with their family physician in a day or two if not feeling better.

    e. Patients who are being transferred to another facility become the responsibility of the accepting physician at the time of acceptance.

The answer is c. A clear, concise, and complete medical record is the best protection against malpractice actions. Documenting follow-up instructions and mental status in patients who refuse treatment and obtaining informed consent are other important steps. Writing inpatient orders probably increases the emergency physician's liability. If it is necessary, clear documentation should be placed on the record that the orders are written on behalf of the attending physician and that the case and general plan were discussed. An order to notify the attending physician at once if there would be any change in the patient's condition should be included. Patients who are transferred to another facility remain the responsibility of the transferring physician until they arrive at the accepting facility.

37. **After several painful years of discovery and pretrial motions, the malpractice case against you finally comes to court. On the witness stand, the plaintiff's expert witness expands his already poorly supported testimony in new and unexpected directions, with attacks upon your competence that his attorney is unprepared to counter. Your expert witnesses patiently explain why the plaintiff's expert is wrong, but the juror's faces demonstrate that the damage is done. You have an option to:**

    a. Personally speak to the judge after court on the day it happens.

    b. Contact the expert's specialty academy.

    c. Immediately declare a mistrial.

    d. Contact the state and local medical societies.

    e. Countersue the plaintiff's expert witness for malicious prosecution.

    The answer is d. The first thing to do is wait for the jury's verdict. When an opposing expert says things that are not true or are unprofessional on the witness stand, an alert defense attorney immediately objects and counters the assertions on cross-examination. If the testimony is a complete surprise, the attorney may not be able to effectively counter it, even with the defendant's on-the-spot medical advice. The next line of defense is the defense expert's testimony, which almost always follows. If this expert went first ("out of order") because of other professional commitments, he or she may need to be brought back to the stand for further testimony. The defense summation is the final chance for a comeback. Talking to the judge personally about the concerns is not appropriate, nor can the judge declare a mistrial except in limited circumstances. The defendant can never declare a mistrial. If the tainted testimony results in a judgment against the defendant, an immediate appeal is appropriate. The defendant certainly should contact the local and state medical societies about the expert, as they may have information on his prior activity, even if he comes from another state. Trial testimony also can be reviewed by medical societies to see if it falls outside the standard for an expert in the defendant's specialty and, in many cases, medical societies have jurisdiction to bring the matter to the state medical board or even to another state board, if the prosecution's expert is from another state. The expert's specialty academy also can review expert testimony if the expert is an academy member and can censure him or her if they agree the testimony fell outside professional bounds. A defendant cannot sue an expert for malicious prosecution; that is only a remedy against a plaintiff's attorney who files a clearly frivolous case.

38. **Defined within law, the term "reasonable medical certainty":**

    a. Means beyond a reasonable doubt.

    b. Indicates at least 95% certain.

    c. Is defined as more likely than not.

    d. Varies from one medical specialty to another; the facts of the case are determinative.

    e. Is determined by the judge on a case-by-case basis.

    The answer is c. Reasonable medical certainty is defined according to the standard in civil litigation, which means 51% probability, even though the word "medical" makes physicians think of a much higher standard. The standard of "beyond a reasonable doubt" probably captures a physician's idea of reasonable certainty, but this is not a legal standard, except in criminal cases.

39. **Which patient can give informed consent to accept or refuse medical treatment?**

    a. A 16-year-old high school football player with a broken ankle brought to the ED by his parents.

    b. Mentally retarded 35-year-old woman who is to be admitted for an elective operation.

    c. A 47-year-old intoxicated man with a blood alcohol of 300 mg/dL.

    d. A 29-year-old, confused, disoriented man involved in a motorcycle accident.

    e. Married, pregnant 15-year-old brought to the ED in labor.

The answer is e. Patient **a** is technically a minor and legally incapable of consenting to his own medical treatment. Patient **b** may be capable of understanding and consenting to her operation, but it would be best to contact her guardian, if she has one, to obtain consent, or seek an evaluation of her competency. Patients **c** and **d** are not capable of understanding and consenting to medical treatment; the legal definition of intoxication has no bearing here. Patient **e** is under the legal age of majority but because she is married she is considered emancipated and can consent to treatment. In a life-threatening emergency, consent would be implied for any of these patients and a signed form is not necessary.

40. **The ED presentation that should prompt inquiry about domestic violence is:**

    a. A 19-year-old homeless woman who is pregnant and complains of headache and pain in her neck.

    b. A 35-year-old married man with bilateral arm pain and obvious ulnar contusions sustained when he "tripped getting out of his car."

    c. A 45-year-old divorced woman who complains of "not feeling quite right" and wants something done this time, unlike the previous 3 times she has visited the ED over the past 4 months.

    d. A 22-year-old lesbian who comes to the ED for closure of a laceration to her forehead, while accompanied by her controlling and protective partner.

    e. All of the above.

    The answer is e. All of these patients have histories or circumstances that raise suspicion of domestic violence. Domestic violence is so prevalent and its potential consequences so severe that it is important to query virtually all adult ED patients about abuse. Failing to inquire about domestic violence will result in failure to identify most of its victims. A high index or suspicion should always be used in such cases and scenarios as outlined in this question.

41. **A 59-year-old woman complains of nervousness and insomnia. You note that she has several contusions of her legs and feet, and scratches on her face at different stages of healing. On questioning, she admits that she frequently is struck by her boyfriend and believes this may be the cause of her nervousness. Her primary reason for visiting the ED is to obtain a prescription for something to help her sleep. Your most appropriate course of action is to:**

    a. Prescribe a minor tranquilizer.

    b. Prescribe an intermediate-acting barbiturate.

    c. Refer the patient to community agencies that assist victims of domestic violence and provide the patient with telephone numbers.

    d. Contact the police as their actions may save the patient's life.

    e. Refer the patient to community agencies that assist victims of domestic violence, provide her with appropriate telephone numbers, and encourage her to make contact (if possible) while in the ED.

    The answer is e. The circumstances requiring a visit to the ED may well create a teachable moment. As such, the patient may be most receptive to initiating the intervention that may stop the cycle of violence. While the patient should be encouraged to act with support, that decision should not be made unilaterally by the emergency physician or other ED personnel, absent a legal requirement to report domestic violence. Depressant medications should not be prescribed because they may interfere with the ability to flee danger or to defend against attack. Patience in presenting these options to the patient is important to get their "buy in" to moving forward with these options.

42. **Legally, performing a procedure without consent is considered:**
    a. Battery.
    b. Negligence.
    c. Unethical.
    d. Assault.
    e. Mayhem.

    The answer is a. Battery is defined as unconsented offensive touching of another person, which would include surgery. Conversely, lack of informed consent is a matter of negligence. Such an act is unethical; however, it is not a legal issue. Assault and mayhem are criminal matters.

43. **A colleague's patient, dissatisfied with the result of a wound repair, wants to know if this constitutes malpractice. Your preferred response is:**
    a. If it looks bad, agree and offer to reoperate.
    b. Sympathize, but withhold criticism until one has had an opportunity to see records and/or discuss the situation with the previous physician.
    c. Stall and say it will get better with time.
    d. Offer no opinion.
    e. Explain and illustrate how it should have been performed.

    The answer is b. The tendency to believe the patient's version of the facts must be avoided. Establish facts by requesting records or consulting with previous surgeons before commenting. At least one-quarter of lawsuits are generated by unfavorable comments by consulting surgeon who may not have all the facts in order prior to making a statement to a patient.

BIBLIOGRAPHY

General Sources

Blaivas M. Lower extremity deep venous thrombosis. In: Ma J, Mateer J, eds. *Emergency Ultrasound.* New York: McGraw-Hill; 2003:335–347.

Danzl D, Vissers R. Tracheal intubation and mechanical ventilation. In: Tintinalli J, Kelen G, Stapczynski J, American College of Emergency Physicians, eds. *Emergency Medicine: A Comprehensive Study Guide.* 6th ed. New York, NY: McGraw-Hill; 2003:108–119.

Dewitz A, Frazee B. Soft tissue applications. In: Ma J, Mateer J, eds. *Emergency Ultrasound.* New York: McGraw-Hill; 2003:363–364.

Flomenbaum NE, Goldfrank LR, Hoffman RS, Howland MA, Lewin NA, Nelson LS. *Goldfrank's Toxicologic Emergencies.* 8th ed. New York, NY: McGraw-Hill; 2006.

Houry D, Abbott J. Acute complications of pregnancy. In: Marx JA, Hockberger RS, Walls RM, eds. *Rosen's Emergency Medicine: Concepts and Clinical Practice.* Philadelphia, PA: Mosby-Elsevier; 2006:2741.

Khandheria BK, Tajik AJ, Taylor CL, et al. Aortic dissection: review of value and limitations of two-dimensional echocardiography in a six-year experience. *J Am Soc Echocardiogr.* 1989;2(1):17–24.

Ma J, Mateer J. Trauma. In: Ma J, Mateer J, eds. *Emergency Ultrasound.* New York: McGraw-Hill New; 2003:78.

Marx J, Hockberger R, Walls R. *Rosen's Emergency Medicine: Concepts and Clinical Practice.* 6th ed. Philadelphia, PA: Mosby-Elsevier; 2006.

Reichman E, Simon RR. *Emergency Medicine Procedures: Text and Atlas.* 3rd ed. New York, NY: McGraw-Hill; 2003.

Roberts JR, Hedges J. *Clinical Procedures in Emergency Medicine.* 4th ed. Philadelphia, PA: W.B. Saunders; 2003.

Sabiston D. The Stomach and duodenum. In: Sabiston D, ed. *Sabiston Textbook of Surgery.* 15th ed. 852–857.

Tayal V, Moore C, Rose G. Cardiac. In: Ma J, Mateer J, eds. *Emergency Ultrasound.* New York: McGraw-Hill; 2003:92–93.

Tayal VS, Graf CD, Gibbs MA. Prospective study of accuracy and outcome of emergency ultrasound for abdominal aortic aneurysm over two years. *Acad Emerg Med.* 2003;10(8):867–871.

Tintinalli J, Kelen G, Stapczynski J, American College of Emergency Physicians. *Emergency Medicine: A Comprehensive Study Guide.* 6th ed. New York, NY: McGraw-Hill; 2003.

LLSA Readings 2006

ACEP Clinical Policies Committee, Clinical Policies Subcommittee on Acute Blunt Abdominal Trauma. Clinical policy: critical issues in the evaluation of adult patients presenting to the emergency department with acute blunt abdominal trauma. *Ann Emerg Med.* 2004;43(2):278–290.

Anderson MR, Klink K, Cohrssen A. Evaluation of vaginal complaints. *JAMA.* 2004;291(11):1368–1379.

Bates SM, Ginsberg JS. Treatment of deep-vein thrombosis. *N Engl J Med.* 2004;351(3):268–277.

Bjornson CL, Klassen TP, Williamson J, et al. A randomized trial of a single dose of oral dexamethasone for mild croup. *N Engl J Med.* 2004;351(13):1306–1313.

Blumenthal D. Doctors and drug companies. *N Engl J Med.* 2004;351(18):1885–1890.

CRASH Trial Collaborators. Effect of intravenous corticosteroids on death within 14 days in 10008 adults with clinically significant head injury (MRC crash trial): randomised placebo-controlled trial. *Lancet.* 2004;364:1321–1328.

Gnann Jr JW, Whitley RJ. Herpes zoster. *N Engl J Med.* 2002;347(5):340–346.

Jagoda AS, Cantrill SV, Wears RL, et al. Clinical policy: neuroimaging and decisionmaking in adult mild traumatic brain injury in the acute setting. *Ann Emerg Med.* 2002;40(2):231–249.

Kidwell CS, Chalela JA, Saver JL, et al. Comparison of MRI and CT for detection of acute intracerebral hemorrhage. *JAMA.* 2004;292(15):1823–1830.

McSweeney JC, Cody M, O'Sullivan P, Elberson K, Moser DK, Garvin BJ. Women's early warning symptoms of acute myocardial infarction. *Circulation.* 2003;108:2619–2623.

Palchak MJ, Holmes JF, Vance CW, et al. A decision rule for identifying children at low risk for brain injuries after blunt head trauma. *Ann Emerg Med.* 2003;42(4):492–506.

Perelman VS, Francis GJ, Rutledge T. Foote J, Martino F, Dranitsaris G. Sterile versus nonsterile gloves for repair of uncomplicated lacerations in the emergency department: a randomized controlled trial. *Ann Emerg Med.* 2004;43(3):362–370.

Sarasin FP, Hanusa BH, Perneger T, Louis-Simonet M, Rajeswaran A, Kapoor WN. A risk score to predict arrhythmias in patients with unexplained syncope. *Acad Emerg Med.* 2003;10(12):1312–1317.

Shah AJ, Kilcline BA. Trauma in pregnancy. *Emerg Med Clin N Am.* 2003;21(3):615–629.

Swartz MN. Cellulitis. *N Engl J Med.* 2004;350(9):904–912.

Thielman NM, Guerrant RL. Acute infectious diarrhea. *N Engl J Med.* 2004;350(1):38–46.

Turner TWS. Do mammalian bites require antibiotic prophylaxis? *Ann Emerg Med.* 2004;44(3):274–276.

Welch RD, Zalenski RJ, Frederick PD, et al. Prognostic value of a normal or nonspecific initial electrocardiogram in acute myocardial infarction. *JAMA.* 2001;286(16):1977–1984.

LLSA Readings 2007

Cardall T, Glasser J, Guss DA. Clinical value of the total white blood cell count and temperature in the evaluation of patients with suspected appendicitis. *Acad Emerg Med.* 2004;11(10):1021–1027.

Costantino TG, Parikh AK, Satz WA, et al. Ultrasonography-guided peripheral intravenous access versus traditional approaches in patients with difficult intravenous access. *Ann Emerg Med.* 2005;46(5):456–461.

Director TD, Linden JA. Domestic violence: an approach to identification and intervention. *Emerg Med Clin N Am.* 2004;22:1117–1132.

Doshi A, Boudreaux ED, Wang N, et al. National study of US emergency department visits for attempted suicide and self-inflicted injury, 1997–2001. *Ann Emerg Med.* 2005;46(4):369–375.

Fesmire FM, Jagoda A. Are we putting the cart ahead of the horse: who determines the standard of care for the management of patients in the emergency department? *Ann Emerg Med.* 2005;46(2):198–200.

Frazee BW, Lynn J, Charlebois ED, et al. High prevalence of Methicillin-resistant Staphylococcus aureus in emergency department skin and soft tissue infections. *Ann Emerg Med.* 2005;45(3):311–320.

Freedman R. Schizophrenia. *N Engl J Med.* 2003;349(18):1738–1749.

Fricchione G. Generalized anxiety disorder. *N Engl J Med.* 2004;351(7):675–682.

Gibler WB, Cannon CP, Blomkalns AL, et al. Practical implementation of the guidelines for unstable angina/non-ST-segment elevation myocardial infarction in the emergency department. *Ann Emerg Med.* 2005;46(2):185–197; WITH accompanying editorial.

Hohl CM, Robitaille C, Lord V, et al. Emergency physician recognition of adverse drug-related events in elder patients presenting to an emergency department. *Acad Emerg Med.* 2005;12(3):197–205.

Knight JR. A 35-year-old physician with opioid dependence. *JAMA.* 2004;292(11):1351–1357.

Mello MJ, Nirenberg TD, Longabaugh R, et al. Emergency department brief motivational interventions for alcohol with motor vehicle crash patients. *Ann Emerg Med.* 2005;45(6):620–625.

Mills AM, Chen EH. Are blood cultures necessary in adults with cellulitis? *Ann Emerg Med.* 2005;45(5):548–549.

Murphy BA, Hansen AR, Howell JM, et al. Clinical policy: critical issues in the initial evaluation and management of patients presenting to the emergency department in early pregnancy. *Ann Emerg Med.* 2003;41(1):123–133.

Sackner-Bernstein JD, Kowalski M, Fox M, et al. Short-term risk of death after treatment with nesiritide for decompensated heart failure. *JAMA.* 2005;293(15):1900–1905.

Sinert R, Spektor M. Clinical assessment of hypovolemia. *Ann Emerg Med.* 2005;45(3):327–329.

Venkat KK, Venkat A. Care of the renal transplant recipient in the emergency department. *Ann Emerg Med.* 2004;44(4):330–341.

Wang CS, Fitzgerald JM, Schulzer M, et al. Does this dyspneic patient in the emergency department have congestive heart failure? *JAMA.* 2005;294(15):1944–1956.

LLSA Readings 2008

Barrett BJ, Parfrey PS. Preventing nephropathy induced by contrast medium. *N Engl J Med.* 2006;354(4):379–386.

Bradley EH, Herrin J, Wang Y, et al. Strategies for reducing the door-to-balloon time in acute myocardial infarction. *N Engl J Med.* 2006;355(22):2308–2320.

Darouiche RO. Spinal epidural abscess. *N Engl J Med.* 2006;355(19):2012–2020.

Eichacker PQ, Natanson C, Danner RL. Surviving sepsis—practice guidelines, marketing campaigns, and Eli Lilly. *N Engl J Med.* 2006;355(16):1640–1642.

Eldelman A, Weiss JM, Lau J, et al. Topical anesthetics for dermal instrumentation: a systematic review of randomized, controlled trials. *Ann Emerg Med.* 2005;46(4):343–351.

Freedman SB, Adler M, Seshadri R, et al. Oral ondansetron for gastroenteritis in a pediatric emergency department. *N Engl J Med.* 2006;354(16):1698–1705.

Freeman TM. Hypersensitivity to Hymenoptera stings. *N Engl J Med.* 2004;351(19):1978–1984.

Godwin SA, Caro DA, Wolf SJ, et al. Clinical policy: procedural sedation and analgesia in the emergency department. *Ann Emerg Med.* 2005;45(2):177–196.

Institute of Medicine. IOM Report: the future of emergency care in the United States health system. *Acad Emerg Med.* 2006;13(10):1081–1085.

Kales SN, Christiani DC. Acute chemical emergencies. *N Engl J Med.* 2004;350(8):800–808.

Kao LW, Nanagas KA. Carbon monoxide poisoning. *Emerg Med Clin N Am.* 2004;22:985–1018.

Koenig KL, Goans RE, Hatchett RJ, et al. Medical treatment of radiological casualties: current concepts. *Ann Emerg Med.* 2005;45(6):643–652.

Levitan RM, Kinkle WC, Levin WJ, et al. Laryngeal view during laryngoscopy: a randomized trial comparing cricoid pressure, backward-upward-rightward pressure, and bimanual laryngoscopy. *Ann Emerg Med.* 2006;47(6):548–555.

Melniker LA, Leibner E, McKenney MG, et al. Randomized controlled clinical trial of point-of-care, limited ultrasonography for trauma in the emergency department: the first sonography outcomes assessment program trial. *Ann Emerg Med.* 2006;48(3):227–235.

Nguyen HB, Rivers EP, Abrahamian FM, et al. Severe sepsis and septic shock: review of the literature and emergency department management guidelines. *Ann Emerg Med.* 2006;48(1):28–54.

Nieman CT, Manacci CF, Super DM, et al. Use of the Broselow tape may result in the underresuscitation of children. *Acad Emerg Med.* 2006;13(10):1011–1019.

Rathlev NK, Medzon R, Lowery D, et al. Intracranial pathology in elders with blunt head trauma. *Acad Emerg Med.* 2006;13(3):302–307.

Spiro DM, Tay K, Arnold DH, et al. Wait-and-see prescription for the treatment of acute otitis media: a randomized controlled trial. *JAMA.* 2006;296(10):1235–1241.

Straus SE, Thorpe KE, Holroyd-Leduc J. How do I perform a lumbar puncture and analyze the results to diagnose bacterial meningitis. *JAMA.* 2006;296(16):2012–2022.

Thomsen TW, Shen S, Shaffer RW, et al. Arthrocentesis of the knee. *N Engl J Med.* 2006;354(19):e19.